June 1996

For Kelli:

With best wishes in using the ideas in this book.

Alan Andreasen

Marketing Social Change

Marketing Social Change

Changing Behavior to Promote Health, Social Development, and the Environment

Alan R. Andreasen

Jossey-Bass Publishers • San Francisco

Substantial discounts on bulk quantities of Jossey-Bass books are available to corporations, professional associations, and other organizations. For details and discount information, contact the special sales department at Jossey-Bass Inc., Publishers.
(415) 433-1740; Fax (800) 605-2665.

For sales outside the United States, please contact your local Simon & Schuster International Sales Office.

 Manufactured in the United States of America on Lyons Falls Pathfinder Tradebook. This paper is acid-free and 100 percent totally chlorine-free.

Credits are on page 348.

Library of Congress Cataloging-in-Publication Data

Andreasen, Alan R., date.
    Marketing social change : changing behavior to promote health, social development, and the environment / Alan R. Andreasen.
       p.   cm. — (Jossey-Bass nonprofit sector series) (Jossey-Bass public administration series)
    ISBN 0-7879-0137-7
    1. Social marketing.   2. Social change.   3. Social problems.
4. Behavior modification.   I. Title.   II. Series.   III. Series:
Jossey-Bass public administration series.
HN18.A629   1995
303.4—dc20
                        95-20785
                        CIP

FIRST EDITION
HB Printing 10 9 8 7 6 5 4 3 2 1

Contents

Preface

Nations around the world are beset with a daunting array of social problems, and have limited resources for combating them. Perhaps five million children die every year of diseases we already know how to treat. In the United States, there are 600,000 homeless people (Cisneros, 1995). Thirteen percent of the U.S. population over the age of twelve uses illicit drugs (Substance Abuse and Mental Health Services Administration, 1993). AIDS—a scourge that once targeted relatively circumscribed populations—now affects an estimated ten million people internationally; as many as twenty-six million could be infected with the HIV virus by the year 2000 (World Bank, 1993, p. 99). Around the world, children are at serious risk:

- Forty-three million children have Vitamin A deficiency.
- Over 700,000 infants in developing countries die each year from tetanus infections contracted during unhygienic childbirths.
- Measles and its complications claim almost 900,000 children yearly.
- One in three children in developing countries is malnourished, a contributing factor in 60 percent of all child deaths.
- Diarrhea-related deaths are the second leading cause of death, killing three million children a year.
- Malaria kills one million children a year in sub-Saharan Africa (U.S. Agency for International Development, 1992, p. 4).

Problems addressed successfully in some countries are cropping up elsewhere. For example, cigarette smoking in the United States has declined significantly since 1979, while tobacco use in other parts of the world is growing and is expected to grow even faster in the next decade. In the face of these persistent and often growing problems, policy makers and practitioners charged with attacking them are continually seeking out novel solutions that have the potential for major impact. Over many decades, many approaches have been tried, ranging from behavior modification to health communications, with varying success.

This is a book about a new, innovative approach to the way in which societies address important problems: *social marketing*. Social marketing is the application of proven concepts and techniques drawn from the commercial sector to promote changes in diverse socially important behaviors such as drug use, smoking, sexual behavior, family planning, and child care. This marketing approach has an immense potential to affect major social problems if we can only learn how to harness its power—while, at the same time, taking care to use it for the good of society and not to advance particular parochial aims.

For the past twenty years, I have been teaching, writing, researching, and consulting on social marketing all over the world. I have found that social marketing really works—but only if it is done properly. In the first place, it provides a framework that social program managers find highly useful to guide their own planning and actions. But more important, social marketing has been proven successful. Campaigns have been improved. Behaviors have been changed. Programs have had major impacts. Because of its compelling logic and its impressive track record, social marketing is now being used and promoted by such diverse agencies as the U.S. Agency for International Development, the Centers for Disease Control, the National High Blood Pressure Education Program, and the National Cancer Institute. It is the basis of the intervention approaches of such major consultants as the Academy for Educational Development, Family Health International, The Futures Group, and Prospect Associates. Advertising and public relations organizations like Porter/Novelli Associates regularly promote their capabilities in social marketing. Programs as diverse as the U.S. Environmental Protection Agency, the American Cancer Society, the National Easter Seals Society, and the U.S. Department of Agriculture want to learn more about it. The acceptance of social marketing has advanced to the point where consulting organizations now have directors of social marketing.

However, despite the growing popularity and influence of social marketing, it remains an approach that confronts three major obstacles. First, its potential is underappreciated. As an integrated approach that starts with target customers and their needs, wants, and perceptions, social marketing is more closely grounded than rival approaches in the reality of the target markets that ultimately decide the success or failure of programs. And because influencing behavior is social marketing's fundamental objective, the discipline can be applied to a wide range of topics and audiences. For example, the social marketing framework is not only valuable in changing the behaviors of ghetto teenagers in U.S. urban centers, farmers in rural areas, and mothers in Bangladesh, it can also be used to influence the behavior of health workers, private physicians, government officials, even the staff of social marketing programs themselves. Although social marketing can be used in all of these areas, few practitioners perceive the depth and range of its potential.

A second obstacle is the fact that social marketing is very often misunderstood. Many people claim they are doing social marketing when they are not. Many do not know how to define it (Andreasen, 1993). Most commonly, social marketing is confused with *social advertising*. While many social marketing programs use advertising and advertising techniques, its core approach is much broader. Social marketing recognizes that influencing behavior—especially behavior change—cannot come about simply by promoting the benefits of some new course of action. Careful attention must be paid to the nature of the behavior to be promoted (the Product), the ways in which it will be delivered (the Place), and the costs that consumers perceive they will have to pay to undertake it (the Price). Promoting the benefits of childhood vaccinations will not lead to the desired behaviors if mothers feel that getting a vaccination means hours of travel and waiting, surly treatment by health workers, and abuse back home when the husband's meal is not prepared and the chores are not taken care of. Social marketing's grounding in these realities—and in a recognition that all of the conditions must be right for behavior to take place—makes it more effective than mere advertising and promotion.

A third obstacle—and the one that is the central focus of this book—is that social marketing heretofore has not had its own conceptual underpinnings. Much of what has been written about social marketing is in the nature of descriptive reports and checklists for carrying out the elements of a sound marketing strategy. Proponents of social marketing have borrowed a number of concepts and buzzwords from commercial sector marketing. Social marketers hold focus groups and pretest ads. They forecast demand and they consider attitudes and values. To date, however, with a few exceptions (for instance, Kotler and Roberto, 1989), no one has attempted to set down a comprehensive conceptual framework for sound social marketing.

The Present Book

The goal here is to outline the basic principles already followed by good social marketers everywhere, while at the same time bringing fresh thinking to the field. Thus, the book has two major audiences. First, it represents a primer for neophytes who have just heard about social marketing. People who know little about social marketing often confuse it with other approaches like health communications, behavior analysis and modification, or social mobilization. Thus, this book is intended for students in business schools and public health programs and for field trainees and funders who have barely heard about the approach but would like to learn more.

Second, because the book offers a new, integrated framework for thinking about and carrying out social marketing, it can help practicing managers achieve behavior-change objectives more efficiently and more effectively. The managers who can benefit from the approach can be found in the fields of public health, environmental management, community development, crime prevention, social work, religious work, education and training, the arts, public transportation, conservation, and agriculture, among others.

The Framework

The central tenet of the book is that all good social marketing starts and ends with the target customer—the person whose behavior is to be influenced. Thus, it is argued that social marketers must always begin by listening to their target market. This listening, in turn, must be guided by some framework that sets out how consumers think about acting and act. Such a framework not only guides listening but also guides eventual courses of action.

The first principle of this framework holds that consumers do not act precipitously in high-involvement decisions such as those that social marketers attempt to influence. Instead, they move toward action in stages. At each stage, different approaches need to be used. At the most crucial stage, where customers are contemplating the desired action, the framework suggests that consumers consider a relatively small set of factors. These factors give marketers clues as to how to intervene. But contemplating—and even deciding positively—is not the same as acting. There are other crucial considerations that marketers must address so that customers will undertake the desired behavior—and stick to it!

The book attempts to explicate this framework and its implications and to show how it can make social marketing programs meet the dramatic challenges and achieve the potential that so many have held for it.

Overview of the Contents

The Introduction provides a general overview of the broad challenges that social marketers address. It defines social marketing and outlines its basic framework, contrasting it with other approaches with which it is sometimes compared. The chapter presents several examples of successful social marketing applications. It concludes by discussing the negative image many people have of marketing—and explaining why this image is the product of bad marketing, not of marketing that follows the approach considered here.

Chapter One starts with the key concept for the approach offered in this book: to put the target consumer at the center of the entire social marketing process. It argues that customers must make the final decision to act and so the only logical and effective way to create a behavior-change program is to start with a thorough understanding of the customers' needs, wants, and perceptions. Adopting such a focus, however, first requires that the managers of social marketing programs adopt a mindset that puts the customer at the center of attention. Chapter One introduces this mindset and shows the reader how to distinguish it from other (wrong-headed) approaches to marketing and behavior change.

Chapter Two then describes the process by which one develops and carries out an effective social marketing strategy based on a customer mindset. It leads the reader through a six-stage process that begins with listening to the customer, then goes on to develop the core marketing strategy based on what is learned in that listening process. This strategy and its principal components are then pretested on target consumers. It is always assumed that the best guide to what will work and what will not is the consumers, who have ultimate control over the outcomes. Pretesting is then followed by the design of marketing structures and systems that can deliver effective programs. Next, the programs are implemented and finally, once again, the customer is studied to ascertain whether the program is having its intended effects.

Three steps of the strategic planning process call for social marketers to carry out research involving their target customers. Chapter Three describes quantitative and qualitative research techniques that present opportunities for listening to customers at all three steps. The chapter also describes a concept called *backward research* that increases the probability that research will be useful to hard-pressed managers. Finally, it suggests ways to complete needed research at reasonable-to-low cost.

Of course, if listening to the customer is central to the design of social marketing programs, then the strongest conceptual foundation for social marketing is a framework for understanding (and then acting upon) consumer behavior. Chapter Four takes up this framework in detail, analyzing the stages customers go through when they approach high-involvement decisions like those involved in social marketing. It describes how people progress from ignorance and indifference in specific steps up to final action and maintenance of that action. At early stages of this behavioral process, education and propaganda are the central technologies that social marketers will seek to bring to bear. However, once the customer reaches the point Prochaska and DiClemente (1983) call the Contemplation Stage, social marketing assumes the central role.

We next turn to the problem of developing a comprehensive marketing strategy—given that one has already gone about listening to target customers. Marketing strategies in the present perspective have two major components. First, they specify the target segments they are going to address. Second, they specify how they are going to address them. Chapter Five focuses on the problem of market segmentation, that is, why one segments target markets and how one goes about doing so.

But, how to address those segments? Here, we turn back to the consumer behavior framework for guidance. Consumers go through stages on their way to new behavioral patterns, and the challenges facing marketers at each of the stages differ. Chapter Six focuses on what Prochaska and DiClemente (1983) call the Precontemplation Stage. This is where target consumers are not considering the proposed new behavior either because they are ignorant of it or because they believe that it is not appropriate or relevant to them, for example for religious reasons. At this stage, the social marketer must rely very much on the tools of the older fields of education and propaganda to move consumers to the point where they begin to think that maybe the new behavior is appropriate for them.

When consumers move on to the Contemplation Stage, social marketing becomes a more central, direct player in the behavior-change process. The tools of private sector marketing are most powerful in dealing with individuals who are thinking about a product or service and in getting them to act both to purchase and to purchase a specific brand, patronize a particular outlet, or use a particular credit card. In such situations, consumers are at least aware of and not opposed to the behavior. In this Contemplation Stage, decisions are typically driven by four sets of perceptions about likely benefits, likely costs, social norms and the wishes of others, and the individual's ability to control the outcome. Chapter Seven focuses on the benefits and costs while Chapter Eight focuses on social influence and behavioral control.

Once the target consumer has decided to act—even tentatively—he or she must actually take the action and, more importantly in many cases, keep up the new behavior. These are referred to here as the Action and Maintenance stages, which are the focus of Chapter Nine.

Social marketing programs, of course, require more than just a lot of good ideas and creativity. Work must be done, people must do it, and the results must be monitored and strategies and programs adjusted as needed. Also, because the ultimate goal is permanent change in a society, attention must be paid to institutionalizing the changes. This is especially important in situations where social marketing technologies are being introduced into countries or cultures not familiar with them. There are too many examples of programs that were wildly successful when outside specialists were there to make them work but that languished badly when the specialists left. These issues of creating strategic partnershs will take up Chapter Ten.

The book concludes with a summary of the major points and some implications and suggestions for those who would like to see social marketing grow and deepen in its ability to bring about dramatic social changes in societies around the world.

Acknowledgments

A great many people have contributed to my education in social marketing over the past twenty years. Although it is difficult to make such judgments, my major mentors among practicing marketers over the years have been Bill Novelli, formerly of Porter/Novelli Associates and now chief operating officer of CARE, and Bill Smith, executive vice president of the Academy for Educational Development. Bill Novelli first introduced me to the field and has helped me tie social marketing concepts again and again back to the commercial sector. Bill Smith has involved me in a wide range of very exciting ventures and, in an astonishing number of instances, has brought fresh and useful frameworks and insights to my own thinking about this field.

But there are many, many others. As will be evident throughout this volume, I have learned much from my academic colleagues, especially Paul Bloom, Martin Fishbein, Jeff Fisher, Bob Hornik, Phil Kotler, Craig Lefebvre, Jim Prochaska, and Everett Rogers. In the practical world of social marketing, my teachers have also included Mary Debus and Michael Ramah of Porter/Novelli, Dan Lissance of Population Services International, Jim Mintz of Health Promotion Canada, Tony Meyer at the U.S. Agency for International Development, Betty Ravenholt and Santiago Plata of The Futures Group, Mark Rasmuson of HealthCom, Tom Reis of the

W. K. Kellogg Foundation, Bill Schelestede of Family Health International, and Sharyn Sutton of the U.S. Department of Agriculture.

This specific book has benefitted from the careful reviews and insightful suggestions of George Balch, Marvin Goldberg, and an anonymous reviewer. Alan Shrader of Jossey-Bass provided useful stimulus and direction and kept the process moving with deliberate speed.

Above all, I must acknowledge the contribution of my wife, Jean Manning, who has provided and continues to provide rich insight into all of my work and is very often the initiator of the new intellectual and practical challenges I have addressed.

Without all of their help, this book would not have been written.

Washington, D.C. ALAN R. ANDREASEN
August 1995

For my wife, Jean Manning,
my source and inspiration

The Author

Alan R. Andreasen is professor of marketing and associate dean for faculty at the School of Business, Georgetown University. He has been a faculty member at the University of California, Los Angeles; the University of Illinois; the State University of New York, Buffalo; California State University, Long Beach; the University of Connecticut; and Claremont Graduate School. Andreasen received his B.A. degree (1956) with honors from the University of Western Ontario, as well as M.S. (1959) and Ph.D. (1964) degrees from Columbia University.

Andreasen is a specialist in consumer behavior and marketing strategy, particularly in the application of marketing to nonprofit organizations, social marketing, and the market problems of disadvantaged consumers. He is the author or editor of nine books and numerous monographs and reports. His most recent books are *Strategic Marketing in Nonprofit Organizations* (fourth edition, with Philip Kotler of Northwestern University, 1991), and *Cheap But Good Marketing Research* (1988c). He has also published more than eighty articles and conference papers on a variety of topics including strategic planning, marketing decision making, consumer behavior, marketing in nonprofit organizations, consumer satisfaction, marketing regulation, social marketing, and marketing research. He is a member of several academic and professional associations, and serves on the board of reviewers of the *Journal of Marketing,* the *Journal of Consumer Research,* and the *Journal of Public Policy and Marketing.* He is past president of the Association for Consumer Research.

Andreasen is an internationally known educator and marketing consultant. He has advised, carried out research, and conducted executive seminars for a diverse set of organizations, including both nonprofits and commercial businesses as well as several government agencies. Among the organizations for whom he has worked are the Academy for Educational Development, The Futures Group, PATH, the National Cancer Institute, the U.S. Agency for International Development, the United Way of America, Boys and Girls Clubs of America, the American Cancer Society, the National Endowment for the Arts, the Foundation for American Communications, the Public Broadcasting System, the American Forestry Association, KitchenAid, Pepsi-Cola, Aspen Highlands Ski Corporation, and family planning and public health programs in Egypt, Thailand, Colombia, Jamaica, Mexico, Indonesia, and Bangladesh.

Social Marketing: A Powerful Approach to Social Change

Changing behavior to improve people's lives is not an easy task. Consider the typical case faced by Lucia, the newly hired program manager for an international health communications program.

> On her first trip to the field, Lucia meets Maria, a thirty-seven-year-old mother of six living in a rural African village. Maria has a husband who leaves the country every summer and fall to earn money harvesting in South Africa. Two of her children have died, one of measles and one of dysentery. Two of her present children are weak and have frequent bouts of diarrhea. She is afraid they will die soon. Twelve children in the village have had measles in the last month and she fears for all her children. Her husband will return soon and will want to have sex again. She does not want more children right now and is also afraid that her husband might have this new disease called AIDS. She would like to go to the health clinic for help but the clinic is twelve kilometers away and she has to take care of the children as well as her family's few animals. Her mother-in-law lives nearby, but can be of little help in taking care of the children because she has four grandchildren already living with her. More importantly, the mother-in-law has great faith in the traditional healer in the next village, and wants Maria to go there and not to the health clinic. Finally, Maria herself does not like going to the clinic because every time she goes, she has to wait three to four hours in a very unpleasant, undecorated room filled with screaming children and with nothing for her and her children to do. Then, when she does get to see the health worker, she is treated rudely by someone who seems to regard her as a very inadequate mother.

Lucia's task in just this one case is a daunting one. She wants to improve the physical and mental health of Maria and her family but she is fighting tradition, community norms, lack of awareness of healthier alternatives, inconvenient and unpleasant health care facilities, and the family-management pressures in Maria's own life.

Tragically, many of the health problems Maria faces are problems we already know how to deal with medically. We know that oral rehydration therapy copes with dysentery and diarrhea. Immunizations prevent measles. Contraceptives prevent or delay conception. But all of these approaches require Maria to change her behavior. Indeed, 70 percent or more of world health problems can be reduced dramatically by relatively straightforward—though sometimes difficult—behavior changes. What is Lucia to do?

The Traditional Approach

Because Lucia is trained as a health educator, her first instinct is to try to educate Maria and other members of the village about better health practices. To tackle the problem of diarrhea and dehydration, she naturally thinks of arranging for a health worker to come to the village to tell the mothers there about oral rehydration therapy (ORT) and how it can save their children from dying of the dehydration that comes with dysentery. She could have the health worker teach Maria and other mothers how to prepare an oral rehydration solution (ORS) at home from boiled water, salt, and sugar. While she is in the village, the health worker could explain about vaccinations and tell the villagers when they can be obtained from the health clinic. She could tell them about AIDS and explain the value of condoms. She could also begin to teach Maria about contraception and explain the alternatives to her. She could leave behind sample condoms.

Lucia also thinks it would be a good idea to develop print materials in Maria's dialect on all of these subjects for the health worker to leave behind on her next visit. In addition, Lucia will consider planning a poster campaign to reinforce the health worker's personal messages and speaking to the Health Ministry about increasing the hours of availability for vaccinations at the health clinic.

Lucia's approach might be successful with Maria. But it is more likely to fail because there will still be conflicting village and family norms, competing time pressures, and an unresponsive medical system. Lucia will also be hampered by her own lack of resources and, many times, by the lack of cooperation she will get from Ministry of Health bureaucrats. It will take many years and many thousands of dollars before traditional education and information programs like Lucia's could make serious inroads into the problems, and many of Maria's children—and perhaps Maria herself—will be dead by then.

The Social Marketing Approach

In the last ten years, a dramatic new approach called *social marketing* has been developed to address the kinds of problems Lucia faces (Kotler and Zaltman, 1971; Lefebvre and Flora, 1988; Novelli, 1990; Andreasen, 1994). In simplest terms, social marketing is the application of marketing technologies developed in the commercial sector to the solution of social problems where the bottom line is behavior change. Marketing is an extremely powerful approach. Marketing has brought the world products that have revolutionized our lives. It has facilitated the development of innovative life-changing products and made them universally available—things like the Sony Walkman, the fast food restaurant, and the microwave oven and a whole range of packaged meals to make use of it. Its new mass markets and vast advertising and distribution networks have brought home computers and software within the reach of every middle class household in every developed country. It has made possible television programming of astonishing variety and coverage, making a reality of McLuhan's Global Village.

Marketing can change lives in both small and large ways. It can persuade us to try new products and switch brands and attend the local department store's One-Day-Only Sale. It can also get us to take up skiing or attending the performing arts. It can induce families that have never left South Dakota to travel abroad or take a Caribbean cruise.

And if marketing can change consumers' lives, surely it can be a powerful tool to improve consumers' physical and mental health and the general quality of our society and its environment.

Marketing in the commercial sector has already begun to have important secondary effects on many social problems, although this has not been its primary objective. As marketers look for new profit avenues, they have contributed importantly to the trend toward buying foods with healthier ingredients and products that are more environmentally friendly. They have helped out major nonprofit organizations by encouraging people to buy products or patronize sellers that contribute to particular charities.

What is still largely untapped is the immense potential to massively improve the quality of people's lives that this approach would have if it were put in the hands of government agencies and a wide variety of nongovernmental organizations and private voluntary organizations around the world. Marketing can help social workers get kids off drugs. It can help workers like Lucia get mothers to immunize their children. It can help get American teenagers to practice safe sex and prostitutes in Tijuana to use condoms. It can help public health services in Thailand and India reduce the number of births through family planning.

The problems faced by marketers in the commercial sector are really not very different from those facing the Lucias of the world. Consider the challenge faced by Ashley, the newly hired marketing manager for the Kellogg Company, assigned to develop the market for breakfast cereals in Japan.

In the first week of her job, Ashley visits the Tokyo home of Miyoshi, a full-time mother of two. Miyoshi's husband works long hours for Sanyo Electronics and delegates household and child-rearing responsibilities entirely to Miyoshi. Ashley learns that the household's breakfast is eaten together and consists entirely of typical Japanese fare: rice, some cooked fish, pickled vegetables, and tea. Miyoshi is aware of dry cereals and her children ask for them sometimes. But Miyoshi does not believe she would ever change her practices. Breakfast has been unchanged since she was born. Her parents, friends, and neighbors all eat the same traditional things. While she has many American products in her household, she feels that eating Corn Flakes or Rice Krispies would simply not be the Japanese way. Besides, her neighborhood market does not carry Kellogg's products and her small refrigerator has little room for extra items like milk.

What social marketers have recognized is that, in very important ways, Ashley's challenge is very similar to Lucia's. In both cases:

- The final objective is to influence the behavior of a target market (Maria and Miyoshi).
- The target behaviors compete with comfortable alternatives.
- Community pressures make it difficult to bring about change even if the target market finds it attractive.
- Critical supporting agencies (the health system and the local retailers) must help out if the behavior change program is to be successful.

Social marketers are convinced that what has made McDonald's and Coca-Cola world-class successes can eventually make Kellogg a success in Japan and can also have a dramatic impact on the problems of high blood pressure, AIDS, drug addiction, child mortality in developing countries, smoking, and heart disease. The applications are not always easy and the social and commercial worlds have dramatic differences (Rothschild, 1979; Bloom and Novelli, 1981). But as we shall see throughout this book, social marketing has already had a number of dramatic successes. Social marketing can have even greater impact if more practitioners, policy makers, and sources of funding understand its principles and its promise.

Fortunately, social marketing is now becoming an established part of the marketing vocabulary in universities, government agencies, private nonprofit organizations, and private for-profit firms. There are social marketing textbooks (Manoff, 1985; Fine, 1981; Kotler and Roberto, 1989), books of readings (Fine, 1990), chapters in mainstream marketing texts (Kotler and Andreasen, 1991), chapters in health education readings books (Novelli, 1990) and a Harvard teaching note (Rangun and Karim, 1991). There have been reviews of the accomplishments of social marketing (Fox and Kotler, 1980; Malafarina and Loken, 1993), criticisms (Luck, 1974; Wallack, 1990), a history of the field (Elliott, 1991), and calls to researchers to become more deeply involved in studies of social marketing to advance the science of marketing (Andreasen, 1993). Major international and domestic behavior change programs now routinely have social marketing components (Smith, 1989; Debus, 1987; Ramah and Cassidy, 1992). Individuals with titles like "Manager of Social Marketing" can be found in private consulting organizations.

Social marketing is a concept whose time has come!

What This Book Is About

This book is designed to introduce social change agents like Maria and her superiors and sponsors to social marketing. It explains what social marketing is and how one goes about doing it in real, practical settings. It points out its advantages and disadvantages in comparison with other approaches with which the reader may be familiar—such as health education or health communications. It outlines the differences between good social marketing and bad social marketing.

But, more important, the book presents a new paradigm for approaching social marketing. Heretofore, books and articles about social marketing have dwelt on selected topics or have adapted standard commercial sector marketing frameworks to this area. What is attempted here is a totally new integrated framework that draws upon work in both social psychology and marketing. As will be shown, it is a serviceable, flexible framework that can guide strategy development in a wide range of social intervention situations.

This is not just a book for those who want to learn about social marketing for the first time. It is also a book for people who are already doing social marketing. A great many researchers and consultants have begun to move into the field from related disciplines like communications and development. And many practitioners have found themselves carrying out projects that have come to be labeled social marketing and so they, too, see themselves as social marketers. This book is designed to furnish a conceptual underpinning for what they do—and a set of guidelines for how to improve what they are doing. As I know from personal experience, there are a great many people out there who mistakenly believe they are engaged in social marketing. They know the jargon and can impress naive listeners, but they have not absorbed the proper mindset and they have employed very limited tools. And they have failed to keep their eye on the behavioral bottom line.

Social marketing can be a very powerful tool for social change, but only if it is done well and only if those doing it appreciate both its potential and its nuances. A great many of those who do not really understand social marketing think of it as *social advertising*. They think that all social marketers really do is bring in so-called Madison Avenue advertising techniques and try to bring about behavior change by inundating markets with slick television or radio commercials, clever product packaging, and a few glossy brochures and posters.

But social marketing is much more—and it is different. It is a way of thinking about the behavior-change process that is different from that adopted by others in the social change business. It is also a process for planning and implementing strategies for change. And, finally, it is a set of concepts and techniques for carrying out various aspects of the social marketing process. To be an effective social marketer who gets the results the approach promises, a social change agent must understand all three. And that is what this book tries to explain.

What Is Social Marketing?

To understand what this dramatic innovation is all about, we first need a definition and some sense of what social marketing is—and what it is not! I begin with a formal definition:

> Social marketing is the application of commercial marketing technologies to the analysis, planning, execution, and evaluation of programs designed to influence the voluntary behavior of target audiences in order to improve their personal welfare and that of their society.

This definition is similar to that of commercial sector marketing (as described in Kotler and Armstrong, 1994). The main difference is that there the ultimate goal is to benefit the sponsoring organization and not—except as a means to an end—the target audience or the broader society. Although it may seem unnecessarily academic, the definition of social marketing contains a number of features that set this approach apart from other technologies with which it is often compared. Here are the key points:

1.   *The ultimate objective of social marketing is to benefit target individuals or society and not the marketer.* This distinguishes it from commercial marketing but makes it similar to nonprofit marketing. It differs from the latter, however, in that it is precisely focused on directly improving welfare. Thus, when we are talking about social marketing, we are not talking about fundraising, lobbying (except to remove restrictions on social marketing), or the election of political candidates.

2.   *The basic means of achieving improved welfare is through influencing behavior, in most cases bringing about a change in behavior.* Social marketers are in the behavior business. (In this book, the phrases "changing behavior" and "influencing behavior" will be used interchangeably to describe social marketing's ultimate objective. Strictly speaking, the former term is a subcategory of the latter, which has broader implications.) Influencing behavior is the bottom line in social settings just as much as it is in private settings. Kellogg will measure its marketing success in Japan on the basis of sales and market share, both behavioral measures. Similarly, social change agents in Egypt will measure the success of oral rehydration programs in terms of the "market share" of episodes of diarrhea that are treated with oral rehydration solutions of some kind. While often very long in coming, behavioral change is central: all other measures of success are only interim measures that offer encouragement on the path toward the ultimate bottom line.

3.   *The target audience has the primary role in the social marketing process.* As will be made clear in Chapter One—and, indeed, everywhere in this book—first-rate social marketing is always totally centered on the target customer. And "customer" is the best word to use; although "client" and "target audience member" can be used more or less interchangeably with it, they are not as effective in calling attention to the active role the target person plays in the process. After all, there is no behavioral influence until the person to be influenced takes an action, and in social marketing this involves doing something just as concrete as buying an airplane ticket or a soft drink. The best social marketers realize instinctively that the customer holds the key to success. It is the customer who must ultimately undertake the action the marketer is promoting. And so everything a good social marketer does starts with the

customer's perspective. As we shall see, this makes all the difference between programs that ought to work and programs that really do!

Alternative Approaches

Before the advent of social marketing, there were a great many other technologies around that sought to induce behavior change. They are still around today, with labels such as: health education (Glanz, Lewis, and Rimer, 1990), health communications (Backer, Rogers, and Sopory, 1992), health promotion (McElroy, Gottlieb, and Burdine, 1987), mass communications (Atkin and Wallack, 1990), media advocacy (Wallack, 1990; Wallack, Dorfman, Jernigan, and Themba, 1993), public advertising (Deutsch and Liebermann, 1985), public communications (Rice and Atkin, 1989; McGuire, 1984), social advertising (Kotler and Roberto, 1989; Weibe, 1951–52), and social mobilization (Minkler, 1990; Glanz, 1990).

These approaches are directed to the same kinds of social problems that social marketing addresses and each of them has useful insights and recommendations that social marketers can use. But they typically start from assumptions that ultimately limit the effect they can have (Hornik, 1992). I shall group them into four alternatives:

- The Education Approach
- The Persuasion Approach
- The Behavioral Modification Approach
- The Social Influence Approach

The Education Approach

The education approach begins with the primary assumption that individuals will do the right thing if only they understand why they need to do what is being advocated and know how to carry it out. The educator's task is to bring the facts to the target audience in the most lucid and compelling fashion possible. It is the approach that underlies the Health Belief Model (HBM) used extensively in the health care field (Hochbaum, 1958; Rosenstock, 1960, 1966, 1974). In the early versions of this model, behavior was seen as driven by four sets of key beliefs:

- Perceived susceptibility to a given health problem
- Perceived severity of the problem
- Perceived benefits from acting
- Perceived barriers to taking the action

Although some authors caution that the HBM "does not presuppose or imply a strategy for change" (Rosenstock and Kirscht, 1974, p. 472), most practitioners conclude that any behavior-change strategy must focus on directly modifying these beliefs. In such strategies, careful attention is paid to using the right channels of communications and the right spokespeople. Messages are carefully assessed for readability to, and understanding by, the target audience.

Changing beliefs can be successful (Janz and Becker, 1984). But this approach is lacking several important components. First, it does not focus on behavior. It assumes that, if one can change beliefs, behavior will follow. Social marketers pay a great deal of attention to how to make that behavior happen and how to sustain it.

Second, it ignores the effects of social pressure. Social marketers recognize that many of us undertake acts even when we personally see no need to or are even actively opposed to them. And many times, we do not act because society or those we respect oppose the action. Inhibiting social norms keep Maria from changing from traditional healers and Miyoshi from switching to Rice Krispies.

Third, delivering facts to change beliefs may have a boomerang effect. Facts have an unfortunate tendency to move action in surprising ways, and *boomerang effects*—that is, results opposite those planned—are not all that rare. Take the case of breast health. Agencies like the American Cancer Society and the National Cancer Institute have tried for many years to get women—especially those over fifty—to practice breast self-examination and get regular mammograms. Many campaigns set out to educate women about the risk factors associated with breast cancer, such as a family history of the disease. It was believed that educating women about risk factors would cause those with higher risk to be especially conscientious in carrying out the desired behaviors, practicing breast self-examination and having frequent mammograms. What the campaigners did not count on was the boomerang effect this message would have on women who did not possess the risk factors. As the National Cancer Institute learned, a great many women concluded that if they did not have the risk factors, they did not need to take precautions. Research has very clearly established that six in seven women who get breast cancer do not have any of the risk factors! Yet over 40 percent of women who decide against having a screening mammogram cite the lack of a family history as their reason. This research is described in detail in an unpublished paper prepared by the American Association of Retired Persons and the National Cancer Institute (cited in Sutton, Balch, and Lefebvre, in press).

The Persuasion Approach

This approach recognizes a number of deficiencies of the education approach and takes it one step further. Adherents to this approach have a fundamental belief that action takes place only if people are sufficiently motivated. Thus, the goal of the persuasionist is to discover the careful arguments and motivational hot buttons that will get the educated consumer to "get off the dime." It is an approach that underlies what Kotler and Roberto (1989, p. 26) call social advertising. Social advertising promotes causes and ideas such as the "Just Say No" antidrug campaign.

The problem is that the persuasion approach is one of getting the consumer to adopt the persuasionist's view of the world. This group knows what is good for consumers and attempts to push this view of the world on them. It is what marketers would call a *selling approach* (Andreasen, 1982), and it is what often gives marketing a bad name because it is organization centered. It tries to sell the new idea or the new behavior to the consumer from the promoter's point of view. Social marketers, by contrast, adopt a customer-centered approach and recognize that change will only come about if one starts with the customers' reality (Sutton, Balch, and Lefebvre, in press) and adapts messages and other program elements to the customers' perceptions, needs, and wants.

❦ The Behavioral Modification Approach

This approach tends to <u>minimize the influence of thoughts and feelings</u> on individual behavior. It stresses very simple principles of learning theory that argue that people do what they do because they (a) learn the techniques necessary for the action and (b) find the outcomes rewarding. Behaviorists emphasize training and modeling of desired behavior and then give careful attention to rewarding the behavior when it occurs (Graeff, Elder, and Booth, 1993; Holland and Skinner, 1961). It is <u>an approach that was used in the frequently cited Stanford Heart Program</u> (Farquar and others, 1985). A basic problem with this approach is that it is <u>very costly</u>. Whereas education and persuasion can be aimed at the masses as well as at individual customers, the behavioral modification approach almost always has to be at the individual level. Social marketers recognize that, to have maximum social effectiveness in a world of very limited budgets, one must focus on changing groups of consumers—not individuals and not mass markets, but carefully selected segments.

❦ The Social Influence Approach

Sensitive to the last criticism, advocates of this approach argue that campaigns directed at influencing community norms and collective behavior are the most cost-effective way to reach and change individuals and families (Wallack, 1990). Thus, they see changing social norms about things like smoking in the workplace or using condoms on a college date as the best way to convince individuals that they must act in the prescribed way or risk social isolation. However, the approach may be limited to situations in which:

- Social issues and norms are well understood and accepted (Miller and Friesen, 1984).
- The pressures to conform are extremely strong (Asch, 1952).
- The behavior to be influenced is socially important and visible.

Thus, the social influence approach might work in Africa for immunization, for example, because community ties are so strong. And there are occasions in more developed cultures where it can work also, as in the revolution in social attitudes toward smoking in the United States and Canada in the last twenty years. However, it is more likely that the more educated and emancipated the individual consumers, the less likely that group norms would have a major role to play in behavior change. Social norms may delay or accelerate action, but this action is more likely to be primarily under individual control. Thus, college women will or will not suggest using a condom on their next date depending on their individual values and beliefs, their own skills and motives, and the nature of the situation and relationship. They may be encouraged to be more vigorous about insisting on condoms if they believe that other young women are doing the same thing—or less vigorous if they feel their personal actions were somewhat unconventional. But getting a particular young woman to act just by convincing her that most of her peers are doing so is not certain. Social marketers recognize that this approach may be worth trying, but certainly would not count on this technique alone.

The Social Marketing Approach

Social marketing has features in common with each of the above approaches. It often attempts to educate. It does seek to motivate individuals to act. It does introduce group pressure when appropriate and it often does employ modeling and rewards to ensure the long term success of its programs. But social marketing is both different and more comprehensive than these alternatives. It has seven features, shown in Exhibit I.1.

First and foremost, like behaviorists, social marketers regard what their customers actually do as the bottom line for judging their success. Unlike educators, who may be satisfied that messages were distributed and received and that people have apparently learned some facts, social marketers argue that learning facts is only important if it leads to a desired behavioral outcome. Expert social marketers would not make the mistake of educating women about the risks of breast cancer without checking to see whether the possession of such information led to increased readiness to practice self-examination and schedule regular mammograms.

Good social marketers recognize that behavior change in high-

Exhibit I.1. Key Features of Social Marketing.

1. Consumer behavior is the bottom line.
2. Programs must be cost-effective.
3. All strategies begin with the customer.
4. Interventions involve the *Four P's:* Product, Price, Place, and Promotion.
5. Market research is essential to designing, pretesting, and evaluating intervention programs.
6. Markets are carefully segmented.
7. Competition is always recognized.

---

involvement situations may take a long time to bring about. Thus they may temporarily focus on achieving nonbehavioral objectives such as a certain knowledge level or a certain attitude change. However, they always keep their eye on the final outcome and make sure that interim measures are always carefully designed to lead directly to the intended goal.

Second, like their commercial sector progenitors, social marketers worry about being cost-effective. That is, they are constantly aware that they are entrusted with limited resources and that they must use them wisely. This makes them willing to make trade-offs, ignore certain markets, seek cooperative alliances, and otherwise leverage meager resources to achieve what are often very dramatic objectives.

Third, as many pioneers in health education have advocated (Nyswander, 1966), social marketers are fanatically customer-centered in their strategies and tactics. They do not seek to persuade target audiences to do what the marketer believes they ought to do. They do not try to make the audience accept the marketer's values and beliefs. Rather, they recognize that customers only take action when they believe that it is in their interests. Social marketing persuasion strategies therefore always start with an understanding of the target audience's needs and wants, their values, their perceptions. Social marketers do not start out with an assumption that their job is to change the customer to conform with the marketer. They recognize that they must often change their social marketing offerings and the way these are presented to meet target customer needs and wants. Respect for the importance of the customer is central to everything the social marketer does.

Fourth, unlike many of the alternative paradigms, social marketers do not rely on one or two program elements to bring about change. Based on their experience in the commercial sector, they recognize that four different sets of factors must be in place before bottom-line behaviors will take place. These four elements are often called the Four P's:

Product: Social marketers recognize that they must propose the right kind of behavioral offering if customers are going to act. Maria is not likely to attend the health clinic if she believes its staff is going to make her wait a long time and then act as though they think she is a very poor and ignorant mother. As Maria might say: she doesn't need to put with that kind of treatment on top of all her other problems. A social marketer would immediately recognize that to have a major impact on target customers like Maria, the health care delivery system (the "product") must be overhauled so that the behavior to be marketed is as attractive as possible. Nordstrom's certainly would not expect to do very well in the retail clothing business if it had surly clerks!

Price: Social marketers recognize that decisions to act are based on considerations of both benefits and costs. In the commercial sector, customers pay costs in money for product and service benefits. In the social sector, customers like Maria pay costs that are not monetary—costs in time away from home, in verbal abuse from unfed husbands, and in concern for the well-being of temporarily abandoned children. Social marketers know that a great many transactions fail to take place not because the benefits were not appreciated but because the costs were too high. They know they must work on both the benefit and cost sides of the equation.

Place: Social marketers recognize that behaviors must be easy to do. This means that health clinics should be made as accessible as possible to women like Maria. It means that condoms should be handy when dates seem likely to lead to sex. It means that oral rehydration liquids should be available at every kiosk and vendor in every village where diarrhea and dysentery are a problem. Social marketers know that great education and motivation programs will fail if products and services needed to carry out behaviors are not readily available to people who want to act. Successful family planning campaigns in rural villages require education, motivation, social pressure—and the availability of pills and condoms.

Promotion: Social marketers, of course, carry out a great deal of advertising where it is appropriate. But they see promotion much more broadly than the production of brochures, posters, TV spots, and public service announcements. Promotion can include what is called personal selling in the commercial sector. Social marketers recognize that a mother like Maria may be much more influenced by a quiet conversation with another mother like herself who has been trained as a village health promoter than she is by any fancy advertising campaign. Promotion can also include tactics that reward consumers for desirable behaviors. A very important component of an ORS social marketing project in The Gambia was a contest that gave mothers a free plastic cup or a bar of soap for correctly mixing oral rehydration solutions.

Fifth, social marketers are almost fanatical about conducting research, even when this research is something as simple as a number of carefully planned conversations with customers. Because marketers know that customers control outcomes, they know that they must understand where customers are coming from before they decide just what to try to sell. Thus, social marketers put a lot of effort into what they call *formative research*. Sometimes this research is fairly costly and involves detailed surveys. At other times, the formative research may be as simple as a number of conversations with groups of consumers to learn their thoughts and feelings about the behavior the marketer is proposing and its behavioral alternatives.

Social marketers also believe research is important to pretest program components before going into the field. Because social marketers start with the customer, they immediately see that is the customer's reaction to the message or the product or the place that is important. They use customers as the touchstone against which everything is measured for potential effectiveness.

Of course, social marketers do not stop researching once a program is in the field. They recognize that a great deal can change as a program goes into a complex field environment, where there can be interference and distortion in what a campaign is trying to do. They know that what is crucial about a campaign is how it is affecting consumers and they are perfectly ready to shift course should mid-campaign data suggest the program is off-track. A good example of this comes from tracking data for an ORS program in Southeast Asia. The promotion component of this program was designed to get mothers to perceive the dangers of dehydration resulting from diarrhea and the possible benefits of using ORS for rehydrating youngsters at risk. The tracking data showed that mothers believed that ORS would cure diarrhea. When it didn't, they lost faith not only in the product but also in the messenger. These data led to a major overhaul of the basic message strategy and a more careful linkage between what the product does and what its effects on the child will be.

A sixth characteristic of social marketing is that, unlike many public education and community motivation programs, social marketers tend not to treat their targets as mass markets. This is a by-product of their customer orientation. Social marketers find that it is difficult to approach markets as masses once they have carried out formative research that inevitably points out all the ways in which customers are different. Social marketers recognize that, although they cannot afford to treat customers individually except in some very well-funded small-scale projects, it is still possible to group customers into what marketers call *segments* for strategic purposes. These segments then become the focuses for distinctive programs, separate budget allocations, and even different emphases over the duration of a project.

The final defining characteristic of social marketing stems from its commercial sector origins. Social marketers place a good deal of emphasis on competition. They recognize that every choice of action on the consumer's part involves giving up some other action. Thus, campaigns must keep in mind not only what the marketer is trying to get across but also what the customer sees as the major alternatives. Many times social marketers can bring about change as much by showing the deficiencies of an alternative as they can by emphasizing the benefits of the approach the marketer favors.

Succeeding chapters will spell out in considerable detail how to translate these unique characteristics of social marketing into specific strategies and tactics. But first, here are several success stories to illustrate how the techniques yield practical results.

Success Stories

What is most exciting about social marketing is that it works. From its beginnings twenty years ago in early public health and family planning programs, social marketing has developed a coherent philosophy and a set of strategies and procedures that its adherents now know can be extremely effective. The success stories that follow not only demonstrate this point very clearly but also outline many of the key elements of the social marketing approach elaborated upon in succeeding chapters.

The National High Blood Pressure Education Program

The National High Blood Pressure Education Program (NHBPEP) is, I believe, the longest-running behavior-change program to use social marketing concepts, processes, and tools in the United States. It is certainly one of the most successful.

The NHBPEP was established in 1972 by the National Heart, Lung, and Blood Institute (NHLBI) after a series of epidemiological, clinical, and actuarial studies made clear that high blood pressure was a major risk factor for stroke and heart disease. The program's objective was to increase awareness of the linkage between these two conditions and to influence those with high blood pressure to obtain treatment for their problem.

When the NHBPEP began, twenty-three million U.S. citizens were estimated to be hypertensive (National Heart, Lung, and Blood Institute, 1992) according to a relatively strict definition. In subsequent years, the definition of high blood pressure was changed to include about sixty million people with blood pressure over 140/90 or taking hypertensive medication. The program evolved over time as the audience changed. Initially, only 29 percent of the public knew of the link between high blood pressure and stroke and only 24 percent knew that high blood pressure causes heart disease (National Heart, Lung, and Blood Institute, 1973). Only about one-half of all hypertensives were aware of their problem. Thus, the behavioral focus in the early stages of the social marketing project was to get people to get their blood pressure checked. The principal approach to achieving this end was educating people about the link between high blood pressure and disease and getting them to their doctors for a checkup.

Ten years later, 59 percent of the population knew the relationship between high blood pressure and stroke and 71 percent knew it caused heart disease. Ninety-two percent knew that it cannot be cured and that a hypertensive person must always stay on a treatment program (National Heart, Lung, and Blood Institute, 1986). Even further progress was made by 1985, when 91 percent knew of the link to heart disease and 77 percent knew the link to stroke (Roccella, Bowler, Ames, and Horan, 1986).

By 1985, the NHBPEP had brought much of the target market into what I shall later call the Contemplation Stage, that is, aware of the problem and actively thinking about doing something about it. According to a 1985 National Health Interview Survey, 94 percent of the population knew whether their blood pressure was high, normal, or low (Roccella, Bowler, Ames, and Horan, 1986). About one-half of those with hypertension had moved beyond the contemplation stage to plan and take action to control their blood pressure. However, almost one-half still had not taken action. The project therefore shifted its focus in 1985 to "aware hypertensives" and securing greater levels of compliance (such as taking efforts to control the problem) from this group. This change in strategy was effective in raising compliance to 73 percent by 1988–1991 (National Heart, Lung, and Blood Institute, 1992).

Other behavior changes have also been manifested. Over 95 percent of hypertensives report cutting salt and sodium in their diets, 89 percent diet to lose weight, and 86 percent exercise (Roccella, Bowler, Ames, and Horan, 1986). However, research has shown that aware hypertensives have trouble staying with their new behaviors and that there remain variations in awareness and compliance across racial and gender groupings. Thus, in recent years, the NHBPEP has emphasized the Maintenance Stage of the behavior-change process and has continued to develop segmented programs for men and women, for blacks and Hispanics, for young, middle-aged, and elderly people, and for people in high-incidence sections of the country. Plans for the decade of the 1990s involve closer targeting of black males over age forty-five (a group where prevalence rates are high and treatment compliance is low), and of hypertensives in the Stroke Belt (the part of the Southeastern United States where the incidence of strokes among hypertensives is 10 percent higher than in any other part of the country).

The program began with—and continues to use—a number of important social marketing principles:

- *It focuses on behavior.* The concern is not with educating and communicating information, but with getting hypertensives to undertake and stay with treatment programs.
- *It works through intermediaries.* It recognizes that the problem is too large for one organization to tackle and that many other health care institutions have an important stake in reducing the incidence of high blood pressure. NHLBI coordinates high blood pressure programs through forty-one partner organizations.
- *It insists on a unified communication approach.* Working in cooperation with Porter/Novelli, a Washington, D.C., social marketing consultant, NHBPEP regularly develops carefully articulated communications objectives and strategies, defines target audiences, and establishes roles for intermediary groups. All messages are designed to reinforce one another.
- *It starts by understanding the customers.* The development of strategy begins with target audience members and their perceptions.
- *It adapts to changes in the audience.* Program strategy follows the target audience as it evolves through various stages of the behavior change process.
- *It avoids mass marketing.* Careful attention was paid to developing differentiated strategies for different market segments.
- *Its message strategies have focused on consequences,* both positive and negative, to the hypertensive person. These consequences include those of going through the treatment regimen (*the*

behavioral process) and also those of being successful in controlling blood pressure (*the behavioral outcomes*).

- *Its message strategies have also focused on social influence.*
- *It emphasized the Place component of the mix.* By making it easy to check blood pressure in homes and shopping malls, the program tore down barriers to implementing behaviors audiences knew were important.

The Pawtucket Heart Health Program

The Pawtucket Heart Health Program (PHHP) is an example of a short-term social marketing program (Lefebvre, Lasater, Carleton, and Peterson, 1987; Lefebvre and others, 1987). It focused on reducing the blood cholesterol levels of residents of the city of Pawtucket, Rhode Island, beginning in 1985 and going on into the 1990s. The program began by studying the characteristics of the target audience and their particular needs and wants. Three groups were targeted. Adults were the major interest. In addition, special focus was given to physicians, who were most likely to treat people with high cholesterol levels, and middle-aged men who had made initial contact with the PHHP. Different strategies were developed for each segment.

The Pawtucket program offered both products and services to its major target market. Program staff developed and pretested a self-help "Nutrition Kit" designed to help target audience members change their diet. They held events where target audience members could get Screening, Counseling, and Referral (SCORE) evaluation. Mass print campaigns were conducted in local media and print media were made available at work sites, churches, and schools. In addition, the campaign used direct mail and telemarketing aimed at middle-aged men. Efforts were made to reduce the costs of getting to the SCORE events by locating them at major life path points such as grocery stores and shopping malls.

Pricing tactics involved a charge of $5 for the SCORE, with a $1 discount to men targeted by the telemarketing and direct mail program. Other promotion features included a kickoff SCORE event during the St. Patrick's Day parade and six weeks of newspaper columns on diet and cholesterol.

The campaign was extremely successful in just its first two months:

Briefly, 39 SCOREs were attended by 1,439 adults, 60 percent of whom were identified as having elevated blood cholesterol levels. Two months after the campaign, 72.3 percent of these persons had returned for a second measurement. Nearly 60 percent of this group had reduced their blood cholesterol level by an average of 29.1 mg/dl. More important than these short-term results has been the integration of the essential components of this campaign into ongoing PHHP activities. This marketing strategy has led to over 10,000 persons having had their blood cholesterol measured in the subsequent two years, all of whom have received information on how to help themselves make dietary changes to manage elevated levels, and many have subsequently been referred to their physician for more intensive treatment. Interestingly, a recent survey of local physicians' attitudes and practice . . . found them to be more aggressive in initiating either drug or diet therapy [due in part to] patient requests for blood cholesterol measurements and/or dietary information [Lefebvre and Flora, 1988, pp. 310–311].

The HealthCom Projects

HealthCom—originally called Health Communications for Child Survival—was a long-term program sponsored by the U.S. Agency for International Development up to early 1995. It applied communications and marketing technologies to increase rates of child survival in selected developing countries. The program worked in seventeen countries in Asia, Africa, and Latin America and focused on immunization, diarrhea control, breast-feeding, nutrition, growth monitoring, and hygiene. While initially described as a health communications project, the managers of HealthCom ultimately recognized that social marketing was the project's organizing principle (Rasmuson, Seidel, Smith, and Booth, 1988, p. 10). Indeed, the full name of the final phase of the project was "Health Communications and Marketing for Child Survival."

Individual HealthCom projects made extensive use of formative research and used a fully coordinated marketing mix that paid attention to the positioning of the sought-for behavior (the Product), the costs that the target audience would have to bear to undertake the behavior (the Price), the locations at which necessary products or services could be obtained (the Place), and both the mass media and personal communications designed to bring about the desired actions (the Promotion). Each project was subject to careful monitoring and evaluation in order to fine-tune tactics and strategies on the run.

Specific HealthCom projects included the following:

The PREMI Project

The PREMI project, carried out in Ecuador between October 1985 and June 1988, has been described as "a milestone . . . in child survival efforts worldwide" (Hornik and others, 1991, p. 2). Working in cooperation with the local National Institute of the Child and Family (known as INNFA) and the Ministry of Health, PREMI focused primarily on promoting increased immunization of young children and the control of diarrhea through the use of ORS packets, with a secondary emphasis on breast-feeding and growth monitoring. The major "product" of the PREMI program was seven *jornadas* or vaccination days where children were vaccinated and sometimes weighed and where mothers could receive ORS packets. These events were backed by both continuing health communications and *jornadas*-specific promotions through mass media and in person through the health system. Cooperative activities by the Ecuadoran Ministry of Health and UNICEF also supported the program.

Immediate results from the program were dramatic. If one uses the very strict standard of verified immunizations (issuing immunization cards marked by health workers), the proportion of children fully immunized by the age of one went from 15 percent before PREMI to 31 percent after PREMI. More generous estimates (adjusting for underreporting) indicate an increase from 22 percent to 43 percent. And if the latter calculation is used for children up to 18 months, coverage rises to 66 percent (Hornik and others, 1991, pp. v–vi). Evaluation research indicated that not only had coverage at least doubled, it was occurring at an earlier age.

With respect to diarrhea control, PREMI could claim not only substantially increased usage of oral rehydration solution (ORS) from about 5 percent of cases to around 20 percent but also increases in awareness and knowledge. After eighteen months of the program, almost all mothers were aware of ORS, 60 percent had tried it, and three-quarters of mothers could prepare it accurately.

The PREMI project also experienced two major setbacks that provide very useful lessons for other social marketing projects. First, the ORS project was not as successful as it could have been because the promotional efforts generated by the *jornadas* and the mass media were not carefully integrated with practices in the Ministry of Health (MOH). About 30 percent of all cases of diarrhea were treated at MOH clinics. Yet, despite the presumed greater seriousness of these cases and despite the apparent commitment of MOH to the PREMI project, only one-third of the children were given ORS. Further, evaluators discovered that there was not full distribution of ORS packets to the clinics, which suggested that future use of ORS after the conclusion of the PREMI project would be restricted.

The second major setback was in the institutionalization of the social marketing methodology in the Ministry of Health. This never materialized. In their evaluation of the project, Hornik and his colleagues offer the following insightful explanation:

> Essentially the social marketing effort was entirely located in INNFA; it received both the funds and the technical advice to support this area. Those activities were run within the broad PREMI framework and reflected many joint meetings with MOH personnel. Nonetheless, operationally they were carried out in isolation. It was clear that these activities were not part of the MOH. Also, it was generally believed that the entire social marketing approach with its heavy emphasis on mass media promotion was also ideologically alien to many MOH personnel, particularly in the health education department. This department historically had emphasized smaller scale community-level promotion efforts; their failure to be incorporated into, or be funded by, or obtain any credit for, the social marketing efforts of PREMI did little to win them over [Hornik and others, 1991, pp. ix–x].

The Philippines National Urban Immunization Program

HealthCom carried out both a pilot test and a national program in municipal centers in the Philippines designed to increase the rate of immunization among children aged twelve to twenty-three months. The project was, in part, in response to President Aquino's pledge to achieve a goal of vaccination of 90 percent of the eligible population. Based on research for the Metro Manila pilot test, managers decided that the program should position itself as a measles campaign. Measles was the most common communicable disease recognized by mothers and was the third-largest killer of infants in the country. Also, the measles shot was the last in the typical childhood vaccination series and mothers seeking measles shots would be forced to get full coverage.

The project used a number of important marketing principles. It sharply focused the campaign on a single day for free immunization each week in order to reduce the cost to mothers who might worry about coming on a day when they could not be served. In addition, sales conferences were held with municipal and regional health care leaders around the country, local mayors, and with the critical local clinical workers to ensure their cooperation. The promotional campaign involved the mass media, four television and four radio spots, and a newspaper announcement, backed with a wide range of promotional pieces including posters, bunting, and welcome streamers for health centers, stickers for local minibuses and tricycles, and T-shirts for health center staff.

The national project took place over a relatively short period of time, six months in the summer of 1990. Even in such a short time, the project reported two significant accomplishments. First, complete vaccination coverage based on both cards and verbal reports went up from 54 percent to 64 percent. Second, more significantly, the proportion of children who had complete coverage by age one increased from 32 percent to 56 percent. Evaluations by the Annenberg School of Communications at the University of Pennsylvania concluded that "the program produced timely vaccination largely by realizing sharp improvements in client knowledge, particularly about the logistics of vaccination" (Hornik, Zimicki and Less, 1991, p. 11). By focusing on the days of free coverage, the campaign may well have increased mothers' perception that they could actually carry out what the campaign and the president were urging them to do. That is, there was an increase in perceived self-efficacy, a concept I shall discuss further in Chapter Four.

Central Java Vitamin A Campaign

The HealthCom Vitamin A (ROVITA) project in Central Java (beginning in October 1988) again points up the value of having a coordinated strategy. In partnership with the Indonesian Department of Health, Diponegoro University, and Helen Keller International, HealthCom carried out formative research, trained health workers, and developed, pretested, and disseminated mass media communications (primarily radio spots). They also developed motivational activities for health workers, and conducted monitoring, evaluation, and professional development activities for health department officials and university staff.

Comparisons of results from one of the two intervention regencies (districts) in Central Java with a control regency indicated clearly that the media campaign was not effective on its own. Only when the campaign was conducted in areas where there was a health post where worker training and motivation were carried out and where Vitamin A products were easily available was there an effect. In the latter cases, Vitamin A capsule coverage of eligible children increased from 24 percent to 40 percent. There were no significant changes in communities without a health post. The project evaluators recommended exploration of additional personal channels of outreach through village leaders and their wives as ways of supplementing the mass media and health worker interventions (McDivitt and McDowell, 1991).

Other Sites

The HealthCom project has also been effective in Lesotho. There, there was a significant increase in the use of oral rehydration therapy both at home and in health centers and, while there was no increase in the already-high rates of immunization, there was an improvement in the age at which the immunizations were given (Yoder and Zheng, 1991). Results in Lubumbashi, Zaire (Yoder, Zheng, and Zhou, 1991), and in West Java (McDivitt, McDowell, and Zhou, 1991) were more modest.

The Stanford Five-City Project Smoker's Challenge

The Stanford Heart Disease Prevention program has frequently been cited as an example of social marketing (Kotler and Roberto, 1989). One component of the lengthy Five-City Project (FCP) in California attempted to reach and influence smokers not highly motivated to quit, who were not being affected by other components of the FCP. The project managers used a great many of the social marketing practices that will be described at length in subsequent chapters of this book:

- They chose a specific target audience for influence: moderately motivated male smokers. (This target audience was in an advanced portion of the Contemplation Stage as discussed in Chapter Four.)
- They set several behavioral objectives for the program:
  Induce a large number of smokers (particularly in the target audience) to sign up for the program.
  Achieve at least a 20 percent quit rate.
  Provide skills for quitters so that they can remain nonsmokers for at least one year.
- They developed an initial product (one six-week quit smoking contest), a product brand (the Smokers Challenge) and a promotional strategy (a contest prize) based on initial needs analysis of the target audience.
- All three elements were pretested on potential target audience members. The contest and label were tested in informal interview settings and alternative incentives were tested in two random telephone surveys of ninety-seven smokers.
- Channels for contest promotion were selected on the basis of experience and media usage data.
- Cooperating organizations (such as the local TV station) were induced to assist in the project in order to stretch the budget and broaden market penetration.
- Attempts were made to minimize both economic and psychological costs of the recommended behaviors.
- Both process and outcome objectives of the smoking contest were monitored throughout the six weeks by means of quitting data and focus group discussions.
- An end-of-campaign evaluation was carried out. It revealed that 501 smokers had signed up for the program, with a higher proportion of men than other FCP projects in the community. Forty-five percent had quit for a short time, and 22 percent "permanently" quit with a one-year maintenance rate of 15 percent (King, Flora, Portman, and Taylor, 1987).
- Revisions in the "product" elements of the project strategy

became the basis of Smokers' Challenge II. As noted in Lefebvre and Flora (1988, p. 312):

> New quitting materials were developed that were more directive and gave smokers a day-by-day set of guidelines for quitting in twelve days. This revised self-help program was supported by a twelve-day radio show that reinforced the principles in the booklet. Based on smokers' preferences for "cold turkey" approaches to quitting, this new guide was titled "Cool Turkey."

> These new guidelines were the only quitting approach advertised in the recruitment materials, which were mailed to all participants requesting them, thus improving access to information about quitting.

> The contest was expanded from six weeks to three months. Smokers could earn chances for both the final prize and for smaller prizes if they sent in monthly "quit cards."

Evaluation of Smoking Challenge II revealed similar enrollment rates as Smoking Challenge I and the same proportion of males participating. However, the revised strategy yielded higher quit rates of 30 percent.

Marketing Image

As just described, social marketing has great potential to help organizations achieve behavior-change goals. However, a great many people are very suspicious, even hostile, toward marketing. This is particularly true of professionals in public service or in private nonprofit organizations. These individuals think of marketing in all its most abhorrent manifestations. They think of marketing as intrusive, gimmicky, and shallow. They see marketers as trying to induce people to take certain actions sometimes against their will and sometimes for the wrong reasons (like the chance to win a radio or a bicycle). They find it offensive to their professional pride to be associated with what they see as craven manipulators (that is, marketers).

They do not like the terms "customers" and "consumers" or even "clients." They think of these terms—which I use interchangeably here—as reflective of a crass manipulating mentality.

The problem is that too many marketers really are bad practitioners. They do indeed use disreputable tactics. They do try to convince customers to do things that are primarily in the seller's interest. (Consider the old standby, "No home should be without a Vegematic!" What home really needs one?) But marketing should not be tarred with the brush wielded by its worst practitioners. Practiced in its ideal incarnation—which this book is all about—marketing can be a win-win activity for all sides. The key, as always in this book, lies in carrying out marketing from the customer's perspective. If the marketer sees the job as meeting customer needs and wants and realizes that it cannot succeed without doing so, this means that, by definition, marketing outcomes must be in the customer's interest.

The difference is seen in a simple example from the commercial sector. Imagine a woman shopper going into a typical clothing store to find a jacket to match a particular skirt. In the typical shop, the customer would be approached by a salesperson who, if reasonably well trained, will find out what the customer is looking for (size, color, and so forth) and then proceed as subtly as possible to convince her to buy one of the items off the store's rack. The shop, of course, would evaluate the salesperson's performance in terms of whether the customer walked out with the store's goods. The salesperson's job is *to sell the store's merchandise.*

Consider, however, a store with a customer orientation—one like Nordstrom's in the United States. In the same scenario, it would not be improbable for a salesperson at Nordstrom's to say to the customer, "We really do not have the item you are looking for. But, on my lunch break, I was in Macy's and I think they might have exactly what you want." If this salesperson worked in the store described previously, she would be fired if she said this. In a customer-centered store, she may well get praise from the boss and even a bonus. The difference is that, in the latter store, the salesperson's job is defined as *helping the customer buy clothes.* The store believes that, in the long run, customers will want to do business with outlets that have the customer's interests at heart first—not their own sales quotas.

This kind of encounter is truly a win-win situation. The store gets what it wants in the long run, more loyal customers, great word-of-mouth advertising (and lower costs), and many sales. And, more importantly, customers get what they truly want, clothes that meet their needs, not the store's. They will return again and again because they know the salesperson is not the enemy but is on the customer's side.

It is this customer-centered mentality that must pervade every nook and cranny of social marketing. In my view, it is the only approach that can prove the critics of intrusive, manipulative marketing to be wrong. It is the best approach to bringing long-run success to social marketing programs while leaving target customers with the feeling—and the reality—that their needs are really the central concern of the social marketers. Good social marketing is inevitably a win-win situation.

Social Marketing Ethics

In my view, social marketers bear a special obligation to behave in an ethical fashion because they are purporting to act in society's interests and not—unlike commercial marketers—in their own (Murphy and Bloom, 1990). They take as their challenge influencing behavior in ways that are good for the individual and for the society. This role, I believe, requires that they pay extraordinarily close attention to the ethics of the goals they choose and the means they choose to get there.

Goals

The question must be asked: who decides what is "good" for the individual or society in a social marketing program that is to improve the society? The Ku Klux Klan believes that the good of the society requires a purification of the race, that is, the elimination of (at least) African-Americans and Jews. There is nothing stopping Klansmen from employing the concepts and techniques outlined in this volume to achieve their definition of the good society. In this sense, social marketing, like atomic physics, is a technology for achieving certain ends. The technology itself does not make value judgments about the ends.

But social marketing practitioners do!

Inevitably, each practitioner of social marketing must answer the question: Do I want to participate in this use of my concepts and skills? Do I think that the end the program seeks is truly in the best interests of humanity? There are no simple answers and in many cases reasonable people will come to different conclusions.

One person may be perfectly comfortable—even excited about—using social marketing concepts and tools to facilitate women's ability to choose abortions should they want them. Another may find this application abhorrent. It is not our place here to list acceptable applications—only to highlight the ethical dimensions of the social marketer's choice of causes.

The most helpful recommendation that can be offered is that decisions to proceed with a controversial application of social marketing, wherever possible, should be made by some sort of societally representative collective. This collective could be a legislature or a government ministry, or it could be a board of directors or an advisory board made up of citizens of diverse backgrounds and interests. Such vetting of controversial projects by broad collectives at least increases the probability that project outcomes will not be counter to popular norms and values, and that they will be ethically sound (Smith, 1993).

Means

Social marketing must also be ethical in its application of means to achieve socially desirable outcomes. Should a smoking cessation program focus on denying people the right to smoke anywhere other than in enclosed space they alone inhabit (like their bathroom or automobile) or that is inhabited only by consenting smokers? Or is this tactic for reducing overall levels of smoking and thereby improving collective health and reducing societal costs of treating smoking too much of an infringement on individual freedom? Is a radio given to induce a sickly woman with a very large family to practice family planning a good tactic even if she isn't really sure that she wants family planning? Should the same family planning program focus efforts on a few ready-to-change, less-poor audiences and ignore the least educated and poorest households because the most behavior change for limited resources will be achieved?

Again, in each of these cases—and others like them—there are no simple answers. One can only apply standards of fairness, honesty, trust, and respect for the individual when choosing among alternative tactics (Smith, 1993). The sole admonition I can offer here is not to avoid thinking about the ethical implications of social marketing actions—and never to assume that good ends always justify the means. Choices are not value free. To use a popular management cliche, the best social marketers are always reflecting not just on whether they are doing things right but on whether they are doing the right things!

This is difficult to do. But I would argue that the focus on the consumer that is so central to this book and to the best social marketing practice is again a very good guide as to what to do. Some argue that a customer-centered approach is unrealistic: many times target audiences just do not know what is best for themselves and so one should not be guided by them! The drug addict or child abuser is sick and needs to be changed—and this is perfectly ethical because the person hurts him- or herself as well as others by the current behavior. The ethical question of ends is clear—the behavior should be changed. But how? Manipulation is seldom the ethical answer.

Social marketing programs will achieve maximum success if they start with the customer's needs and wants. For the high-involvement behaviors with which social marketing is typically involved, manipulation with extrinsic rewards will ultimately fail if the target behavior is done only for the reward. It is only when the behavior is intrinsically rewarding that it is likely to be permanent, that is, only when it truly meets the target's basic needs and wants. This is what the best social marketing tries to do. For this reason, its customer rationale is most likely to generate programs that are not only ethical in their ends but also ethical in their means: they are ultimately honest, fair, trusting, and respectful of the individual.

Summary

Social marketing is a powerful new approach to a wide range of social problems in health, crime, the environment, and social welfare. It draws upon proven concepts and processes from the commercial sector and applies them to challenges such as AIDS, malnutrition, excessive population growth, and recycling. The challenges are not fundamentally different from those in the private sector. They involve influencing the behavior of a target market that has alternatives with which they are comfortable. Community norms and other pressures inhibit change. Supporting agents and service people must help out if the program is to be successful.

But social marketing can only be successful if it is done well. The purpose of this book is to provide readers with a framework for effective social marketing. It describes a way of thinking, a process, and a set of concepts and techniques that underlie sound social marketing programs. Social marketing is different from alternative approaches to behavior change such as education, persuasion, behavior modification, and social influence, although it incorporates many of their principles. Social marketing emphasizes behavior as the bottom line for everything it does. It does not settle for merely changing awareness or attitudes. It is fanatically customer-centered. It uses a combination of influence factors to bring about change, factors that have analogies to the Four P's of the commercial sector (Product, Price, Place, and Promotion). Social marketers are also fanatical about conducting research before, during, and after their influence efforts. They segment their markets rather than treating them as masses.

The success of social marketing is now well established both by specific program experiences and by the way in which social marketing thinking has become commonplace in government agencies such as the Centers for Disease Control and Prevention, the U.S. Agency for International Development, and the U.S. Department of Agriculture, as well as such nongovernmental groups as the American Cancer Society, the Academy for Educational Development, and the Futures Group. However, the field still has to overcome a certain external prejudice against it and its terminology ("customers," "segments," "positioning"). And it also has internal ethical issues it must address if it is to be not only powerful but also honorable!

Finally, while a number of books and articles on social marketing are now appearing, and social marketing topics are covered in many basic university courses, the field lacks a solid conceptual framework for those who wish to understand and undertake social marketing programs. The objective of this book is to provide such a framework.

Part One

Preparing for Social Marketing

Chapter One

Putting the Customer First: The Essential Social Marketing Insight

As I have noted, social marketing is, in simplest terms, the application of commercial marketing technology to a special class of problems. It is designed to help social change agents influence people to take actions that improve their own welfare or that of the broader society. However, to be an effective social marketer, it is not enough to know the tools and processes. One needs to develop the instincts and mindset that distinguish a first-rate marketer from one who merely knows the moves. One objective of this book is to demonstrate to readers how they can become professional social marketing managers. The place to begin is with the proper orientation—or philosophy—toward marketing, what it is, what it does, and how it does it.

The Marketing Mindset

The marketing mindset is, in some sense, a philosophy. That is, it comprises "a system of principles for guidance in practical affairs." In this chapter, I will set forth the basic premises that good social marketers bring to their programs. There are many approaches that masquerade as social marketing but lack either the right mindset or the right process. It is good social marketing that is our concern here. The core of this preferred approach is the premise that _all social marketing decisions must emanate from a consideration of the target customer_. This premise has not always been at the center of marketing in the commercial sector. And in all too many cases, it remains unappreciated in organizations that are otherwise very sophisticated in their approaches to finance, production, and personnel management.

In my years of consulting, I have listened to innumerable marketing executives claim they are "customer oriented." They tell me about the fancy consumer studies they have done and the products and services they have developed that have been wildly successful. To them, this activity and these sales results prove that they are truly customer driven. But further conversation and investigation inside and outside the organization make clear that they have learned the words of a customer orientation but they haven't learned the music! A customer orientation has more to do with how one thinks than with what one does.

In the commercial sector, organizations can often get away without being terribly customer driven. They may have a great product or no competition. They may have hit the right cultural moment for their innovation. With limited marketing skills, they can do very well. But in social marketing, almost everything is different. First, most field practitioners have had little experience with any kind of marketing, so they often copy what looks to them like the best practices of the commercial sector without recognizing that the premises that drive these practices are often fatal in social marketing. The main reason that run-of-the-mill marketing is so dangerous in social marketing is that we are almost always dealing with high-involvement behaviors for which target customers often have very ambivalent or very negative feelings.

High-involvement behaviors are those about which individuals care a great deal, where they see significant risks, where they think a lot before acting, and where they frequently seek the advice of others (Celsi and Olson, 1988). In the commercial sector, a great deal of focus is on low-involvement behaviors about which consumers care relatively little—choosing a detergent, a fast food outlet, a T-shirt. In such markets, consumers can be greatly influenced by modest interventions such as simple price changes, clever jingles or celebrity testimonials, coupons, and so on. Much of this strategy—and the thinking that goes behind it—is not very transferable to high-involvement social marketing settings.

Social marketing often involves very high-involvement behaviors. Smokers and drug users are not eager to quit. Gay men are extremely concerned that tenuous relationships will be sundered by the mere mention of safe sex or condoms. Mothers with busy lives often see the admonitions of health workers to treat their children differently as simply one more imposition on a life that is close to overwhelming.

Because social marketers must work on such important behaviors at such a deep level, they cannot risk approaching their task casually or without careful thought about the complex motivations involved. As we shall see, the chances of going wrong are especially great in the social marketing world in part because of the kinds of problems it deals with and in part because of the kinds of people who have chosen to tackle them.

The "Wrong" Mindsets

In my experience, most organizations go through three distinct stages in their approach to marketing. This evolution is predictable. The problem is that too many organizations get stuck in a mindset that is less than ideal. It is crucial that this not happen to those who wish to practice the very best in social marketing application.

The first orientation that most organizations adopt is one that was probably the most common in the earliest days of modern marketing. It is called a *product mindset*. Managers with a product mindset believe that the best marketing is that which focuses on developing superior products and services that will beat the competition and capture great shares of the consumer market. This can be described as the "build-a-better-mousetrap" approach, and it is perhaps a natural one for organizations convinced that they have a really good idea that the world has been dying to have. It has characterized the early days of a great many computer and software companies and many pioneering neighborhood entrepreneurs. It is a mindset that says "Offer it and they will come!" All the marketing that is really needed is sensible pricing, a modest amount of informative advertising to tell everyone how good the product or service is, and careful attention to keeping the product or service as up-to-date technically as possible. It is an orientation that can be effective for a very long time if the product or service has a clear advantage and little competition. Many firms, indeed, adopt a management style that they call "sticking to your knitting" and do quite well at it (Peters and Waterman, 1982).

The product orientation is one that is also found in a great many so-called social marketing organizations at the early stages of their careers. They develop a new product or a new service, or they introduce an existing set of products or practices into a new community, and are immediately successful because of the existing pent-up demand. Families are eager for a way to space children. Mothers want something to combat epidemics of diarrhea. In such cases, the major problems social marketers face are often just getting enough supply into the field and telling consumers about the availability of needed goods and services. Marketing at this stage consists mainly of getting enough condoms into the shops, hiring enough health workers to conduct needed vaccinations in the field, and making sure there are appropriate informational posters everywhere that the target audiences might be found.

But this approach can only go so far. Eventually the pent-up demand will be satisfied. Or early success may lead to a backlash, as when the cigarette industry attempts to fight antismoking campaigns. At this point, most organizations will realize that a product mindset will no longer suffice. They then switch to a _selling mindset_. The selling mindset views marketing as basically a powerful tool of persuasion that can be brought to bear to convince reluctant consumers that the organization's offering is infinitely superior to the competition (that is, sticking to the old behavior patterns).

Unfortunately, it is commercial sector organizations dominated by a selling orientation that are the principal culprits responsible for the poor reputation marketing has acquired among many social change specialists. This is because, in its ugliest manifestations, the selling mindset leads to high-pressure sales tactics, gimmicky advertising, and a willingness to aggressively promote trivial differences to make a sale. It is selling refrigerators to Eskimos. But there is a more fundamental problem with a selling mindset. Along with the product mindset, the selling orientation conceives of the customer as a target whose behavior is to be shaped to fit the organization's goals. However, modern marketers recognize that an organization is only successful if customers agree to undertake the recommended behavior. They say that the selling and product mindsets have the influence equation backwards. Organizations should not lead customers: customers must lead organizations!

The "Right" Mindset

Those who practice the very best modern marketing approaches in both the commercial and nonprofit sectors put the target audience in control of the transaction. They adopt a *customer-centered mindset* that develops their strategy beginning with what the target audience needs and wants, not with what the organization needs and wants. The organization is led by its customers and does not try to make customers serve the organization's purposes. It makes the organization what Whitely and Albrecht call "truly customer driven" (Whitely, 1991; Albrecht, 1992). A customer-driven orientation, as we shall see, is particularly appropriate for social marketing organizations.

The selling orientation is very often seen in programs that call themselves "communications" programs—health communications programs, for example. In these programs, the objective is to tell target audiences about the benefits of a particular new behavior and motivate them to act. But the mindset that drives such programs is focused more on what the organization wants than on what the consumer wants. The latter is what the social marketer must instinctively put first. But this is not easy!

The Organization-Centered Mindset

In my experience, the vast majority of social change programs have adopted a selling or a product orientation. What they have in common is that they are *organization centered*. In many respects, an organization-centered mindset is one that it is very easy for a social behavior-change specialist to fall into. Unfortunately, this "natural" mindset is one that can be severely damaging to any really effective social marketing program. It is critical that social marketers learn the symptoms of this wrong-headed, inside-out approach and move beyond it to the proper outside-in, customer-driven approach.

What then are the symptoms of an organization-centered mindset? There are seven basic clues (Andreasen, 1982).

1. *The organization's mission is seen as inherently good.* Wrong-headed social marketers cannot imagine why anyone would not wear seat belts, practice birth control, or give up smoking. They expect everyone to appreciate the benefits of immunizing a child against measles and polio and to want to give blood to the Red Cross. Of course, there is nothing wrong with being enthusiastic about one's product or service. It is the driving force behind many great organizations. However, where this enthusiasm becomes problematic is when it creates what Levitt calls "marketing myopia," the inability to see beyond one's own particular offering.

Social marketers are particularly prone to this affliction. In many ways it is what makes them great. They have a passion for their cause—they desperately want everyone to stop smoking and wear seat belts. But too many times this passion slips over the edge into obsession.

One explanation for this is that most social marketers are underpaid. They could command significantly higher salaries and a working environment that is dramatically less problematic if they worked in the commercial sector. But they care about an issue or a social problem and they sign on with an agency or a program at some economic sacrifice, and this can lead them to an unconscious assumption that everything they do is justified and that everyone else should appreciate it.

2. *Customers are the problem.* Where organizational myopia can cause the most trouble is when it leads to this second characteristic of a selling organization–centered marketing strategy. Believing passionately in a product or a program is one of the most endearing traits of social marketers. They want absolutely everyone to wear seat belts or prevent forest fires or get their kids immunized. What often happens, however, is that in their zeal these committed marketers find it hard to believe that anyone would not do these obviously good things. Every teen should stay away from drugs and every sexually active teen should practice safe sex. Every mother in Niger should have her children fully vaccinated by the age of two.

This zeal becomes dysfunctional when the marketer sees the customer as an adversary, as someone who has the wrong habits or the wrong ideas or is just plain ignorant or unmotivated. In this wrong-headed mindset, the customer is seen as standing in the way of program success. The goal of the program then is to change the customer to do what the social marketer knows is the right thing to do.

When the organization-centered social marketer has only limited success in achieving his or her program goals, the customer is seen as the source of the problem. The customer is seen as deficient in one of two ways.

- *Ignorance*. Because the social marketer knows what a good idea it is to practice safe sex or put campfires out carefully, he or she assumes that the reason other people don't do this is that they simply do not know how desirable the marketer's favored behavior is. Customers who are not complying are just too ignorant of the virtues of the proposed action.
- *Lack of motivation*. Every once in a while, social marketers who are convinced that customer ignorance is the main source of their lack of success are confronted by research data showing that customers are not at all as ignorant as the marketers thought. They then turn to their backup explanation: the real problem must be a character flaw.

Many of those involved in early stop-smoking campaigns believed that the reason people continued to smoke was that they did not know how bad it was for them. As a consequence, the National Cancer Institute and the American Cancer Society spent a great deal of money and time producing ads detailing the horrific consequences of continued smoking.

But a careful look at customer research on smokers revealed a troubling set of findings. First, a very high proportion of smokers had already tried to quit. Of the remainder, perhaps the overwhelming majority wanted to quit. When asked why they tried to quit or wanted to quit, respondents said it was because they knew smoking was bad for them. Clearly, the years of antismoking ad campaigns, school health programs, and the like had produced an educational effect: people knew that smoking was bad for them!

When confronted with this information, antismoking marketers were forced to give up their first assumption about the cause of their lack of success; consumers clearly weren't ignorant. So they turned to their backup explanation, which runs something like this: well, if people know that smoking is bad and they continue to smoke, then they must have character flaw! They must be too cowardly to quit. Or they are just too weak to stand up to peer pressure. Or they are just too vain about gaining weight to try to quit.

The sensitive reader will note the patronizing tone in the preceding analysis. Customers are seen as ignorant, weak individuals in need of shaping up by the helpful marketer. And the inexorable logic of this view is that a good social marketing program is one that tries to overcome these problems.

3. *Marketing is seen as communications.* If one sees the problem in securing behavior change as one of either customer ignorance or customer lack of motivation, then clearly the implication is that one needs to provide information and then persuasion to act. This inevitably forces the marketer into an advertising-and-promotion implementation scheme. Organization-centered marketers tend to adopt an approach to customers that says: "I know this is a good idea. Let me tell you why it is a good idea. Once you appreciate its good features, then let me urge you to act."

This is the approach used by practitioners who refer to what they do as *communications*. The problem is that it leads many to be satisfied with communications objectives such as reduction of ignorance and increased motivation—even when there is no behavioral change. A good example of this problem is the experience of the Centers for Disease Control and Prevention (CDC) in the early 1990s, as described by Fred Kroger in Exhibit 1.1.

The communications-centered approach has a number of correlates.

4. *Marketing research has a limited role.* In general, those with a selling orientation are often likely to accord marketing research a relatively limited role in the marketing and persuasion process. Formative research (before the campaign gets underway) is typically limited to finding out the extent of consumer ignorance or apathy. Pretest research on communication instruments may also be undertaken to make sure that informational items are under-

Exhibit 1.1. Fred Kroger on HIV Prevention: Communications Success, Marketing Failure.

"America Responds to AIDS" is the campaign banner for the Federal government's campaign to inform the American public about HIV and AIDS. Campaign planners have employed marketing techniques which have resulted in its messages being seen or heard by more Americans and with greater frequency (e.g., more than 7 billion audience impressions estimated for 1993) than for any government sponsored public service health campaign to date. Yet, its CDC sponsors consider it more a health communications program than a social marketing effort.

In 1993, a panel of health communications experts external to the CDC was asked to assess its national efforts to promote HIV prevention, and to recommend strategies for improvement. The principal elements of the effort have been a national media campaign, national toll-free hotline services, a national clearinghouse for distributing materials and managing databases on HIV services and programs, grant programs for national partnership development, grant programs to support state and local information activities, and communications research and evaluation.

The panel gave favorable marks for the program's marketing efforts to media gatekeepers and for its success in nurturing effective collaborations among its many and diverse national partnerships. Aggressive, sustained interaction with national and local public service directors helped place HIV prevention high on their list of concerns. The national partners advised CDC on its "product" development processes, but also became its sales force in delivering materials and programs to constituencies at organizational and community levels. The communications program was recognized as an integrated system that allows information to flow bi-directionally, and that had mass, institutional, community and individual elements to it.

Its shortcomings, however, fell within two dimensions that most social marketing practitioners consider essential—audience segmentation and product definition. Undergirding these two deficiencies, the fifth "p" of government-based marketing programs, "politics," was described as the major impediment to effective marketing in HIV prevention.

Audience Segmentation. Congress had been clear in designating the general public as the primary audience for CDC's mass communication efforts on AIDS. An informed and supportive population is recognized by behavioral scientists to be an important ingredient for causing healthy behaviors to be initiated and sustained. The "America Responds to AIDS

Exhibit 1.1. Fred Kroger on HIV Prevention:
Communications Success, Marketing Failure (*continued*).

Campaign" was criticized by the AIDS Action Council, the Gay Men's Health Crisis in New York City, by other AIDS advocacy groups, and by the review panel for not meeting the needs of high risk audiences, such as gay men, by not providing sexually explicit behavioral messages.

Product. "American Responds to AIDS," though viewed by some as a public service advertising and pamphlet distribution campaign, was designed to be a sophisticated communications system that includes on-line computer databases; toll-free, live telephone hotline services; and a network of national organizations to mediate and deliver education programs and materials. The product was seen by campaign planners as value-free, technically accurate information. AIDS activists called for condoms promotion as the principal product. Congress and media critics expected proof of prevention effects. In assessing this confusion over product specificity, the review panel called for a more behaviorally focused product—i.e., "health information with an attitude." Disease preventing behaviors, including condom use, should be aggressively promoted.

Evaluation efforts have been undertaken to position the HIV prevention "product" in more consumer relevant terms. Just as athletic footwear is sold as aids to "soar through the air, slam dunk, in your face" feats of athleticism, rather than as canvas covers for the feet, such prevention products as condoms, monogamy, or abstinence still lack similar, consumer-oriented positioning.

The awareness task has been judged by experts to be complete. It has been accomplished primarily through communication tools. Can the adoption of risk reducing behaviors now be sold to persons at highest risk, and will the body politic be supportive? This more challenging goal will require better application of core marketing principles. Will the second decade of HIV prevention marketing improve upon the first? Stay tuned.

Used with permission of Fred Kroger of the Centers for Disease Control and Prevention.

stood by consumers or that they raise motivation levels. And post-project evaluations will look at communications—rather than behavioral—objectives. Thus, they may look at process measures such as the number of posters printed, brochures distributed, advertisements run, workshops held, lectures given, and face-to-face meetings held. Or they may look at outcomes measures such as number of target consumers reached, extent of message recall, degree of attitude change, and changes in intentions to act.

But they do not look at what customers want, what they actually do, or what is keeping them from acting. The customers' reasons for inaction may have little to do with knowledge or motivation; people who can't get to the recommended products or facilities or can't cope with resulting problems (such as withdrawal symptoms from addiction) won't act no matter what they know or what they think they ought to do.

5.   *Customers are treated as a mass.* Because organization-centered marketers tend to see the problem as one of persuading people to do what the marketer knows is right for them, and because formative research is often very superficial, selling-oriented social marketers tend not to see the need for segmenting consumers into meaningful subgroupings. They may use relatively gross criteria such as demographics. But this decision is often driven by the fact that media can be chosen on the basis of demographics or by the fact that the problem of ignorance tends to be associated with basic demographics such as education, ethnicity, and income. Seldom do they consider more important determinants of behavioral responsiveness, such as individual readiness to change or stages in the decision process. They tend to treat customers as a mass, saying things like, "We want to reach everyone with our program," or to divide their customers into two or three elementary segments (men and women, rural and urban, young and old) and treat them essentially all alike with "the one best approach."

6.   *Competition is ignored.* Because selling-oriented marketers think they know the basic problem, they seldom really get inside the heads of their target customers as I will recommend here. As a consequence, they tend to ignore a fact that is very fundamental in the commercial sector, namely, that every attempt to change behavior faces competition. Now, if you mention this to a persuasion-

oriented marketer, the response will probably be something like, "Well, our competition is the consumer's ignorance and lack of motivation." But this attitude both misses the point and is patronizing to consumers.

Target consumers in most behavior-change situations have very good reasons for maintaining the behavior patterns they have held—often for a lifetime. As experience has shown, a great many of these behavior patterns are not the result of ignorance but of conscious choice. For example, the woman urged to boil her water to prevent the spread of bacterial disease may argue that this runs counter to the teachings of her village elder and she does not wish to risk ostracism from her group by changing to the new Western ways.

7. *Staffers are drawn from those with product or communications skills.* Given their view of the problem, organization-centered marketers tend to choose staffers who either are very knowledgeable about the behavior itself (the product) or are good at communicating. Thus, they might put a nurse in charge of hospital marketing or a public health administrator in charge of a national health change program. Alternatively, some managers think that the real marketing challenge is to do a better job of getting the story out. This is likely to lead them to put advertising or public relations specialists or journalists in key marketing roles (MacStravic, 1977; Kotler, 1979).

What is Different About the Customer-Centered Mindset?

The approach that a good social marketer with the right mindset takes to each of these topics is virtually a mirror image of the organization-centered mindset. Whereas the latter thinks first of the organization and its objectives, the customer-centered social marketer starts with the customer and his or her objectives (and perceptions and wants and attitudes). The organization-centered marketer keeps track of how the organization is doing; the customer-centered marketer keeps track of how the customer is doing. Let us go down the list.

1. *The organization's mission is seen as bringing about behavior change by meeting the target market's needs and wants.* Social marketers, like organization-centered marketers, health communicators, and

other so-called behavior-change specialists, begin with a behavioral objective they wish to achieve. However, good social marketers are not so blinded by the desirability of their goal that they neglect to see that, from the consumer's perspective, the behaviors the marketer wants may not be desirable or even possible. The social marketer, rather than thinking that the customer is somehow wrong for being reluctant to change, knows that the change program must start with where the customer is now. The social marketer says, in effect, "Maybe I am the one who will have to change what it is that I am proposing and how I propose it." The social marketer recognizes that it is much easier—and, ultimately, much more effective—to change the marketing program and the marketer than it is to change the customer to fit the program. This does not mean that the customer does not eventually have to change. Indeed, that is the social marketer's mission. But expert social marketers recognize that the way to get where they want to go is to start with where the customers are now! For example, getting college students to worry about condom use when they are worried about getting a date simply ignores the target's reality.

2.   _The customer is seen as someone with unique perceptions, needs, and wants to which the marketer must adapt._ The first-rate social marketer does not consider the consumer at fault for the marketer's lack of success. If a program is not meeting its goals, a well-trained social marketer will not blame the consumer but, rather, will ask: "What is it about the consumer do I not understand well enough so that I can bring the consumer to want to do what my program recommends?" The social marketer thinks of further research and program changes—not browbeating the poor consumers with louder and more insistent messages urging that they "get with the program!"

The social marketer's first goal is to get inside their target market's psyche and understand why these people are doing what they are doing and what their perceptions are of the costs and benefits of the behavior change the marketer is attempting to achieve. The assumption is made that customers have very good reasons for doing what they are doing. The marketer's challenge is to figure out how to adjust the marketing program to respond to these reasons. The customer is always the figure who drives the program—not vice versa.

Good social marketers see consumers as making choices about action based on their perceptions of the balance between benefits and costs of present and proposed actions. Thus, they need to know what these perceptions are and what must change in their program so that the balance turns in the marketer's favor.

3.   *Marketing is seen as more than communications.* Because social marketers do not automatically see their problems in terms of overcoming ignorance or lack of motivation, they inevitably recognize that their behavior-change program must have many more elements than communications. If they learn that consumers do not get their children immunized because of long travel times, then they know they must provide vaccinations closer to the consumer, perhaps through mobile clinics, or they must find ways to transport consumers to clinics more expeditiously. The communication specialist's approach might be just to urge a target customer more vigorously that she really should make this sacrifice because it is the right thing to do for her children. What the marketer would argue is that the Place element of the marketing mix needs adjustment.

Or—to continue the same example—suppose that the marketer discovers that a customer neglects to go to the public health clinic for vaccinations because the last time she was there she was treated very shabbily and she vows not to subject herself to such indignities again. The problem here is that the Product needs a good deal of work before the marketer goes out to promote it.

Or finally, suppose that the marketer learns that the target customer will not go the clinic because of the many obligations she has at home. She is concerned that she would have to neglect her garden and her housecleaning and food preparation duties. She would have to leave her other children behind. She would not be home when her husband returns from the factory. All of these are important perceived costs; the marketer needs to reduce the Price for the immunization transaction to take place.

Note that in none of these cases was the problem one of communication or Promotion, the fourth key element of the marketing mix. The social marketing paradigm insists that all programs have coordinated strategies because the consumer requires it. And even when the social marketer thinks about the communication component, other communications options often take precedence over just getting the facts out about the benefits of the particular behavior. For example, suppose that in attempting to promote the use of oral rehydration therapy, the social marketer learns that many consumers simply do not know how to administer it properly. The marketer will realize here that what needs to be transferred to the consumer is not information but skills. The mother must learn how to mix ORT solutions and how to feed them to uncooperative offspring.

Or suppose the marketer finds out that the target customer is very much influenced by some important people in her family or community. The communications challenge here is not at all to tell the consumer about the benefits of the action but to indicate that others are doing it and so should be emulated.

4.   _Marketing research is vital._ Because social marketing programs revolve around consumers, good social marketers try as hard as they can to understand their market. Further, they realize that what they need to learn is not just about consumer ignorance and lack of motivation (although these can sometimes play a role) but also about the barriers consumers perceive to behaving in the desired way, the role of significant social pressure groups in accelerating or retarding adoption of the new behavior, and the consumer's own perceived self-efficacy—that is, belief in his or her ability to carry out the recommended behavior. Understanding all of this is essential to crafting a fully rounded marketing mix.

Social marketers know that one need not spend an inordinate amount of money on this kind of research and it need not be excessively sophisticated. Nor do they think that they need to rely on surveys and questionnaires. They are adept at using such tools as focus groups, depth interviewing of small samples of representative potential targets, careful observation, and digging into available secondary sources to learn simple facts that will have significant impact on where they are going and how they are going to get there.

Their interest in research goes well beyond that needed at the start of a program. The social marketer recognizes the essential role that tracking information can play in monitoring program success and indicating needed corrections. But here, unlike communications specialists, social marketers look for measures of behavior change or measures of process that are expected to lead to behavior change. Social marketers are very bottom-line (behavior) oriented and so pay relatively less attention to process measures (such as number of persons reached) unless it can clearly be demonstrated that such measures are, indeed, good predictors of behavior.

And in evaluating overall programs, good social marketers look to long-run behavioral impact and not to such potentially transient factors as information learned (an education objective) or attitudes changed (a persuasion objective). Further, social marketers, especially in recent years, have paid a great deal of attention to making sure that the impacts they have are lasting. Ideally, they focus on system changes, changes in norms, administrative changes in partner institutions, and similar deep changes that give some assurance that there will be effects lasting well beyond the limited span of the social marketing program or campaign.

5.   *Customers are grouped in segments*. Commercial sector marketers have long appreciated the benefits of aggregating consumers into meaningful groupings for the purposes of strategy. Because of their customer-first orientation, they begin with the principle that the more closely tailored a marketing program is to the needs and wants of a given individual, the more likely that individual will respond positively. Ideally, this would mean one-on-one contact with each customer so as to learn about the customer's unique needs, to present alternatives, and to receive feedback to adjust the individualized campaign to reach the desired goal.

But commercial sector marketers are also realists. They know that resources are limited and that individualized approaches are often not cost efficient. On the other hand, they recognize that mass approaches are also often ineffective because they must inevitably be too broad to speak to anyone in any great specificity. Wise marketers therefore choose a middle ground by focusing on market segments.

Selling-oriented marketers also use segmentation. However, they typically do not segment the market finely enough, being content with gross classifications such as men versus women, urban versus rural, or old, middle-aged, and young. In addition, they tend to use segmentation criteria that do not provide an explanatory link between marketing programs and consumer behavior. Marketers who do not carefully explore consumer characteristics prior to implementing a marketing strategy will very often opt to segment markets based on obvious demographics. Sometimes they do this because they believe these demographics are somehow related to the behaviors at issue. Often they choose demographic criteria because the choice allows them to allocate resources in some seemingly rational fashion. By contrast, as I shall spell out in further detail in Chapter Four, social marketers try to get inside the heads of consumers and understand what they need and want and what sort of marketing intervention they are likely to respond to. Only then do they try to link these factors to more readily observable traits such as demographics. Very often their research leads them to conclude that consumers are better segmented by such factors as past behavior (such as adoption of some earlier new behavior or attendance at a health clinic) or what are called *lifestyle factors* (such as participation in religious life in a community or attendance at sporting or musical events).

6. *Competition is seen to be everywhere and never ending.* Once they get inside target consumers' minds and hearts, expert social marketers quickly recognize that, for every new behavior they want to propose, there is one or more alternative behaviors they will be fighting against. Life for everyone is a matter of minute-by-minute choices. Individuals do what they do at any given time because they think that the net consequences will be better for them than some other course of action, including doing nothing.

This insight comes naturally to a marketer accustomed to fighting for shelf space in supermarkets or for consumer awareness amid television clutter. In the social realm, it alerts marketers to the fact that, first of all, they must identify their competitors for each key market segment. Second, they must learn not only what consumers find appealing or unappealing about the social behavior being proposed but also what they find appealing and unappealing about its competitors. Third, they must develop strategies that take account of the fact that consumers will always be comparing their proposal, consciously or unconsciously. Sometimes, a marketer will have to not only market the proposed behavior but *de*market the alternative. Thus, social marketers promoting oral rehydration therapy must convince mothers that during episodes of diarrhea (a) doing nothing (thereby drying the child out) is potentially lethal; (b) using folk remedies (such as applying ashes to the sunken fontanelle) is ineffective; and (c) using an oral rehydration solution—preferably with some food (such as a bit of rice)—will have the best consequences for their children's health. They also have to convince the mothers that using ORT is worth the costs it inevitably incurs—even if the solution is free, the mother will have to spend a lot of time to get the proper amount of liquid into the child, and that time is a genuine cost.

Finally, they will have to recognize that competition is always there and it is typically always changing. A good example is the tobacco industry. Antismoking social marketers are constantly faced with new competitive techniques from tobacco marketers— from college giveaways to promoting Joe Camel to sponsorships of sports events to lobbying attacks on Capitol Hill. Elections change the extent to which legislators are friendly or antagonistic to regulatory anti-smoking interventions. Predicating a strategy on an assumption that your competitor will stand still is not good marketing in either the commercial or public sectors.

Those with a selling orientation are much more likely to focus on simply promoting the benefits of their option. Because they do not have the in-depth understanding of the consumer psyche and the appreciation of the role of competition in consumer decision making, they are much more likely to push their product and ultimately lose to the competition because they do not understand the battle they are in.

7. _Marketers are chosen for their knowledge of consumers_. When Apple Computer looked for a new CEO in the late 1980s, most observers thought the company would turn to someone in the computer hardware or software industries for the candidate. Someone from IBM seemed to be an obvious choice. But Apple chose John Sculley, who at the time was a senior executive at the Pepsi-Cola Company. The rationale they offered at the time was that, although Sculley did not know a lot about computers, he certainly knew a lot about consumers. For years, he had been convincing consumers to buy his brand of colored sugar water over a competitor's colored sugar water with great success, mainly because he understood "the Pepsi Generation" and how to speak to them. "Think of what he could do with great products like the Apple and Macintosh."

This is the same approach good social marketers take. They believe that a CEO can always turn to others who know the product (as Sculley could) or who could turn out first-rate advertisements and brochures (as Sculley could). But what is unique to the social marketer is his or her understanding and empathy for customers. In choosing social marketers, the most important criterion should be: Have they assimilated the appropriate consumer mindset? Do they automatically look for the consumer's perspective when thinking about what course of action to take? Do they think that customer research—even if it is relatively informal—is usually necessary before embarking on new campaigns? Do they try to keep in touch with customers as campaigns unfold? If things are not going well, do they think that the main reason is that the organization has failed to understand the consumer thoroughly enough?

Other Characteristics of a First-Rate Marketing Approach

Commercial sector marketers bring a number of other characteristics to the social arena that distinguish their approaches from others. The more prominent of these distinguishing characteristics are discussed in this section.

Willingness to Change the Offer

A customer-oriented marketer, while convinced of the desirability of the behavior being promoted, is totally open to the possibility that many customers may not agree. The social marketer realizes that the behavior being promoted, the *offer,* is not an objective reality; it is only what the customer thinks it is. Changing the offer thus means changing these perceptions (Shimp and Bearden, 1982).

Sometimes the perceptions of reluctant or antagonistic customers are deadly accurate and changing the offer requires the marketer to make fundamental, real changes. If seat belts really are uncomfortable and consumers are not just using this as an excuse for personal bravado, then seat belts must be redesigned. If oral rehydration solutions—which are really just clean water plus salt and sugar—cannot safely be prepared from scratch by typical households, then premixed ORS packets must be provided and adapted to accommodate the best local liquid measure available (perhaps a Coke or Pepsi bottle). Efforts to convince

consumers that they should persist in learning a technique—
home preparation—that they truly believe is impossible will be ill-
considered.

Of course, there are other times when consumer perceptions
do not reflect reality. In that case, it is the marketer's challenge to
understand what has led to the misconception and how to alter it.
Many mothers still feel ORS can induce vomiting, so they believe
that two spoonfuls are enough for a small, sick child. Social marketers do not assume that it is the mother's ignorance or apathy
that is at fault when she does not take action. They do not see the
problem as just having to convince the target audience that they
are wrong and that the behavior promoted is really highly desirable. Rather, they assume that it is more likely that the marketer
has inadequately understood the target market's perceptions and
their needs and wants. Mothers want to avoid any chance of vomiting, so marketers must make it clear that ORS must be given
slowly with a spoon. Mothers believe two spoonfuls are enough
because they've been told that ORS is a medicine. If marketers
reposition ORS as a tonic, perhaps this will change consumers'
understanding of the product and its benefits and, ultimately, their
behavior. It is much easier for marketers to change their own behavior than try to change the target customer.

Commitment to Planning

As part of their sense of responsibility for the bottom line, good
marketers believe very strongly in the need to take reasoned action.
This encourages them to systematically think through major steps
they undertake, both in determining long-range strategy and in
making specific tactical decisions (Kotler and Andreasen, 1991).
This, of course, does not differentiate them from those in education or propaganda who also make plans. However, both the contents and objectives of their plans will be very different. For
example, marketers' plans will have detailed evaluations of competition, will incorporate extensive customer research before
moving forward, will require frequent field checks of tactical effectiveness after implementation, and will emphasize careful coordination of all elements of the Four P's.

Willingness to Take Reasoned Risks

Marketers recognize that they are operating in a battleground for target audiences' minds. And while they attempt to use research as much as possible to understand where those minds are now and how those minds might respond to a course of action under consideration, the marketers recognize that minds are imperfectly knowable. This is especially so when one is dealing with important social behaviors about which consumers have complex, sometimes guilty feelings.

This recognition has two consequences. First, marketers realize that some proportion of their actions will fail. Good marketers are rarely immobilized by that prospect—unlike those less accustomed to living with day-to-day risk. Marketers routinely take reasoned risks, often incorporating some formal calculation of inherent risk into their initial decision-making processes.

Second, because they know their environment is in many ways unknowable or at least unpredictable, good marketers are by nature experimental. They rarely make major irrevocable commitments to "one best strategy." When they do select a course of action, their bottom-line and research orientations make them vigilant for any signs of failure. And because they have anticipated this risk, good marketers will have designed contingency plans.

In many cases, risk-prone managers who recognize the unpredictability of their environment will often try several strategies at once, and simply wait to see which one works best. They say to themselves: "I don't know everything here. Trying out other variations will not cost me much. I'll let the market tell me what works best." They will also stay alert through careful monitoring for changes in the environment that inevitably make existing strategies obsolete. This is far different from the one-best-strategy typical of marketers with a selling orientation.

Specialized Skills

Marketing specialists bring to the area of social behavior change a number special competencies. There are seven technical areas in which marketers are probably more skilled than any other type of change agent:

- *Marketing research:* Marketers have developed an extremely wide array of expensive and inexpensive techniques to probe the minds of large numbers of target consumers. They use surveys, focus groups, experiments, and mall intercepts to gather rich lodes of data. If necessary, they can apply highly sophisticated techniques to extract very subtle meaning from seemingly bland data bases. They have pioneered such analytic concepts as lifestyle (Plummer, 1974) and trade-off analyses (Green and Wind, 1975), multidimensional attitude modeling (Wilkie and Pessemeir, 1973), and panel analysis (Sudman and Ferber, 1979). They know when to use research and when not to. They know when sophisticated research is important and when something simple like a few carefully designed conversations with representative target customers will do just fine. The better marketers have learned to take very few steps without such information.
- *Creation, positioning, and enhancement of brands:* Marketers have been responsible for many of the brand name artifacts of our daily lives—from Tide to Apple to Taurus to Holiday Inns. They have been able to associate qualities, even personalities, with simple words. They have done it for products, services, and (some would say) political candidates. They know how to create a brand and how to change it when it needs changing (Assael, 1971).
- *Packaging:* Marketers recognize that how an offer looks is often as important as what it actually is. Over the years, they have become highly imaginative in package design and construction. Packaging concepts have even been extended to services, where they are labeled *atmospherics* or image management.
- *Distribution:* Marketers are extremely effective at bringing masses of merchandise to remote locations of even the poorest countries. They know how to store, warehouse, and transport goods efficiently and how to provide incentives that persuade retailers and wholesalers to help achieve their distribution goals.
- *Promotion:* Marketers know better than most how to use other techniques besides advertising to market to mass audiences or large market segments. They are extremely adept at direct mail and telemarketing, the use of contests, coupons, and

giveaways, and the use of point-of-sale materials and corollary literature like brochures and package inserts. They are effective users of trade shows and trade advertising to get others to participate in their marketing programs.

- *Creation and placement of advertising:* The advertising industry now produces over $200 billion (U.S.) in billings yearly worldwide. Advertisers are extremely skilled at designing television and radio commercials, print ads, posters, and billboards that change behavior. Because they must make a profit, they are good at designing messages that work. They are therefore not only highly creative and technically efficient in producing ads but are also thoroughly trained to keep their eye on the impact of those ads. This extends not just to the creation of the ads but to placing them accurately and at the lowest possible cost in front of key target audiences.

- *Global marketing:* The major commercial sector marketing organizations are now global enterprises. They and their staffs have accumulated extensive experience in what works and what does not work in many highly diverse cultural settings. They know how to study and adapt to local markets. They know when and how to obtain economies by duplicating strategies in multiple settings. More importantly, perhaps, they also know when not to standardize programs—that is, when standardization will have serious negative effects on overall performance (Wind, Douglas, and Perlmutter, 1973).

The Special Nature of Social Marketing

Although commercial sector marketing has a lot to offer social marketers in meeting the challenges they face, it is extremely important to point out that these challenges are qualitatively different from the ones faced by private sector marketers (Kotler and Andreasen, 1991; Bloom and Novelli, 1981; Rothschild, 1979). This is because social marketers must deal with a number of characteristics unique to their field.

- *Negative Demand.* It is rare for a private sector marketer to be asked to market a product or service for which the target audience has a clear distaste. Yet, as Kotler and Andreasen note: "[Social marketers] must try to entice 'macho men' into wearing seat belts, timid souls into giving blood or taking medication around which swirl rumors about devastating effects on sexual potency, or aging citizens to finally admit they are infirm or otherwise need assistance" (1991, p. 28). Within these behavioral domains, social marketers must be especially careful not to exaggerate their potential contributions.

- *Highly Sensitive Issues*. Most of the behaviors that social marketers are asked to influence are much more highly involving than most of those found in the private sector. Asking parents to begin to limit family size or rural mothers to regularly weigh their children and expose the fact that their families have little food is much more serious than asking them to buy a bicycle or a new sofa. One consequence of this very high level of involvement is that it often makes it very hard for social marketers to carry out the customer research that they need to be effective. As Bloom and Novelli (1981, p. 80) have noted: "While people are generally willing to be interviewed about these [social marketing] topics, they are more likely to give inaccurate, self-serving, or socially desirable answers to such questions than to questions about cake mixes, soft drinks or cereals." Special efforts must be made. As Ramah and Cassidy (1992, p. 3) note: "Because HIV infection and AIDS produce fear in people, and because one's sexual and drug habits are difficult to talk about . . . [p]eople [in research encounters] must be enabled to think and speak frankly about private acts" (p. 3).

- *Invisible Benefits*. Whereas in the private sector, it is usually relatively clear what benefits one is likely to get—it is easy to imagine a Hilton hotel room or a new Xerox machine—social marketers are often encouraging behaviors where nothing happens. Immunization is supposed to prevent disease in the future. Hypertensives are told their blood pressure will be lowered if only they take their pills. Women are promised that taking a birth control pill means that a baby will not come. In each of these cases, absence of outcomes is a sign of success. The trouble is that the consumer will have difficulty knowing whether the behavior worked! Often the consumer who agrees to the behavior has the nagging feeling that the same outcome would have occurred without the recommended course of action. It is much harder to market behaviors that lack visible consequences than behaviors that have them.

- *Benefits to Third Parties.* Some behaviors advocated by social marketers have payoffs for third parties such as poor people or society in general and not to the person undertaking the behavior. This is the case, for example, for energy conservation and obedience to speed laws. In these cases, most individuals will regard slowing down or turning down the heat as a personal inconvenience but many will still do so because they feel it is in their society's interests (Kotler and Levy, 1969). It is much more difficult to motivate people to take actions when they do not benefit (even invisibly) than when they or their immediate families are the direct beneficiary.

- *Intangibles That Are Difficult to Portray.* Because the consequences of social behavior change often are invisible or apply only to others, they are much more difficult to portray in promotional messages. Marketers must be highly creative to develop advertising that describes the benefits to families and the country of carrying out family planning or growth monitoring of their children. Because symbols in communications are often used to communicate intangibles, there is often the risk of sending the wrong signals, as when rural consumers in developing countries are alienated by promotions that seem too Western.

- *Changes That Take a Long Time.* Because many of the proposed behavior changes are highly involving or entail changing individuals from negative to positive demand, the process for achieving behavior change can take a very long time indeed. This will be because: (a) often very large amounts of basic information will have to be communicated; (b) basic values will have to be changed, and (c) a great many outside opinion leaders and support agencies will have to be brought on board. For example, to create widespread use of ORT, target consumers must learn that dehydration *per se* is life-threatening, that modern remedies are better than folk remedies and can be trusted, and that packaged, branded products are safe and reliable. Simultaneously, physicians, pharmacists, and public health workers must be educated about the problem and given or sold supplies to distribute. Marketers accustomed to short-term objectives such as found in consumer packaged-goods markets can find the complications and length of time involved in social marketing very frustrating. In many cases, they will have to settle for objectives that are short of ultimate behavior change—although they must be careful to choose interim objectives that are likely to have a direct link to behavior.

- *Culture Conflict.* As Jean Manning and I have pointed out elsewhere (Andreasen and Manning, 1987), many social marketing organizations may be infected with a basic conflict between two or more cultures. Many social marketing organizations are founded to achieve a basic social service mission. They want to eliminate homelessness, reduce child abuse, or improve the physical and mental well-being of the very elderly. They care deeply about this mission and are often willing to overlook waste, misdirection, and inefficiency in a good cause. Those with what we called a *social service* orientation frequently come into conflict with social marketers who come from a corporate culture. The latter often enter the organization many years after its founding and attempt to increase the efficiency and effectiveness of its often dramatically growing programs. The concerns of those in the corporate culture are often seen by the social service people as heartless, uncaring, even immoral. For their part, the corporate people often see their counterparts as ill-focused, wasteful, and impractical. Such conflicts can have highly debilitating effects on social marketing programs if not resolved. Chapter Two returns to this problem, and offers some solutions in Exhibit 2.1.

- *Public Scrutiny.* Because social marketers have as their goal the improvement of the welfare of the target audience or the general society, it is typical that some form of formal or informal public scrutiny will be accorded their performance. This scrutiny may be by the government, a funding source, or the general public as represented by the press or academic researchers and critics. This scrutiny, among other effects, makes it more difficult to take risks in social marketing and increases the importance of politics and public relations in the social marketing mix.

- *Limited Budgets.* Traditional marketers are used to working with relatively generous budgets to meet a given challenge. Social marketers typically have severely restricted budgets, in part because there is not enough to go around in some government or nonprofit agencies or some foundations. Sometimes budgets—or components of them—are restricted because watchdog groups think that an organization that pays too high salaries or "wastes" too much money on advertising or sales commissions is somehow not being frugal with taxpayers' money or donations. As a consequence, social marketers must spend much time and effort leveraging their meager budgets by engaging the assistance of distributors, advertising agencies, broadcast or print media, business firms, unions, and other social marketing organizations to carry out their programs. This is a point we shall turn to toward the end of the chapter.

 • _Multiple Publics._ The constant need for ongoing outside assistance and the constant oversight by other individuals and agencies increases the need to market not only to target customers but also to those who are giving assistance or regulating activities. This only adds more burden to overworked social marketing managers.

 • _Absence of a Marketing Mindset._ One of the most important correctable weaknesses in many organizations is the absence of a pervasive marketing mindset. If the organization is not committed to a bottom line of behavior change, if management does not put customers at the center of all its intervention planning, if the organization sees customers as the problem and in need of changing (rather than changing the organization), if there is a reluctance to bother with marketing research, then the social marketer has a great deal of internal training and attitude change to undertake if the social marketing program is to be at all effective and lasting. And this may be especially difficult if the organization is caught up in a social service mentality.

 • _Few Opportunities to Modify Products._ If business people or consumers want a faster, more flexible computer, Apple will invent one. If a commercial marketer cannot satisfy a customer with one product, he or she simply creates another. But if women want a diarrhea remedy that stops the diarrhea as well as prevents dehydration, or they want an effective male contraceptive, such products cannot be easily developed. Years of research are needed. Responsiveness to consumer demand is limited by science. Products such as ORS, which meet important public health criteria for effectiveness, must be marketed despite existing inherent disadvantages from the consumer's point of view.

How to Develop a Customer-Centered Marketing Approach

In most organizations that have adopted social marketing as a new approach to behavior change, it is typically relegated to a secondary role. Social marketing may be carried out by a department or a simply by a single individual. In still others, social marketing may be carried out by a lowly subsidiary group or division within a broader communications department. This may reflect the relative newness of the field and the lack of familiarity many people have with this new concept. However, in my judgment, all of these approaches are very shortsighted.

In the first place, as noted in this chapter and throughout this book, good social marketing is not a special case of communications. Rather, the reverse is true. Communications is simply one of the components of a fully developed and well-coordinated strategy to achieve behavior change.

More critically, I would make the somewhat arrogant contention that, for any program or organization whose basic objective is to achieve social behavior change—as opposed to merely educating and influencing (that is, changing attitudes and values of a society), social marketing should be the paramount guiding philosophy for the specific program and for the entire organization. This means that the adoption of a customer-centered mindset should start with program directors and CEOs of organizations whose mission it is to achieve social behavior change. These individuals should be social marketers themselves, or at the very least be able to think and act like social marketers when it comes to behavior change. I would argue that the mindset outlined in this chapter, when combined with the processes and concepts outlined in the rest of this book, provide the best comprehensive framework for CEOs carrying out that mission. I argue this for five reasons:

1. *Social marketing forces the manager to be market driven.* It gets him or her out of the office and, at least conceptually, into the field. As every first-rate private sector CEO knows, you cannot be successful unless you truly understand your customers. A good CEO is one who has an excellent gut-level feel for what customers need and want. Such CEOs are not driven by donors or even their

own missionary zeal. They do not run off in wasteful and unproductive directions, pursuing what they or any noncustomer groups think is the right course of action. They respond primarily and deeply to their customers.

2. *A customer focus makes it much less likely that the organization will lose its way or will miss trends.* It will have its ear to the consumer ground, so to speak, so that very little will develop without its knowledge.

3. *Social marketing forces the organization and its program managers to focus firmly on the critical bottom line, behavior change.* It ensures that they do not get sidetracked (or at least not for long) pursuing potentially wasteful avenues such as elaborate education or persuasion campaigns with no clear linkage to behavior change. Social marketing provides an iron rod (behavior change) to measure the worth of every program component.

4. *Social marketing forces the organization to think about all the tools that can be used to achieve behavior change.* It keeps managers from getting caught up in the glamour of fancy media campaigns and award-winning posters that promote the benefits of the behavior but ignore Place, Price, and Product aspects of the influence process.

5. *Because social marketers are alert to competition, they are compelled to be much faster on their feet.* Competitive environments change rapidly, so those with a marketing orientation train themselves to be more flexible and in touch with market developments. Again, this discipline makes it much less likely that the organization will rest contentedly with a program or campaign long after it has passed its prime.

The Universality of Marketing

A more global reason for a social program manager to adopt a social marketing orientation is that the social marketing technology does not apply only to target consumers. It should be remembered that, basically, social marketing is an approach to bringing about behavior change. Therefore, it is an approach one can use whenever the objective is to get someone else to act in a certain way. And a great many of the tasks that face a manager beyond target marketing involve behavior change. The following behaviors are only some of the critical behaviors a manager will want to influence in order to be successful:

- Contributions by individual and corporate donors
- The awarding of grants by government agencies or private foundations
- Contributions of services by cooperating agencies and organizations (such as advertising agencies)
- Supportive media coverage by newspapers, magazines, radio, and television
- Contributions of time and effort by volunteers
- Job performance by volunteers
- Cooperative behaviors by intermediaries essential to carrying out programs (such as government health workers)
- Approvals by boards of directors for planned actions
- Granting of waivers or other actions by government agencies necessary for program success
- Job performance by paid staff and other managers

In all of these cases, the same social marketing principles that I develop in this book apply. For example, if a manager wishes to recruit more volunteers, he or she can be most effective by first understanding, even in a general way, the perceptions, needs, and wants of the target audience (the potential volunteers). By conceptualizing the prospective volunteers' behavior as coming about as the result of their choices among alternatives, the manager can understand how to change the perceived benefits and costs in order to get the targets to volunteer. The manager will try to understand the nature of the competition and what might be done to lessen its vigor. The manager will recognize the need to track volunteer satisfaction in order to adjust incentive programs or to diminish costs of participation.

It is all just good social marketing!

Summary

To be an effective social marketer, one must have the proper mindset—a philosophy or orientation for action. This mindset is one that starts every program and every action by first considering customer needs and wants. Too many organizations that think they are practicing social marketing are really mired in an organization-centered mindset that sees their mission as inherently good and their lack of success as their customers' fault. They think that marketing is really just communications, that research is seldom necessary, that customers can be treated as a mass, and that competition can be ignored. But good social marketers are guided by a very different mindset. For them the basic mission involves responding to customer needs and wants. It recognizes that lack of success is usually the organization's fault and not the customer's. It sees marketing as much more than communications. It knows that research is vital, that markets must be segmented, and that competition is everywhere.

The essence of the social marketing mindset is that it is incessantly customer-centered. It looks to customers for what to do. It pretests programs and tactics with those same customers and then monitors customer reactions constantly when programs are initiated. Because marketers are customer-driven, they know they must also be flexible risk-takers, willing to change their offerings if customers change or if the strategy is wrong. They know that this takes careful planning and agile footwork.

One cannot, however, adapt commercial sector approaches to social issues without careful attention to the subtle differences between the two worlds. Social marketing is different from commercial marketing in that it often involves negative demand, highly sensitive topics, invisible benefits that are sometimes only available to third parties, intangibles that are hard to portray, changes that are a long time coming about, public scrutiny, multiple publics to satisfy, an absence of co-workers with the proper mindset, and few opportunities to modify products.

Once someone learns to use a social marketing framework, its points of application are myriad. Because the bottom line of social marketing is influencing behavior, the framework and concepts outlined in this book can be applied to influence volunteers, government agents, donors, staff members, and a range of potential intermediaries and other cooperating organizations.

Chapter Two

The Social Marketing Strategic Management Process

A proper marketing mindset is the first requirement for developing an effective social marketing program. The second requirement is a serviceable process for developing and carrying out social marketing programs. This applies whether one is planning a short-term campaign or the overall thrust of a social marketing organization over three, ten, or twenty years.

There are many approaches to this task. The process outlined in this chapter is simply one possibility. However, it is one that has served me extremely well in a wide range of social marketing consulting environments. It is comprehensive and contains all of the central elements that distinguish most process models. It can serve as a road map for those about to undertake any strategic planning exercise. While it serves very well in the commercial sector, it is extremely well adapted to social marketing.

It is important to keep in mind during this discussion that strategies do not evolve and get implemented on their own. They require effective leadership. Some of the most impactful social marketing programs in the world today are those that have had strong, charismatic leaders driving them to success. For example, Mechai Viravaidya, a charismatic leader and master of publicity, is considered by many to be one of the main reasons his Population Development Associates in Thailand has had so much impact on the birth rate in that country and now on the impact of the AIDS epidemic. Everett Koop, former Surgeon General of the United States, has lent both visibility and direction to antismoking and AIDS efforts in the United States (Snyder, 1991).

In this chapter, I describe processes and procedures that each leader can use to implement social marketing programs effectively. Ultimately, however, processes and procedures are only as good as the people who will carry them out. I will assume that some sort of broad organizational mission and strategy already exists and that a manager is charged with developing a strategic plan. Here, my focus will be on the process of planning and not on detailed contents. In subsequent chapters, I shall consider how one carries out specific elements of the strategic plan such as understanding customers, segmenting markets, and developing the elements of the marketing mix.

The Terminology of Strategic Marketing

Marketers make a number of distinctions when they think about planning marketing programs. First, they distinguish between *strategy* and *tactics*. A strategy is the broad approach that an organization takes to achieving its objectives. For example, Apple Computer has a strategy that involves making its products extremely easy to use, what they call "user friendly." IBM, on the other hand, has a strategy that emphasizes technical competence, product support, and the reliability of its equipment. Tactics, on the other hand, are the detailed steps that an organization takes to carry out its strategy. Thus, Apple may choose a warm and friendly spokesperson with a just-folks manner for its advertising as a tactic in keeping with its user-friendly strategy. IBM, on the other hand, may choose an all-business, no-nonsense spokesperson as a tactic to emphasize its strategy of technical competence.

The second distinction is between *long term* and *short term*. Long term typically refers to three to five years (or twenty to fifty years if you are planting trees for a paper business). Short term typically refers to one year or less. Strategies are usually designed for the long term and tactics are things one does in the short term.

The final distinction is between *strategies* and *plans*. Strategies, again, are the big picture of how the organization is going to achieve its goals. Plans are the guidebooks that spell out the steps that will be taken to carry out the strategy to achieve the goals. Plans, too, can be short term or long term.

In the social marketing world, organizations speak of *programs* and *campaigns*. Programs are ongoing coordinated activities designed to achieve an organization's mission. They may include one or more specific campaigns (Rogers and Storey, 1988). Both programs and campaigns can have strategies, plans, and tactics. By definition, programs are long term. Campaigns may be short term, as in campaigns in Thailand to promote vasectomies on the King's birthday. They can also be long term, as in the "Just Say No" antidrug campaign or the Smokey Bear fire safety campaign in the United States.

I shall begin by considering the broader issues of program planning and then turn to campaigns. Much of the material will be drawn from conventional commercial sector marketing approaches. Throughout, however, I shall pay attention to how conventional marketing thinking needs to be altered to accommodate the special circumstances one faces when trying to change social behaviors.

Organizational Advantages of Planning

The preparation of a sound strategic plan is critical to any successful social marketing program or campaign. Without it, the enterprise is rudderless. An operation with only a vague sense of its strategy can career dramatically from program to program or campaign to campaign, trying this, trying that. Such a course will demoralize staff and discourage supporters from providing necessary funds and cooperation. On the other hand, the actual process of preparing the strategic plan can have a very salutary effect on a program, organization, or campaign if all of those who must implement it participate in its development. Despite the often long hours the preparation process entails, there are a number of benefits:

1.   *Those who must implement the plan will have ownership of its contents.* It is they who will have decided where to go and how to get there. The plan will not be something handed to them by higher-ups. As a consequence, they will be strongly motivated to achieve

their own objectives, will understand deeply both what is stated and what is implied by the plan, will recognize points of weakness and uncertainly that need careful monitoring, and will consider eventual judgments about their own performance to be fair and equitable because they set the standards for themselves.

2.   *The process of working together to develop the strategic plan has significant effects on group cohesion and mutual respect.* The process tends to break down barriers between organizational levels, which can be particularly valuable in cultures where such barriers are the norm and are often very rigid.

3.   *Individual staffers and volunteers have the opportunity to express their own desires for the program and for their personal participation in it.* This venting of ambitions typically leads to one of two outcomes, both valuable to the program. The majority of the staff or volunteer contingent will come to feel that their personal goals are more aligned with the program and its activities. By contrast, a small minority will conclude that the program is not going in ways that will meet their personal needs and they will decide to drop out. Managers who have seen the latter happen are extremely grateful for two reasons. First, the parting is usually amicable because both sides realize that there is not a good fit. But second, it also significantly reduces the internal friction within the organization. By weeding out those whose personal goals are incompatible with the program, the director is left with a group that agrees at the most fundamental level on the desirability of the approach and the intended outcomes. And while there will be vigorous debates about tactics and even specific campaigns within the overall strategy, these debates will rarely sink to the level of personal animosity that can destroy an organization's working environment. Members can disagree with others without implying (or feeling) that there is a fundamental conflict in basic means and ends.

4.   *Assumptions about the marketplace and the competitive environment are made explicit—and tested.* Programs that do not do formal strategic planning are very often caught proceeding down a pathway that is simply not supported by the true market situation. A case in point is the antismoking campaigns of the 1960s and 1970s that were based upon the assumption that people continued to smoke because they did not know how bad it was for them.

5.   *Program managers and staff are forced to look ahead.* One of the

maxims a professional marketer brings to the strategic marketing process is the simple notion that strategies are implemented in the future. This means that the relevant environment is not today's environment but tomorrow's environment. In my experience, a major failing of a lot of organizations, even when they attempt to develop strategic plans, is that they assume the environment will stand still. This can very dangerous for social marketing programs, especially those that must be implemented in developing countries with volatile governments. To establish a program that works through a health ministry that is today very sympathetic to the program is very shortsighted if there is even a modest chance that a supportive Minister of Health (who is usually the only person who counts) will be replaced. In such cases, a strategic plan will only be sound if it plans a program that either ignores the Ministry or that has developed specific contingency plans in case the climate changes.

Strategic Social Marketing

There are many ways of going about carrying out strategic social marketing. One approach that has had considerable success in the nonprofit environment is that outlined in Figure 2.1. This process has been adapted from earlier work for the United Way of America (Andreasen, 1990) and for the American Cancer Society (Andreasen, 1992). It also reflects in many ways the thinking of William Smith of the Academy for Educational Development (Smith, 1993). It divides the strategic marketing task into six stages:

1. *Listening.* Conducting extensive background analysis, including listening intently to target customers.
2. *Planning.* Setting the marketing mission, objectives, and goals, and defining the core marketing strategy.
3. *Structuring.* Establishing a marketing organization, procedures, benchmarks, and feedback mechanisms to carry out the core strategy.
4. *Pretesting.* Trying out key program elements such as the core marketing strategy.
5. *Implementing.* Putting the strategy into effect.
6. *Monitoring.* Tracking program progress (including more listening to customers) and adjusting strategy and tactics as necessary.

Figure 2.1 Strategic Social Marketing.

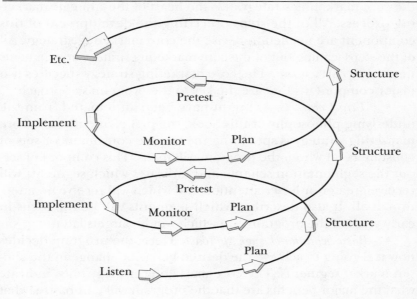

Two features of this process must be noted:

1.   *The process is really continuous, not a one-way activity with a neat beginning and end.* It is more like an upward spiral (Smith, 1993) where planners listen, plan, structure, pretest, implement, listen (that is, monitor), plan, structure, pretest . . . and so on indefinitely. The process is iterative, ratcheting upward at each revolution. With good strategists, this spiral or recycling is an unending process. Indeed, the willingness to constantly try and experiment and adjust is a key characteristic of the way commercial sector marketers approach marketing. As General Motors puts it, there is no finish line in this race.

2.   *Customers are central.* Customers are constantly a part of the process. The process starts by studying customers and their needs, wants, and perceptions. It develops strategies that are heavily influenced by what is learned. It then tests key program elements with the customers it is supposed to influence before going ahead with full-scale implementation. And finally, implementation is always followed by efforts to monitor how strategies and tactics are actually influencing those they are designed to reach.

The central component around which the process revolves is the core marketing strategy. It is the heart of the strategic marketing process. All of the steps preceding the development of this component are needed to devise the core marketing strategy. All of the steps leading out of the core marketing strategy are elements needed to carry it out. The core marketing strategy specifies two major components that are the key to the program's approach:

- *Target markets.* As might have been anticipated from the underlying philosophy of this book, the first element of the core marketing strategy is specifying the precise consumers or sets of consumers on whom the program will focus. This component sets out the segmentation scheme and indicates which segments will receive greater or lesser attention and which will receive no attention at all. It also describes which segments will be the focus in early years of the program and which will be targets later.

- *Basic behavior-change approach.* Here, the program decides how it is going to achieve the desired behavior change in the chosen market segments. The core marketing strategy must indicate what the major benefits are that the program will emphasize, what costs it will seek to reduce, what social pressures it will bring to bear, what distribution system will be necessary to deliver needed products and services, and what communications will be employed to tell the target market about the behavior and its benefits. There are seven characteristics that distinguish an effective from an ineffective core social marketing strategy (Kotler and Andreasen, 1991, pp. 165–166). These characteristics are set out in Exhibit 2.1.

Stage 1: Listening

Quite obviously, every organizational undertaking—whether it is social marketing or not—must begin with some assessment of the environment in which the undertaking is to take place. Traditional planning models tend to divide up the environment into two broad areas labeled the internal and external environments. The *internal environment* refers to the organization that will carry out the strategy and the strengths and weaknesses it brings to the new enterprise. The *external environment* is the world outside the organization that can present opportunities and threats having an effect on the success of the enterprise. Among the key elements of the external environment are economic, social, political, legal,

Exhibit 2.1. Characteristics of a Sound Core Marketing Strategy.

1. *It is customer centered.* It has as its principal focus meeting the needs and wants of its target audiences. It is not designed to sell a program that the social marketer thinks needs to be sold.

2. *It is visionary.* It articulates a future for the program that offers a clear sense of where the program is going and what it will achieve when it meets with its expected success.

3. *It differentiates the program from its key rivals.* The social marketer will stand out, and will offer target markets unique reasons for undertaking the actions it seeks.

4. *It is sustainable for the long run and in the face of changing market and competitive conditions.* Strategies are not implemented in a vacuum. If they are to be successful, they must anticipate change and be prepared to respond to it.

5. *It is easily communicated.* The central elements of the strategy will be simple and clear so that both target audiences and the program's own staff will have an unambiguous understanding of just what the strategy is and why it should be supported.

6. *It is motivating.* A successful core strategy is one that has the enthusiastic commitment of those who must carry it out. A strategy will not be motivating if it is either merely "business as usual" (just one more program like many other programs) or unrealistic in its aspirations.

7. *It is flexible.* The core strategy should be sufficiently broad that it allows for diversity in the ways in which staffers and campaigns implement it. It must not be so rigid and uncompromising that it is not adaptable to unforeseen contingencies.

---

technological (sometimes), and competitive (sometimes) factors (as described in Kotler and Andreasen, 1991, Chapter Three).

But the single most important environmental feature in social marketing programs is the external factor called *customers*. As the Introduction made very clear, what distinguishes the present approach from its competitors is its slavish attention to customers at all stages of the process. This is perhaps most crucial at the outset, when social marketers are gathering information to guide their basic plan. It is therefore natural to begin here our consideration of the strategic marketing process.

Listening to Customers

Good social marketers begin by saying: "I need to know everything I can about those whom I am supposed to influence." They then proceed to begin collecting the necessary data, which can come from both secondary and primary sources. Secondary research seeks out available information on potential target customers and insights gained by past marketers and researchers, and can be a fast and inexpensive way to get a feeling for the market. However, primary research is almost always essential at some point, despite the additional effort involved.

Secondary research is typically out of date, and it often does not define the problem in the way the social marketer might wish. For example, for a contraceptive social marketing program, secondary data may be available—say, from a government health ministry—on general contraceptive rates in a given population and on condom distribution for recent time periods. Such data, however, do not indicate who is using condoms and how often, information that is key to knowing how to make changes. In addition, secondary data are very rarely attuned to social marketing needs. Thus they do not provide the depth of insight one needs to develop message strategies or product and package designs. They usually do not have the segmentation characteristics a marketer wants, such readiness to act or media habits.

Primary research that is carried out before a social marketing campaign is undertaken is usually defined as *formative research*. Formative research can take many guises, as I discuss in the next chapter. However, two important points must be made about this kind of consumer research:

Formative research need not be expensive. A great many of the techniques described in Chapter Three can be carried out on a small scale, with volunteer (but trained) help, in relatively convenient locales. The crucial objective is to get out and talk to potential customers. The very best managers in the commercial sector pride themselves on their abilities to get close to their customers. This means going out and sitting and chatting with customers in the coffee houses, the village centers, the churches, the workplaces. It means being open to hearing what they have to say and not simply waiting for reinforcement of one's prejudices. Good managers are open to learning about what customers really think and feel. They come to know what customers fear and what they don't understand, what they want and hope for, what they listen to, and whom they respect. They understand their media patterns and their shopping habits. They know how they get along with their families and neighbors. And—eventually—they begin to get a good idea of what might be successful in getting them to adopt a new course of action.

But they are also aware that even informal research must be planned research. They are careful to get representative cross-sections and are alert for possible selection biases and biases in responses. They know that small samples may be unique and that they must always temper what they hear with experience and judgment. But they also know that the alternative is not necessarily large, sophisticated studies that drain valuable resources and time.

Formative research must be based on a model of consumer behavior. A series of random conversations and nice chats about life and the behavior to be influenced does not constitute research. And certainly, a formal study that simply measures everything anyone can think of that might be relevant is not good research—except by chance—either. As I have pointed out in other places (Andreasen, 1988c), the only useful formative research is research that helps mangers come up with a good strategic plan. Sound decisions are most likely to be those based on some notion of what strategies and tactics will work on what target customers. To know this, we must have some understanding of how target customers come to adopt new behaviors. This understanding is what is meant by a model. A model is simply a representation of the way in which target audiences make critical decisions.

The present book is organized around a consumer behavior model that I have found useful for developing strategic social marketing plans. This model will be outlined in Chapter Four; for the moment it is enough to assume that it exists.

Listening to the Organization

Kotler and Armstrong have defined strategic marketing as "the process of developing and maintaining a strategic fit between the organization's goals and capabilities and its changing marketing opportunities" (1994, p. 334). Thus, a critical requirement of good social marketing strategic planning is listening to the organization's own goals and capabilities. Sometimes these goals and objectives are not what they should be—problems revealed by the presence of one or more of the following characteristics:

• *Nonbehavioral Objectives.* As I have noted, social marketers have a bottom line behavioral orientation that may conflict with organizational objectives. The organization may have defined its objectives in terms of "raising awareness" about the need for behavior change or "changing values" that affect the behavior in question (for example, getting mothers to agree that child spacing is not against a particular religion's tenets). The social marketer would argue that these objectives are only important if they lead to behavior change.

• *Conflicting Objectives.* Social marketers sometimes face situations in which organizations want to have it all. They want all children under five in Lesotho to be perfectly healthy. This leads them to embrace such objectives as improving the prenatal care of mothers, making children immune to infectious diseases, increasing the frequency and length of breast-feeding, effectively treating disease episodes when they occur, and supplementing rations to maintain proper rates of physical growth. It is impossible to achieve all of these objectives at once. Indeed, some may conflict. Focusing on breast-feeding may make it more difficult for mothers to take older children to the clinic for proper medical treatment. Focusing on supplementing household food rations with Vitamin A may discourage mothers from breast-feeding. In such circumstances, the social marketing practitioner must require that the organization sort out its priorities first, before embarking on any marketing program. The social marketer should ensure that his or her programs are not challenged to achieve two or more mutually exclusive outcomes.

• *Hidden Objectives.* It is not uncommon for the stated objectives of an organization to be very different from the objectives the organization is really pursuing. In my experience, this is a relatively common occurrence in social marketing. It appears in two areas. One is the political sphere, where a social marketing program is undertaken by a government agency. Very often the cognizant bureaucrat has personal political objectives that can sabotage or at least distort well-intentioned social marketing programs. This often shows up in proscriptions against certain activities (such as embarrassing advertisements on television) or an emphasis on certain politically important populations (such as corporate employees in urban areas). In other organizations, social marketers may find the case to be that certain strategic approaches are preferred (such as the use of many consultants) because a real goal is to increase the organization's capabilities for future projects.

• *Nonquantified Objectives.* In all well-run organizations, objectives have to get translated into measurable goals against which progress and eventual overall achievement will be assessed. But many organizations avoid precision because they either think it is somehow grander to have a vague general objective such as "healthier children by the year 2000" or are afraid to be held to anything that is objectively evaluated. Social marketers should insist that nonquantified objectives such as increasing the rates of immunization be translated into specific goals such as the statement that "from now to the year 2000, 15 percent more children under two will be immunized each year than the previous year."

• *Unrealistic Objectives.* While some have very negative attitudes toward social marketing, others expect too much of it. In such cases goals may be set at unrealistically high levels. In commercial markets, marketers are often given responsibility for improving market shares a few percentage points or launching a new product or brand that will yield the firm a reasonable return on investment. In social marketing, the challenges may be for complete eradication of a problem or the universal adoption of some desirable behavior. Though it may seem counterproductive at first glance, social marketers must spend at least some of their time working to reduce the goal expectations of key oversight publics. It is important that those individuals and organizations approving and funding social marketing programs do not have unreasonable hopes for their accomplishments. Social marketers can often achieve dramatic changes in behavior that overshadow most accomplishments in the commercial sector—for example, as in the high blood pressure education program described in the Introduction—but results take time to get, and impatient funders can make the work much harder at every stage of the process.

Other organizational weaknesses can be identified through a thorough "marketing audit" (Kotler and Andreasen, 1991, pp. 80–88). For example, distribution systems can be weak in serving the poorest customers. Staff can have attitudes that are far from customer friendly. Inventories may be chronically out-of-date. All of these shortcomings can cripple efforts to achieve ambitious objectives.

Listening to the Competition

As I have noted, social marketers very naturally think of competition when they think about the external challenges facing them in the area of social behavior. Further, they realize that this competition is best defined from the consumer's standpoint rather from the marketer's standpoint. Consumers always have choices—if only to continue with their existing behavior. This can be very compelling competition.

In most program areas, it will be important for the social marketing manager to understand both what consumers see as the program's competition and how that competition might change in future. Sometimes the competition is relatively uncomplicated. Take binge drinking by high schoolers—a major source of automobile fatalities among teenagers. Any program seeking to moderate or eliminate this destructive behavior must recognize that it meets important needs and wants of the target audience. To effectively change the behavior, the social marketer must understand those needs and wants and show how the proposed behavior can either also meet those needs and wants or can meet other needs and wants that are superordinate. Thus, while binge drinking can help a young person feel accepted and valued by peers, elimination of the behavior can be shown to also get the young person accepted and valued by different but equally desirable peer groups (it never works to say that the nerds will think you are cool to stay dry). Or elimination can meet other needs, such as getting dates with desirable members of the opposite sex or increasing the chances of getting better grades and going to a good college.

It is never enough to talk about what you want the audience to do. Expert social marketers also talk (implicitly or explicitly) about how the behavior is better than what the competition offers. A useful framework for understanding this competition is to see it at four different levels, each of which can be addressed by a marketing strategy tailored to meet it.

- *Desire competition.* These are alternative immediate desires the consumer might wish to satisfy by not adopting a proposed social behavior, for example, the desire to please a spouse by being at home after work rather than going to a clinic to get a child immunized so as to live a healthier life.

If the marketer believes that the most serious competition is at the desire level, then a program designed to get mothers to take more actions benefiting their children rather than their husbands might be appropriate—but difficult.

- *Generic competition.* These are alternative ways in which a single desire of the consumers can be satisfied, for example, seeking to improve a child's health by spending time growing vegetables to improve the family diet rather taking the same time to get immunizations against infectious diseases.

If the marketer believes that the most serious competition is at the generic level, then a program designed to promote immunization over (or perhaps along with) other methods of improving a child's health might be appropriate.

- *Service form competition.* These are alternative ways in which a generic need can be satisfied, for example, to keep the child from acquiring a communicable disease by using homeopathic or traditional medicine instead of immunization.

If the marketer believes that the most serious competition is at the service form level, then a culturally sensitive strategy designed to promote immunizations over traditional healing might be appropriate.

- *Enterprise competition.* These are other enterprises offering the same service form, for example, public health services, pharmacists, midwives, some nongovernmental organizations (NGOs), and private physicians all offering immunization services.

If the marketer believes that the most serious competition is at the enterprise level, then a strategy promoting the use of a particular NGO instead of (presumably less hygienic) local midwives might be appropriate. Alternatively, partnering with established competitors may be the best way to achieve program objectives.

Listening to Scientists, Politicians, and Your Local Demographer

There are a number of other sources of information in the external environment that the social marketing manager will want to investigate prior to forming a specific social marketing strategy. At the outset of the planning cycle, social marketers should listen to scientists, politicians, economists, demographers, and other social commentators in order to develop a best estimate of the kind of future in which their marketing plan will work itself out. Planning a strategy that is best for today's situation may be very dumb for tomorrow's environment. For example, many AIDS programs in the United States planned condom promotion and distribution programs in 1993 on the assumption that the U.S. government and its principal agency (the Centers for Disease Control and Prevention) would continue to avoid direct promotion of condom use. Their efforts turned out to be seriously misdirected, given the change in government policy that took place in early 1994.

Stage 2: Planning

Once the social marketer has spent an intense period listening to customers, the organization, competitors, and assorted politicians, economists, and the like, the next step is to use this information to create a specific marketing strategy. The strategy must first set out broad guidelines about where it wants to go (in the form of a mission and specific marketing objectives and goals) and then set forth a prescription for how it is going to get there. This latter is what is called the core marketing strategy. I will discuss each of these briefly, using the HealthCom child survival program of the Academy for Educational Development as an example.

It should be pointed out, however, that the two steps of listening and planning are not discrete steps. The listening process continues through planning. Good managers are always keeping an eye and ear to the marketplace and directly or indirectly matching emerging planning ideas to the reality they might encounter when they are actually tried out. Environments seldom stand still while managers think about influencing them.

The Marketing Mission

The marketing mission statement is typically a simple sentence or two or a paragraph that gives broad guidelines to staff about where the strategy is designed to go and communicates this information to the outside world, in particular the various agencies and institutions that must assist to make it happen. Perhaps the two most important characteristics of the marketing mission statement are that it *focuses on behavior change* and it *differentiates the social marketer from competitors*—including other social marketing organizations with which it must compete for attention and resources. A generic social marketing mission statement would be the following:

> The mission of the [program] is to bring about changes in the [specific behavior] of [target population(s)] using [description of approach] in order that the lives of the target individuals and the welfare of society as a whole will be significantly improved.

Thus, a mission statement for the Academy for Educational Development's HealthCom social marketing program would be:

> The mission of the HealthCom program is to bring about changes in the behavior of mothers of children under five years old through the use of social marketing techniques so as to increase the life-chances of those children and to improve the quality of their lives and those of their family members.

Goals

Goals translate the marketing mission into specific behavioral outcomes. Thus, the HealthCom program might specify the following goals:

- Increase the number of mothers getting their children fully immunized by the age of two years.
- Increase the number of mothers who breast-feed their children.
- Increase the frequency with which mothers serve their children foods with Vitamin A.
- Increase the usage of oral rehydration solutions by mothers in serious cases of childhood diarrhea and dehydration.
- Increase the general quality of meals served to children under five.

Objectives

The function of objectives is to *quantify* the goals. Again, the feature that distinguishes the social marketing approach is its emphasis on behavioral objectives. Thus, each objective should specify a behavioral outcome, a target population, and a time frame for the objective's achievement. To pursue the HealthCom example, representative objectives might include the following changes for a specific population (say, Manila, the Philippines) for the period from January 1, 1993 to December 31, 1994:

- Increase the proportion of children who have been immunized by the age of two from 80 percent to 95 percent.
- Increase the proportion of mothers with children under five years reporting that they breast-fed their youngest child at least six months after birth from 30 percent to 50 percent.
- Increase the proportion of mothers claiming to have served at least one portion of food high in Vitamin A (or one Vitamin A pill) to her children under five the previous day from 15 percent to 40 percent.
- Increase the proportion of times in which the last case of serious diarrhea of a child under five was treated with some form or oral rehydration therapy (preferably with a food supplement) from 20 percent to 35 percent.

While each of these goals implies some sort of direct measure of mothers' behavior, in many of these cases, market data on sales or distribution of products (such as oral rehydration solutions or Vitamin A pills) may be substituted. The source of the numbers may range from pure speculation, experience in other countries or other settings, or formative research of some kind.

Core Marketing Strategy

The next challenge is to specify exactly how the social marketing strategy is going to achieve the behavior-change objectives and goals. As noted earlier in this chapter, this requires that the social marketer spell out the market or markets to be targeted, and also specify a detailed approach that is to be employed to bring about the desired change in the target market or markets.

A core marketing strategy statement for a hypothetical child health program not unlike HealthCom might contain the following components:

> *Target markets:* Targets will be (a) women between the ages of sixteen and thirty-nine who have one or more children under the age of five and live in urban centers and nearby areas in selected African, Caribbean, and Southeast Asian countries; (b) health workers in public health centers in these communities; and (c) village or community leaders.

Note first that this program will not start out to target rural areas. The premise is that the marketers need to walk before they can run and that a limited budget will have more impact if concentrated in smaller geographical areas than if spread thinly across an entire country. Note, second, that the program targets multiple target groups, including two that we will see in later chapters can have important influences on mothers' behavioral choices and that play a part in the program's positioning statement below. Finally, note that the program does not target women who do not yet have children—that would be pure education, with no measurable behavior requirement, and social marketing's priorities lie in behavior change.

> *Strategy:* Behavior change will be brought about by (a) employing messages tailored to the target market's stage of readiness;

(b) reducing the costs of the desired behaviors (including making access easier); and (c) bringing to bear social influences on target consumers by working through community leaders and national celebrities. The program to carry this out will consist of the elements listed below.

- *Product Development.* Vitamin A, ORS, and new highly nutritious food products will be developed to meet local taste preferences and packaged in containers that use colors and symbols appropriate to the culture. Products will be branded to signal quality and to enhance the sponsor's reputation so it can expand markets and services later. In the case of immunizations, efforts will be made to make the service setting attractive and the service encounter rewarding. Training sessions will be designed to train health workers in immunization techniques (and record keeping), and in the value of breast-feeding, Vitamin A, oral rehydration, and more nutritional feeding of children. They will also be trained to be more customer-friendly.

- *Cost reduction.* Costs to mothers will be reduced by having vans available to transport them to health care centers for immunization or training. Health workers will be trained to be supportive of mothers and not patronizing. Babysitting services in communities will be provided for children left behind on days that mothers go to the clinic. Food, ORS, and vitamin products will be provided at minimal cost (but not free, to ensure that they are used).

- *Improved accessibility.* Vitamin A, food, and ORS products will be made widely available in each community. They will be distributed in kiosks, by community health volunteers (who can make a small profit), midwives, pharmacies, and so on. Workshops on breast-feeding, ORS preparation skills, Vitamin A cooking techniques, and other aspects of nutrition will be held in local areas and taught by trusted local authorities wherever possible. Training for health workers will be held at their places of work on company time.

- *Promotion.* Communications strategies will focus on tailoring messages for mothers to their stage in the behavior-change process. For those in early stages, posters and radio messages will explain the benefits of the various behaviors. For those later on, messages in the same media will emphasize how to acquire products or services and how to acquire necessary skills. Those at final stages will have messages directed at them urging action and, for those who are actually trying out the behavior, providing verbal rewards and other support for their actions. For this last group, the media will shift from impersonal to personal sources. At the same time, messages will be directed at health workers to encourage them to support program initiatives. Finally, personal interventions will be designed to recruit important community leaders and train them in intervention techniques that will support the rest of the program.

Note that this is clearly not just a communications program! It recognizes that women in developing countries have complex lives and are often intensely connected to social networks that are important to them. Thus, the behavior-change program focuses on making the behaviors easier for them to perform when they are ready to do so. It also recognizes that women will differ in the extent to which they are ready to act. Some mothers may need more information. Some may have the information but need to practice skills. Others may have the skills but need their own costs reduced even further. And social networks will have to be brought to bear on the behavior change, recognizing that even if mothers are personally willing and able to undertake the behavior, they may not do so unless they perceive neighborhood women and key elders are supportive, even encouraging.

Stage 3: Structuring

Once the core marketing strategy has been determined, the next steps involve putting in place the mechanisms to carry it out. These involve designing an organizational structure, a set of benchmarks, and a tracking system to keep in touch with how the program is going. Benchmarking and tracking are relatively straightforward. *Benchmarking*, as the term is used here, means the establishment of indices that will indicate, when measured, whether the organization is moving toward a particular goal. For example, in the case of the hypothetical child survival program mentioned above, one benchmark might be the number of units of some essential product (such as ORS or Vitamin A packets) sold or distributed in a month. The *tracking system,* then, might comprise monthly reports from a sample of outlets who are paid to report on sales or other types of offtake each month (Andreasen, 1988a).

Alternative Organizational Structures

The design of the *organization structure* of the social marketing operation itself is a more complicated decision than the benchmarking and tracking system design. In many programs, the marketing department may well be one person. In others, it may include several individuals. In some organizations, the marketing department may be placed in some illogical or undesirable organizational niche such as under the communications or public relations director. Preferably, the marketing department will be situated very high in the organizational hierarchy and, in the best of possible structures, given control of all organizational elements that affect its abilities to implement its strategies.

Assuming the latter is the case, the marketing manager then has to decide how to organize and staff the activities within the department. There are three broad types of organization structure that a social marketing program can adopt. The department can be organized by function, by program, or by customer group. Each of these approaches has its own virtues.

• *Functional organization.* There are a number of functional activities that must be carried out in order to design and implement a social marketing program. Someone will have to design products and packages. Someone will have to create and run advertising. There will be a need for marketing research and for management of distribution systems. If a field force of some kind (such as community health workers) is involved, someone will have to manage it. Someone else will be needed to manage public relations, using the popular media to further the organization's objectives. Each of these tasks is called a function. Each can have a separate person in charge of it—or several related functions can be combined under one person in organizations with limited staff. This approach provides economies of scale and useful skill synergies, and it matches staffers' natural affiliations.

Functionally based organizations work well if programs are relatively homogeneous and if the marketplace has limited volatility.

If this is not the case, there is a real danger that the functional specialists will ignore programs or customer groups that do not interest them. Functional people will busy themselves worrying only about the advertising or the marketing research and how they are being designed and implemented. If the market changes, they may simply not notice—and, in a sense, it is not their responsibility to notice. A program could go seriously off-track while having excellent advertising and research!

There are other disadvantages to this approach, the most important of which is that bottom-line responsibility is diffuse. Functional managers can always blame each other if behavior-change goals are not met. ("It wasn't the radio ads that were at fault, it was the lousy packaging.")

- *Program-centered organization.* In a program-centered organization, one person is given responsibility for coordinating all of the functions with respect to a given program. Thus, the Vitamin A program manager might have his or her own advertising, marketing research, and distribution managers. The same would be true for the immunizations program manager and the manager of the diarrheal disease program. This clearly assigns bottom-line responsibility. It ensures that someone will keep in close touch with market dynamics. In addition, the program manager approach, while not giving the manager a lot of training in any one skill, does develop general management skills that may be valuable to the organization as a whole later on. A final virtue for this approach is that it tends to promote competition within the organization as program managers vie to outdo one another in meeting bottom-line objectives.

In my experience, a unique danger for social marketing in this organizational form is that it encourages CEOs to select managers who know the program content area rather than people who are good at understanding customers. As noted earlier, this can lead to an organization-centered mindset that can be fatal to overall success!

- *Customer-centered organization.* An organizational alternative that is consistent with the overall theme of this book is to structure the staff by customer group. Social marketing organizations with multiple programs may consider developing specialists in particular populations. Thus, in the hypothetical child survival project, one might have separate managers for mothers and for health-care workers. Customer group managers would have the responsibility of understanding their particular market as thoroughly as possible and of introducing programs to the group whenever appropriate.

Whatever the organizational framework that is ultimately chosen, it is important to recognize that, to be truly effective, marketing must pervade the entire organization. As Albrecht (1992), Albrecht and Zemke (1985), and other authors point out, to be fully effective, organizations whose mission is to influence behavior must make sure that everyone who touches upon a target audience is infused with the proper marketing mindset. It is not only the CEO or the marketing department that must understand marketing and what it means to be customer-driven. Every clerk, secretary, service-giver, custodian, and accountant who deals with customers must learn to put the customer's interests ahead of the organization's. People who sense that an entire organization is truly working in the customer's interests first will be well disposed to accept the organization's recommendations for action, to repeat initial pleasant encounters, and to encourage family, friends, neighbors, and co-workers to do the same.

Using Alliances

More and more social marketing programs in the 1990s are taking on partners in strategic alliances to achieve program ends. These alliances can involve commercial sector firms such as distributors, advertising agencies, and marketing researchers. They can involve government agencies, such as a health clinic system or an army of public health workers. They can involve nongovernmental organizations in local areas that have closer ties and often greater credibility among local citizens. Alliances can make programs significantly more effective.

Such collaborations are not new. Indeed, one of the oldest social marketing programs (although it was not called that at the time) was the Nirodh condom marketing program in India in the 1960s and 1970s. A central feature of this government-sponsored program was the use of commercial sector marketers such as Lever Brothers and Brooke Bond Tea Company to distribute condoms in the remotest parts of that vast country. The government decided early on that it did not have the capability to reach distant communities with products on a week-to-week basis—although it could reach the communities with campaign messages (via radio) and once-in-a-while product delivery through health services. But private marketers were routinely packing merchandise into these remote areas—often in backpacks or on donkeys—and would be willing to help in the program in return for the goodwill it would build for their other contacts with the government.

Stage 4: Pretesting

Once the strategy is set and the organization and tracking systems put in place, the social marketer's attention then turns to implementation. But a good social marketers recognize that, even though they have carefully listened to customers up front in Stage 1, this doesn't mean that the newly designed strategy is on target from the customer's standpoint. Thus, it is time to go back and listen to customers to see if what is planned is what will work! This is the virtue of the customer-driven mindset introduced in Chapter One. Social marketers' pervasive customer mindset forces them to realize that the ultimate arbiter of the quality of programs is the target audience. This inevitably leads them to undertake a great deal of pretesting of key elements of their core strategy before going into the field. This is a step that can often save a campaign from misdirected approaches. Take this example from the field of AIDS prevention:

> In the spring of 1989, a proposed AIDS prevention headline concept intended for Caribbean audiences began: "Stop AIDS!" When tested among focus groups, however, this headline was scrapped in favor of another: "Protect yourself." Researchers made the change in response to comments by members of the focus group among whom they had tested their headline concepts. These respondents had emphasized two things. First, they found the phrase "Stop AIDS!" misleading. To some, it implied that a cure was in sight—yet they knew it was not. To others, it suggested that humans were overstepping the boundaries of their capacities, for only God could stop AIDS. Second, participants kept returning to the issue of protection and agreed that it was a priority. Analyzing this event one step further, I suggest that people were more motivated with the close-

up and accessible concept of personal and familial safety—"Protect yourself!"—than with what must have appeared as a cosmic abstraction, "Stop AIDS!" [Ramah and Cassidy, 1992, p. 8].

Stages 5 and 6: Implementing and Monitoring

The final steps of the social marketing planning process are implementing and monitoring the program. The critical factor here is monitoring, not implementing. It is assumed that, if the core strategy is sound and well thought through, the challenge of implementation is a matter of:

- Clear delegation of responsibility, defining who does what and when
- Careful specification of tasks to be accomplished and a time line for their accomplishment
- Dedicated attention to detail
- Consistent follow-up to ensure that what is planned is done and is done on time

But good social marketing managers know that things will never turn out as planned. Strategies and tactics will not be carried out to the letter. The competitive environment will change. Governments will add or subtract programs or support. Customers will not respond as intended. And so on. But to a well-trained social marketer, all of this is perfectly normal. The capacity to change is always built into social marketing programs because they are going to be wrong—one hopes in small ways—but wrong. The marketer's objective, then, is to find out as soon as possible when things are going wrong or aren't living up to expectations. With that information, the marketer can act to change strategies and tactics (redirect the spiral) as rapidly as possible.

This is why going back again and again to listen to customers in the form of monitoring is so crucial to sound social marketing programs. Good monitoring systems keep the organization's finger on the pulse of the market and allow it to be very quick on its feet. And the most central element of that monitoring must be some tracking of customer reactions. As we shall see in the next chapter, monitoring can be done with routine surveys, periodic focus groups, intercepts at appropriate locations, or even periodic one-on-one conversations with target audience members. It is important to recognize that such monitoring need not be unbiased. What managers are looking for are two things:

• Are things going wrong or are they below expectations in some important way?
• Are things changing in ways that suggest the program is moving in the right direction (and so should do more of whatever is working) or is moving in the wrong direction?

In the first case, what is needed is market probes that will identify problems. One need not have a representative sample to discover problems. One only needs broad coverage of the target group. But having ten or twenty people report something that suggests that something is amiss is often quite enough. The manager does not need to know that the problem is experienced by 32.67 percent of the marketplace. It's a *problem*.

In the second case, the important first step is to establish a baseline methodology, even one with biases, and to repeat the same methodology on a regular basis. Assuming the biases are constant, what will appear will be major changes in program success. It is this that the manager needs in order to adapt rapidly to changing markets. It is what keeps Coca-Cola ahead of Pepsi and allows Apple to catch up with IBM!

In all monitoring, it is necessary to temper results with judgment and experience. Data can be deceiving. Savvy social marketers always look to be sure that distressing data are reporting real problems and not methodological artifacts. And they are cautious in making mid-course corrections based on questionable data. In all instances, their commitment to the strategy spiral ensures that they will subsequently pretest any corrections to confirm that they have their intended effects.

Most behavior-change programs have some sort of summative evaluation at their conclusion (Bossert, 1990; Hornik, Zimicki, and Less, 1991). But it is important to recognize that a summative evaluation is no substitute for monitoring (which, of course, is also evaluation but which takes place regularly within programs to keep them fast on their feet). Summative evaluation is usually done at the end of a program to answer very profound questions such as whether the program had the impact it was supposed to have and, if not, why not. Such evaluations are major undertakings and require careful attention to issues of validity and reliability. They are as needed in social marketing programs as any others. But they should not be considered satisfactory for monitoring purposes because they usually come much too late for desirable changes to be implemented.

Evaluation is a normal step in most social change programs—if nothing else, funders usually require it—but monitoring is often neglected. It is not uncommon for the social program manager and the program staff to figure out what to them is their very best strategy. They conscientiously implement it and stick with it until such point as the project is done and the evaluation team comes along to see if they were correct in their strategic choices. This is not good program management and certainly not good social marketing. One of the many valuable contributions of the customer-driven mindset is that it makes marketers realize that if they do not keep continually checking their progress with customers, their programs will surely get off track. If necessary mid-course corrections are not made, all a final, formal evaluation at the end of the project will tell you is: (a) you screwed up and (b) it is too late to fix it.

The Strategic Marketing Process Is an Oscillating Spiral

It is the monitoring function that makes the social marketing process an upward spiral. But monitoring is just the last step in an oscillating process within the spiral. Good, customer-driven social marketers oscillate between going into the field to observe and talk to customers and going back to the office to think about how best to influence them. They begin by listening to the marketplace, then devise programs and structures, test them, and then implement them. But they know that programs are always works-in-process. If—as is almost always the case—monitoring suggests that there is something amiss with a program, the good marketing manager goes back to Stage 1 and once again listens to customers—this time, more carefully. This is the spiral at work. When programs are not going as well as expected, social marketers assume that they didn't understand things well enough. So they listen some more and the program then moves to Stage 2 again and devises a new strategy—or, more often, some new tactics. Although social marketers are often eager to immediately replace the strategy or tactic that is not working so well, the good social marketer does not bypass Stage 4 (Pretesting), recognizing that there is no point in making the same mistake twice. The new implementation then leads to more monitoring and, one hopes, improved results. But this is never certain—and good social marketers are ever vigilant, ever moving up the spiral. Figure 2.2 gives a bird's-eye view of the concept, looking down on the spiral to reveal the oscillations in the loop.

Summary

Once a social marketer adopts the appropriate mindset, the next challenge is to develop a systematic approach to carrying out specific programs. The approach recommended here involves six

Figure 2.2. Strategic Social Marketing Reviewed.

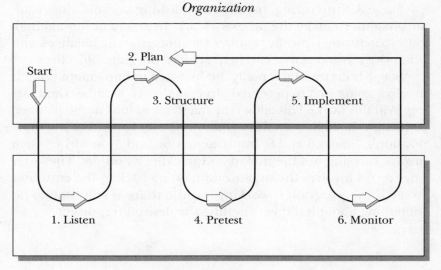

stages: (1) background analysis including listening to potential target customers, (2) planning, (3) structuring the organization and its systems, (4) testing program components prior to implementation, (5) implementation, and (6) monitoring. The process has three features: it is really a spiral in that it repeats and recycles over time; it places the customer at the center of the spiral; and it oscillates between going out to customers for insights and going back to the office to turn those insights into programs.

Stage 1, Listening, involves listening to four features of the marketing environment. First, the social marketer must listen to customers with both formal and informal research. Such research should be organized around the model of consumer behavior presented in Chapter Four. Second, the marketer must listen to the sponsoring organization and clearly understand its objectives and goals, its strengths and weaknesses. Next, the marketer must become aware of competition at many levels. And finally, the marketer must investigate other aspects of the social, political, economic, and technological environment in order to understand the future in which the planned strategy will play itself out.

Stage 2, Planning, requires careful specification of a program's mission, objectives, and goals, and its core marketing strategy. The latter comprises a careful specification of the target market and a specific strategy for influencing its behavior.

Stage 3, Structuring, involves establishing organization, staff, and systems to make the program work. In an era of limited budgets, structuring typically requires forming effective alliances with other organizations that can help achieve program objectives.

Stage 4, Pretesting, is really the first step in implementation. It involves going first to potential target audience members and asking: Will this work? This allows the marketer to look at the planned campaign through the target audience's eyes instead of the organization's. Stages 5 and 6, Implementation and Monitoring, then involve carrying out the design and tracking its results. The latter once again involves the organization going back to the customer to see if the program is working—while there is still time to do something about it if it isn't getting the desired response.

Chapter Three

Listening to Customers: Research for Social Marketing

As we have seen in the previous chapters, customer-driven social marketing relies on constant listening to consumers to ensure that strategies are well designed, well implemented, and effective. Consumer research is the lubrication that sets the strategic social marketing spiral spinning.

Research, of course, is common to a great many types of social interventions. Most major funded projects involving social change require "needs assessments" at their start and formal evaluations at their conclusion. Typically, both involve some form of survey research with careful samples and (often) elaborate questionnaires. Smaller projects with limited funding are at the other extreme. Because they have limited budgets, managers typically do without any research at all, going with past experience and their gut feelings and relying on simple activity measures (such as brochures delivered or clients seen) to gauge their performance.

The approach that social marketers take to research is different in a number of ways. First, in contrast to most large-scale projects, social marketers (a) rely on a much wider array of methods than survey research and (b) use research over the life of the project, not just at the beginning and end. Second, in contrast to small-scale projects, social marketers believe that research is very often justified in some form even if one has to do it very inexpensively. Social marketers believe that tough calls that they must make—both great and small—can always be improved by listening to target consumers.

And finally, social marketers are very much concerned that their research be genuinely useful. They try not to do research (other than that mandated) that does not have a direct impact on their decision making!

This chapter will discuss some of the techniques that social marketers use to listen to customers at three stages of the strategic process:

- *Formative research* to study markets while in the strategy development process
- *Pretest research* to test strategy elements before they go into the field
- *Monitoring and evaluation research* to find out how projects are doing so they can be fine-tuned to improve efficiency and effectiveness

Before discussing these alternative approaches, we must first address the issue of making research useful.

Useful Research

Social marketing projects typically have limited resources, particularly in relationship to the immense social problems they usually face. Thus, managers are reluctant to spend any more on research than they have to. This is sometimes difficult to do because there is often considerable pressure from funding agencies to do extensive studies, especially needs assessments and evaluations. Further, there is a long tradition in fields like health communications to do elaborate surveys whenever one goes into the field. So, on the one hand, the social marketer worries that research will cost too much. Yet, on the other hand, he or she knows that listening to customers is the only (relatively) fool-proof way to make sure that a project is on the right track.

How, then, does the social marketing manager avoid wasteful and unnecessary research while, at the same time, finding time and money to carry out necessary research?

The answer to both questions is simple: *Conduct research only when it helps make a better decision!* Managers are constantly faced with choices. Focus on Market *A* or Market *B*? Use advertisements or interpersonal communications to get commitment to action? Delay action or move ahead now? And so on. Research can help make these choices.

But surprisingly, a lot of research does get done that does not help with decision making and is clearly wasteful.

Curiosity. The most common scenario for wasteful research is when managers conduct research because they are simply ignorant about some aspect of the environment and want (as opposed to need) information about it. A great deal of wasted research follows from statements like: "I really do not know very much about [subject X—some specific datum like the average age of women who use health clinics]. This is an important customer characteristic for our immunization project. Let's find out." The difficulty here is that the research will be done, the manager will say "Ah, now I know more about the subjects—their average age is thirty-three years and three months," but then have to add, "Well, now that I know that, what should I do?" If the manager has not thought through how the information is likely to lead to decisions, then there is a very high probability that the research will be wasted. Curiosity should not be the basis for research expenditures!

Impracticality. A related scenario is one where the research provides interesting but useless findings. Suppose a manager has read about research that identified a type of consumer who could be labeled a "Hypochondriac." Such a person didn't trust doctors and self-medicated with a lot of over-the-counter drugs. The social marketer might think: "Aha! I'll bet that this kind of person is a great prospect for Oral Rehydration Therapy or Vitamin A." The social marketer might then decide to carry out the research to see if such a segment existed and, indeed, if they were above-average users of ORT or purchasers of Vitamin A. Suppose the research concluded that the hypothesis was true! The problem is: what do you do with such a finding? The difficulty is that there is no obvious tie to the marketplace—no hypochondriacs' magazine, no hypochondriacs' TV or radio program—no way, in short, to get at hypochondriacs without blanketing the general population. As a result, the research—although very interesting and probably acceptable to an academic journal—has no practical value to a social marketing decision maker. Spending on it is another waste of resources.

Irrelevance. Another very common wasteful research scenario is where managers collect information that is unlikely to change their decision at all. There are a great many scenarios in which managers have strong assumptions about the world and intend to act on the basis of those assumptions unless some research shows that the assumptions are way off base. Thus, a manager may believe that the best way to reach Hispanic U.S. teenagers with a safe-sex message is though MTV. Research could be conducted to see whether, indeed, Hispanic teens watch MTV and whether they see and are affected by social ads they see there. But if the only circumstance under which the manager is likely to abandon MTV for program messages is if, say, no more than 15 percent of Hispanic teens watch MTV at least once a week or it turns out that less than 1 percent of those who do watch MTV recall any social advertising. If the manager thinks that the research is highly unlikely to come up with this decision-changing result, the best thing to do is abort the research and just go ahead with the decision. The money wasted on such research could be better utilized to buy more ad placements.

Bias. Biased research can often be wasteful. As I will suggest below, bias may not be a serious problem in ongoing monitoring. However, in one-time studies, bias from sample selection, interviewer influences, or respondent lying or distortion can be a very serious problem. It is most serious when management cannot estimate what the direction and scope of the bias might be. Thus, if there is evidence from other studies that condom usage by males is underreported and by females is overreported, then actual (biased) results can be interpreted in this light. On the other hand, suppose research is to be undertaken, say, to gather data about how men and women talk about sex so that managers can construct personalized promotional messages. Further suppose that the market culture is known to be highly secretive about sexual matters. In such cases, the manager may simply not know how much to rely on what is learned. Such research, again, is likely to be wasteful.

Reassurance. Another major source of wasted research is that which is done to meet the manager's personal insecurities. I have personally seen wasteful research done to make a manager more comfortable with a decision or to provide ammunition to justify a course of action to colleagues and others. I have even seen research projects initiated to imitate projects conducted by other respected program managers, even though the particular kind of research has nothing to contribute to the program in hand.

Fishing. Finally, a common source of wasted research is the *fishing expedition.* This description may apply to an entire study or to many of the sections within it. The fishing expedition asks questions in the hope that something will show up that will lead to some action. This not good management nor a good use of research funds.

Backward Research

How then does one go about conducting research that is not wasteful? An approach I have developed to deal with this problem is what I have called *backward research.* While it is described in detail elsewhere (Andreasen, 1985), it is useful to recap the steps involved:

1. Determine what key decisions are to be made using research results and who will make the decisions.
2. Determine what information will help management make the best decisions.
3. Prepare a prototype report and ask management if this is what will best help them make their decisions.
4. Determine the analysis that will be necessary to fill in the report.
5. Determine what questions must be asked to provide the data required by the analysis.
6. Ascertain whether the needed questions have already been asked.
7. Design sample.
8. Implement research design.
9. Analyze data.
10. Write report.
11. Implement the results.

The secret here is to start with the decisions to be made and to make certain that the research helps management reach those decisions. For example, in 1992, I agreed to undertake a social marketing study for the Environmental Protection Agency funded through the private nonprofit group, American Forests (Andreasen and Tyson, 1993). The objective was to determine potential strategies that could be used to encourage builders of single-family residential homes to plant or save more trees on the properties where they built. More trees would have important environmental benefits in reduced pollution, lower energy costs, and improved aesthetics. In a typical research scenario, researchers would have a few discussions with the funders and then go off and conduct what seemed to them a sensible study, write a report, present it, and hope that the findings would be of use. In this study, we proceeded *backward* instead. Here is a detailed discussion of how the process worked:

The first step was to ascertain what decisions were to be made as a result of the report that would be eventually written and to ascertain who was to make them. It was determined that organizations such as American Forests (AF), local forestry extension specialists, the National Association of Home Builders (NAHB), and the Environmental Protection Agency (EPA) wanted to know what messages and what incentives should be used to influence builders' behavior and how these options should be communicated. Discussions with AF and NAHB staff indicated that one of the implementation options they were considering was a series of magazine articles that would motivate builders to plant and save more trees.

In step two, we held meetings to learn what information would help AF and NAHB decide what to say and where to say it. In the latter case, it was clear that information was needed on where builders got their information on new and desirable building practices. It was further clear that questions about information sources needed to include more than just magazines to test the assumption that magazines would present the best aperture to reach builders when they were ready to be influenced. It was further decided that, in order to write persuasive messages, we needed to understand how builders made decisions about new practices so that AF and NAHB would know how to intervene. Focus group discussions with representative builders at this point helped significantly in determining what should be investigated.

At step three, we held discussions about what types of data presentation would be most helpful. This generated a recognition that simple frequency counts—say, magazines read—would be less useful than tables that cross-tabulated readership with measures of receptivity to AF and NAHB persuasive messages. Among other tables, it was suggested that a table showing readership by intentions to plant or save more trees in future would be very helpful.

Step four involved designing the analysis to fit the proposed report. The preceding discussions made clear that much of the analysis would have to be in the form of cross-tabulations. But it was also clear that AF and NAHB staff members were not afraid of fancier analysis techniques and so, we made plans to look at multiple predictors of intentions (to plant or save more trees) using a technique called stepwise regression.

With step five, we turned our attention to what questions would best provide data for the proposed analysis, and a large number of options became clear. For example, because we were going to use stepwise regression to analyze predictors of intentions, the technique required that the measure of intentions be one that had what are called *metric* properties. This just means that, when we asked respondents to indicate how likely they were to plant or save more trees, the numbers representing their answers had to have certain relationships to each other (see Andreasen, 1988c).

Step six was relatively easy, as there were no prior studies of the type we were planning. However, my co-researcher and I did look at other studies for ways of asking key questions.

Design and implementation—steps seven and eight—were relatively conventional. The National Association of Home Builders assisted with sampling, a questionnaire was developed, and two mailings were sent to a random sample of NAHB members.

Responses were then analyzed at step nine, including some approaches using the fancier analytic techniques.

For step ten, we wrote a report addressing the decisions that AF, NAHB, and EPA were considering. We made several suggestions about vehicles for carrying motivational messages. Recommendations about the messages themselves reflected the framework outlined in succeeding chapters of this book. The findings suggested three possible message strategies:

1.   *A Benefits-Based Strategy.* Focusing on benefits to builders, this strategy involved increasing builders' awareness of customers' demand for trees and thus presenting tree-saving as sound

business. It also proposed impressing upon builders their responsibility for helping the environment through better tree management. Overall, it sought to increase builders' perceptions of the benefits of trees, including increased land and property values, increased desirability of the physical space for customers, and increased energy savings, which could be marketed to customers.

2.   *A Social-Influence–Based Strategy.* This would indicate to builders that being assertive about saving and planting trees is a way to show innovative leadership in the community. It might well involve organizing awards programs, which are excellent ways of rewarding desired behavior.

3.   *A Self-Efficacy–Based Strategy.* This would work to persuade builders that they could preserve or provide trees without inordinate effort. It would attempt to decrease builders' concern about the difficulty of getting county officials to cooperate to help save trees—while, at the same time, working with them to encourage more cooperation. It would also increase builders' factual knowledge about proper tree handling practices through lectures, manuals, videotapes, and the like, and would teach builders how to avoid damage during replanting and generally maximize the chances that trees will survive the construction process.

Step 11—implementation of these results—was delegated to AF and NAHB staff. The research report was printed and bound and is sold to builders, developers, government officials, and others who might find it valuable.

Low-Cost Research

The backward approach is helpful for managers assessing whether a given project is worth doing and making sure that, when it is done, it is to the point. But how should social marketers think up projects? In my experience, not only do a great many social marketing projects waste money and time on research they did not need, they also ignore myriad opportunities to do more research. The sources of the latter problem are threefold:

•   *Managers tend to think of research in terms of surveys,* whereas there are many simpler techniques such as focus groups, observation, and experimentation that can make the difference between a good decision and a better one.

- *Managers tend to think of research as expensive.* Thus, when they are trying decide among various messages, they may think that they can't afford the careful study that would really make it clear what to do. Yet there are many inexpensive approaches that, while not leading to certainty, at least improve the manager's decision to a degree that justifies the cost.
- *Managers tend to think that research takes a long time* and so will only slow things down.

The solutions here are relatively straightforward. First, managers need to become aware of the wide range of low-cost research alternatives (Andreasen, 1988c). Second, they need to understand a simple principle of what is called *decision science.* Decision scientists point out (in their rather technical language) that one should undertake research whenever the expected value of the best course of action after research exceeds the expected value of the best course of action before the research by more than the cost of the research. To take a simple example, this means that, if a proposed research study would make it likely that a new message strategy or a relocated health center will convert thirty more people to a new practice than would be the case without the change and the new behavior will yield revenue to the marketer of, say, $100, then the manager can spend up to $3,000 on the research! When put in this light, a lot more research will make sense than is typically the case now. Many decisions about which the manager is unsure will benefit from a little bit of research if it makes the outcome a little better—and the increased value of the outcome is more than the cost of the research.

Managers also need to be aware of opportunity costs of not doing research. Some managers shy away from doing research because they think it is time consuming and will delay getting on with the real job. But they need to think about what would happen if they neglected research, moved ahead, and took the wrong turn. The costs in lost "sales" and in having to correct the strategy could be substantial. Suppose in a given case there is a 10 percent chance this would happen and the cost would be $200,000—then, according to decision science, research that could avoid such a scenario is worthwhile if it cost $19,999 or less (that is, less than 10 percent of $200,000).

Carrying out low-cost research can be habit forming. Just a little practice at doing some cheap-but-good small studies will show the conscientious manager that there are many, many opportunities to improve the effectiveness and efficiency of social marketing programs with only a little more information at the formative, pretest, and monitoring stages.

Formative Research

Formative social marketing research is designed to help develop effective strategies to achieve important social change goals. Generally speaking, all marketing research falls into two broad categories, quantitative and qualitative, though some only use the term formative to refer to the latter. *Quantitative research* is carried out when one needs hard numbers about a target market or some aspect of a marketing strategy. It provides counts and measures of various kinds to tell managers how many people know certain information, engage in certain practices, or feel positively about some organization or product. Quantitative research is carried out using formal sampling procedures and careful field controls to ensure that the results are representative of the population under study. Quantitative research permits investigators to use high-powered statistical techniques to assess relationships, similarities, and differences that can help decide between alternative courses of action.

Quantitative research is usually relatively expensive. It is also the kind of research with which those trained in disciplines other than marketing are most familiar.

Qualitative research, on the other hand, does not involve representative samples and thus its results are not projectable to general populations. It sometimes involves counts and measures—but very often it does not. It may be as simple as a series of structured conversations with target audience members or as complex as a combination of observation, case study, and focus groups. Analysis of qualitative research is more often impressionistic than statistical. Qualitative researchers look for insights and trends, not statistically verifiable numbers.

Qualitative research is usually less costly for field work—although it can eat up substantial amounts of time and cost in analysis and interpretation. It isn't always less costly on a per-respondent basis.

At the formative stage, both quantitative and qualitative research can prove very useful. At this stage, the key decisions that will have to be made on the basis of the research results are basically of three types:

- What target markets should we address (and how should we segment them)?
- How should each chosen target market be addressed?
- How much resources should be allocated to each program component?

Taking the backward research perspective, the next step is then to ask: What information will help managers make the best decisions? As I will make clear in subsequent chapters, the necessary information, in most cases, must come primarily from listening to customers to learn answers to the following questions:

- What is the extent and nature of the behavioral problem?
- Who are those most affected? Where are they? What are they like?
- How can they be reached?
- What beliefs do customers hold about both the perceived benefits and the perceived costs of the proposed behavior?
- What do they perceive that other people who are important in their lives want them to do?
- Do they think that they can carry out the behavior and, if necessary, stick with it? Do they have the skills? Are the necessary products and services easily available?
- What is the major competition to the proposed behavior?
- What factors are likely to influence them to shift to the new behavior and stick with it?

The next step backward considers the appearance and content of the final report. The most basic issue here is: Does the manager need projectable numbers and measures of associations or differences, or will impressions be enough? This will determine whether one needs quantitative or qualitative information.

Quantitative Formative Research

Quantitative formative research can help managers make all three kinds of decisions—that is, decisions about targeting, behavior-change strategy, and resource allocation. Quantitative research is best at yielding statistically reliable estimates of the following kinds of information:

How many people are not doing the desired behavior? This will help the manager determine what resource level would be necessary to try to eradicate the problem.

Which subgroups of the population are more affected by the problem? Which subgroups are more likely to respond to potential interventions? As will be demonstrated in Chapter Five, this will help managers decide how to allocate resources across target segments.

What is the level of awareness of the new behavior and what are people's feelings toward it? This will also help managers estimate the resources necessary to the task. Obviously, if awareness levels are low and feelings or attitudes negative, then many more resources will be necessary than otherwise—or managers may have to scale back their objectives or narrow their targets.

What are the characteristics of the subpopulations we are likely to target? This begins to give managers a picture of the demographics and perhaps lifestyles of target audiences that will help them choose courses of action.

What are the media habits and travel patterns of the target audiences? This information will present what Wells (1989) calls "apertures" through which one can reach target audiences. One needs to reach audiences in times, places, and circumstances where they have the greatest receptivity to intervention—not just when they are physically present. (For an example, see Sutton, Balch, and Lefebvre, in press.)

One of the most common quantitative techniques used in social marketing for gathering the above kinds of data are so-called KAPB studies. These are comprehensive surveys of a representative sample of the target population designed to secure information about the social behavior in question and on the current status of the target audience's:

- Knowledge
- Attitudes
- Practices
- Beliefs

KAPB studies are relatively common in social marketing environments, especially in the area of health. They are very often carried out routinely by local governments, the World Bank, or the United Nations. For this reason, they are sometimes available to social marketers as part of a secondary database. Unfortunately, these studies typically are not designed by a social marketing specialist. As a consequence, they often do not contain the kind of information a social marketing campaign manager needs. For example, they rarely provide lifestyle information. As with all study results, they require careful assessment prior to use. For some guidelines on the topic, see the Quality of Completed Research section, toward the end of this chapter.

The kind of insight that qualitative formative research can give a project is indicated in the following comment about a KAPB study in Mexico:

> An AIDS prevention social marketing project undertaken by AIDS-COM (AIDS Public Health Communication Project) and local collaborators in Tijuana, Mexico, targeted female sex workers for increased condom use. The first task was to determine the KAPB of the sex workers regarding AIDS and condom use. Research findings showed that women were not motivated by the idea "I want to live." They felt that the need to put supper on the table was far more important than the possibility of dying of AIDS five years down the road. On the other hand, the research revealed that many of the women had children and were deeply concerned for their welfare. Because they were responsible parents, they responded to the query, "If something happens to you, what will happen to your child?" Accepting this finding, communications experts designed a small comic book distributed inside a two-condom pack, which features "Barbara" explaining to her sex worker friend one reason why she uses condoms: *"Quiero cuidar a mu hijo, por eso no expongo mi salud."* (I want to protect my child, so I take no chances with my health.) [Ramah and Cassidy, 1992, p. 7].

Where a serviceable KAPB formative study does not exist, social marketers may have to carry one out themselves. This requires careful attention to issues of sampling, interviewer training, questionnaire design, and statistical analysis that are beyond the scope of this book. General sources of research guidance include Andreasen, 1988c, and Kinnear and Taylor, 1991. Assistance on sample design is available in Sudman, 1976, and on questionnaire design in Sudman and Bradburn, 1972, and in Baume, 1993.

Research Compromises

Very often (perhaps always) social marketing programs will not have the resources to carry out an extensive quantitative study. In such cases, compromises will have to be undertaken. There are basically three ways in which one can compromise:

1. *Reduce the quantity of data.* Here, there are several possibilities:

- Reduce the scope of the planned primary research. Here, management would reduce the sample size, the number and sophistication of the questions, and/or the extent of analysis.
- Append a core set of key questions to someone else's primary research. There are two possibilities here—piggybacking key questions onto somebody else's study (such as a study by a cooperating utility, convenience goods marketer, or advertising agency), or adding key questions to an omnibus survey carried out by a single research organization for multiple clients (see Andreasen, 1988c).
- Sample only primary target audiences, that is, those groups determined to be especially important on some *a priori* grounds.

2. *Reduce the quality of the data.* Here, there are also a number of possibilities:

- Reduce the quality of the sample. If one cannot do a representative sample, one can do a *convenience sample.* This involves asking all the key questions, but of a sample of individuals who are easily encountered (such as mothers attending a series of meetings or workers in a set of workplaces). Alternatively, one could use *snowball sampling.* This approach involves first inter-

viewing a convenience sample and then asking the people in the sample to suggest others like them who could be interviewed. This technique can yield matched populations alike in many respects (same socioeconomic status (SES), age, place of residence, and so on) but different in behavior.
- Substitute informal for formal interviewing. As described in the next section, instead of a survey, one could conduct depth or focus group interviews with small selected groups of potential target segments, again asking them in an informal way about their objective characteristics, sources of information, problem exposure, and so on.

3.   *Use available secondary data, that is, information collected by some other source.* Secondary data can be misleading, out-of-date, not exactly on point, and insufficiently documented. However, they can also be very valuable. There are several possible sources of such data:

- Unrelated studies of the proposed targeted audiences. This would include studies of local communities on topics related to the target social marketing behavior but only generally so. An example would be a local study that shows that men read more national political news in the newspaper and women read more practical homemaking news. Such data would encourage a family planning marketer to create (a) messages directed at men that refer to national impact and appear toward the front of the newspaper and (b) messages directed at women that refer to immediate household impact and appear in the newspaper near other homemaking news.
- Related studies of target audiences in other locations. This source comprises social marketing studies on the behavior in question but in some other country or even some other hemisphere. An example might be a finding from a social marketing study in Canada that young women are more accepting of condom use than men think they are (Zaichkowski, 1990). Such a finding might recommend a strategy that tells men what women really think while reinforcing women in their present beliefs.
- Unrelated studies of only generally related subject matter.

These would include research articles in sociology, social psychology, or marketing on subjects like choosing ideal spokespeople, segmenting markets by lifestyle, increasing self-efficacy, and so on. This source is the most problematic because it is the most general. Managers would need to have some rational basis that would allow projection of such data to the immediate context. For example, a manager might decide to assume, based on research done by cultural anthropologists, that female spokespeople will be highly effective for child health messages in egalitarian societies but should never be used in strongly patriarchal societies. Or, based on a study of cognitive processing in other cultures, a manager might be willing to conclude that a village that has only just recently learned of a new desirable health practice will need educational information whereas another, more advanced village will need how-to information (Rogers, 1962, 1983; Robertson, 1967).

Qualitative Formative Research

Quantitative research is valuable in providing broad, projectable parameters for a social marketing program. The difficulty is that the portrait of the market it offers is relatively shallow. Qualitative techniques, on the other hand, can provide significantly more depth. They allow marketers to get "up close and personal" with the target audience to learn what they are really like, what they are thinking, what worries them, what turns them on, who they listen to, what words they normally use in talking about the behavioral topic, and so on. There are three broad types of qualitative research used in social marketing to gain this information:

- Ethnographic studies
- Depth interviews
- Focus groups

Ethnographic Research

Ethnographic research can provide the deepest penetration into the potential market (Coreil and Mull, 1988). As an anthropological discipline, its broadest objective is to understand a total culture (Good, 1987; Eisenberg, 1977; Brokenshaw, MacQueen, and

Stess, 1988). Typically, it involves extensive immersion in the target market by a researcher or team of researchers and careful recording of behaviors, social relationships, status patterns, norms, taboos, language, and so on. It can be nonparticipant or participant. *Nonparticipant observation* requires that the researcher remain invisible as much as possible to avoid influencing the behavior under observation. It typically takes a very long time because it requires that the local culture accept and eventually ignore the observer.

Participant observation is the opposite—and the approach most often used in social marketing. Indeed, in social marketing, there is now considerable interest in developing what is called *rapid ethnography*—that is, ethnographic conclusions based on participant research that goes into a culture intending to observe it and come out with useful insights in a relatively short period of time. Participant observation makes no pretense of anonymity. The researcher will ask questions of individuals, groups, and key informants, and will record observations on the spot, often in a relatively formal way.

In rapid ethnographic studies, the immersion, observation, and questioning are not random (although the trained anthropologist is always looking for the serendipitous insight). The research goal is clearly stated and the process typically moves more or less in a linear pathway. An ethnomedical ORT study in Nigeria and Zaire (Yoder, Oke, and Yanka, 1993) provides a useful example of how the process works.

Project managers wanted to understand how ethnic groups in these countries classified illnesses, diagnoses, and possible causes and treatments, that is, to find out what the community "knew" about disease. The following principles guided the collection and analysis of the data:

- Interview small groups of individuals.
- Follow a progression of questions—going from the general to the specific.
- Select certain illnesses for more detailed questioning on symptoms, causes, and treatments.
- Organize data on the illnesses of greatest interest into analytic tables.

- Compare the responses of different groups to each illness.
- Write an interpretation of the daily results estimating the degree to which specific knowledge about illnesses is shared.

Groups of mothers were selected to be relatively homogeneous with respect to age, social status, and language. The researchers noted that, "Asking questions of three or four people simultaneously guaranteed discussion among all the participants. An interview of approximately 45 minutes was sufficient to obtain a solid amount of information. In this way, one researcher could interview four or five groups every day, and up to 40 groups (possibly from several villages) in ten days" (Yoder, Oke, and Yanka, 1993, p. 18).

The research revealed a number of differences in illness categories and treatments that affected program communications strategies. In both countries, researchers could identify the terms mothers used to label specific conditions associated with dehydration and diarrhea for use in messages. They also learned the nature of alternative native treatments for conditions like dysentery and general diarrhea. In Nigeria, they found differences in classifications between groups speaking Nupe and groups speaking Hausa. For example, it turned out that Hausa lacked a term for the symptoms of dehydration, which meant that the eventual Hausa communications strategy would need to start by creating a way to talk about the problem. For the groups speaking Nupe, on the other hand, the communications strategy could go straight to treatment issues.

In Zaire, six distinct illnesses were characterized by loose and frequent stools. As the researchers note: "Thus, a prevalence [meaning KAPB] survey in Swahili that had asked only about the biomedical equivalent of diarrhea (maladi ya kuhara) would have missed important information. It would have missed one half of the illnesses related to diarrhea" (Yoder, Oke, and Yanka, 1993, p. 21). Once the six disease names were identified, subsequent print messages and face-to-face interventions could then be designed to focus on all the primary illnesses, as could training sessions for health workers. Results from the Zaire rapid-ethnography study also contributed to the wording of a later quantitative KAPB study in the country.

Depth Interviews

When a project wishes to study individuals rather than cultures in depth, this can be carried out individually or in groups. Individual depth interviews are of two types:

In-Home Depth Interviews. These are face-to-face interviews conducted in privacy. They are particularly useful for subjects where one seeks information on the sensitive topics that social marketing often involves. Among the latter would be family planning (especially in developing countries), AIDS (especially among gay and bisexual men), drug and alcohol abuse, obesity, and breast health.

Out-of-Home Depth Interviews. These often take the form of street or market intercepts or workplace interviews. They are particularly useful for subjects that are in some way related to the site of the interview. This would include studies of AIDS among sex workers in brothels or among gay men in bars, studies of childhood health care among parents visiting hospitals or clinics, and studies of the use of contraceptives and other pharmaceuticals among people intercepted in front of retail outlets.

Focus Groups

Focus groups are, in some sense, depth interviews conducted in groups. The technique has extremely wide use in commercial sector marketing. It is used for:

- Formative research on needs, wants and perceptions
- Development of questionnaires
- Pretesting of product or service concepts
- Pretesting of communications themes
- Pretesting of message executions
- Assessment of customer satisfactions and dissatisfactions

The focus group approach has two major virtues. First, it is relatively inexpensive because the researcher interviews several people at once. In addition, the resulting data are even richer than data from one-on-one in-depth studies. The reason for the latter is inherent in the focus group format. Focus groups are typically made up of six to ten individuals who are relatively homogeneous in standard demographics and lifestyles and who are unknown to each other before they are recruited for the session. The session is held in a relatively natural setting such as a simulated kitchen or living room and takes an hour and a half to two hours. During the session, a trained moderator guides the discussion but leaves the talk among the participants unfettered and free to flow. The advantages of this approach are:

- *Synergism.* Because each group member can respond to, elaborate on, criticize, modify, or otherwise react to the comments of other group members, focus groups can significantly increase the total volume of information gleaned over what would be the sum of six to ten individual interviews.
- *Minimal interviewer effects.* Although the moderator will act to stimulate the group at times or to move the discussion in a particular direction (that is, to focus it), participants will most often be responding to the remarks of others like themselves. For this reason and because focus group members are usually actively caught up in the discussion, respondents are less likely to try to guess the purpose of the study or try to please or impress the moderator. The process will be less intrusive.
- *Increased spontaneity.* In an individual interview situation, the respondent has to pay attention and answer all questions. In a group situation, participants usually feel they needn't speak if they don't want to. The lack of pressure tends to make respondents feel less uptight and more spontaneous and enthusiastic in their participation.
- *Serendipity.* Because there are several interviewees in the group, many more questions, perspectives, and comments may be introduced than the researcher or moderator would ever have thought of alone.
- *Higher quality interviewing.* Because several people are interviewed at once, the research organization can afford a more expensive interviewer than they could if hour-long interviews had to be conducted one by one.
- *Natural setting.* A one-on-one interview situation is usually highly artificial. In a focus group, one can create an atmosphere of a bunch of people sitting around chatting about a product, service, or social problem, or a set of advertisements. This will seem to participants very much like the real world. Their comments and

reactions therefore will have much more projectability to that real world.

Guidelines developed by Mary Debus of Porter/Novelli for choosing between focus groups and depth interviews are presented in Exhibit 3.1 and suggestions for soliciting focus group responses are presented in Exhibit 3.2.

Here are some guidelines for effective groups:

Keep the group size from six to ten. Groups smaller than six tend not to generate enough data and run the risk of being dominated by one or two individuals. Groups larger than ten are likely to find some members bored or frustrated because they do not have enough time to talk.

Make the atmosphere as nonthreatening and natural as possible. Pick a setting that will suggest the sort of place where the group members would normally gather to talk—without regard to what the interviewer will find most comfortable.

Hire the very best moderator the budget can afford. The moderator must be able to guide the discussion without seeming to do so, catching subtle points and hidden meanings and bringing them out through elaboration. A good moderator will draw out shy or inhibited participants, and be able to quiet or distract those who wish to dominate the group. A good leader will encourage participants not to criticize the thoughts of others but to react to them. Participants should learn to talk to each other and not to the moderator. Finally, the moderator is the one who must summarize the major findings of the focus groups after the last session ends.

If possible, tape record or videotape each session. This allows the moderator to focus on group dynamics rather than on note taking. It also permits multiple reviewers to interpret the session results.

Have clear objectives for each session and a hidden agenda of topic sequences. It is typical in focus groups to begin the discussion generally (with a universal interest like male-female relationships) and then gradually narrow the topic to the researcher's specific interest (such as use of condoms in specific encounters). It is this approach that led to the term *focus* group.

Conduct multiple groups wherever possible. Make sure that all the major demographic groups in the eventual target audience are included. Replication allows researchers some insight into the

Exhibit 3.1. Which to Use: Focus Groups or Individual Depth Interviews?

Issue to consider	Use focus groups when . . .	Use individual depth interviews when . . .
Group interaction	interaction of respondents may stimulate a richer response or new and valuable thoughts.	group interaction is likely to be limited or nonproductive.
Group/peer pressure	group/peer pressure will be valuable in challenging the thinking of respondents and illuminating conflicting opinions.	group/peer pressure would inhibit responses and cloud the meaning of results.
Sensitivity of subject matter	subject matter is not so sensitive that respondents will temper responses or withhold information.	subject matter is so sensitive that respondents would be unwilling to talk openly in a group.
Depth of individual responses	the topic is such that most respondents can say all that is relevant or all that they know in less than ten minutes.	the topic is such that a greater depth of response per individual is desirable, as with complex subject matter and very knowledgeable respondents.
Interviewer fatigue	it is desirable to have one interviewer conduct the research; several groups will not create interviewer fatigue or boredom.	it is desirable to have numerous interviewers on the project. One interviewer would become fatigued or bored conducting the interviews.
Stimulus materials	the volume of stimulus material is not extensive.	a large amount of stimulus material must be evaluated.
Continuity of information	a single subject area is being examined in depth and strings of behaviors are less relevant.	it is necessary to understand how attitudes and behaviors link together on an individual pattern basis.
Experimentation with interview guide	enough is known to establish a meaningful topic guide.	it may be necessary to develop the interview guide by altering it after each of the initial interviews.
Observation	it is possible and desirable for key decision makers to observe "firsthand" consumer information.	"firsthand" consumer information is not critical or observation is not logistically possible.
Logistics	an acceptable number of target respondents can be assembled in one location.	respondents are geographically dispersed or not easily assembled for other reasons.
Cost and timing	quick turnaround is critical, and funds are limited.	quick turnaround is not critical, and budget will permit higher cost.

Source: Debus, n.d., p. 10. Used with permission.

Exhibit 3.2. Suggestions for Soliciting
Responses in Focus Groups.

1   *Build the relevant context information*—What are the experiences or issues that surround a product or a practice that influence how it/he/she is viewed?

2   *Top-of-mind associations*—What's the first thing that comes to mind when I say "family planning"?

3   *Constructing images*—Who are the people who buy Panther condoms? What do they look like? What are their lives about? (Or) Where are you when you buy condoms? Describe the place. What do you see? What do you feel? What do you do?

4   *Querying the meaning of the obvious*—What does "soft" mean to you? What does the phrase "it's homemade" mean to you?

5   *Establishing conceptual maps of a product category*—How would you group these different family planning methods? How do they go together for you? How are groups similar/different? What would you call these groups?

6   *Metaphors*—If this birth control pill were a flower, what kind would it be and who would pick it? If this group of products were a family, who would the different members be and how do they relate to each other?

7   *Image matching*—Here are pictures of ten different situations/people. . . . Which go with this wine and which do not? Why?

8   *"Man from the moon" routine*—I'm from the moon; I've never heard of Fritos. Describe them to me. Why would I want to try one? Convince me.

9   *Conditions that give permission and create barriers*—Tell me about two or three situations in which you would decide to buy this chocolate and two to three situations in which you would decide to buy something else.

10 *Chain of questions*—Why do you buy "X"? Why is that important? Why does that make a difference to you? Would it ever not be important? (Ask until the respondent is ready to kill the interviewer!)

11 *Benefit chain*—This cake mix has more egg whites; what's the benefit of that? (Answer: "It's moister.") What is the benefit of a moister cake? (Answer: "It tastes homemade.") And why is homemade better? (Answer: "It's more effort.") And what's the benefit of that? (Answer: "My family will appreciate it.") And? (Answer: "They will know I love them.") And? (Answer: "I'll feel better; they'll love me back.")

12 *Laddering (chains of association)*—What do you think of when you think of Maxwell House Coffee? (Answer: "Morning.") And when you think of morning, what comes to mind? (Answer: "A new day.") And when you think of a new day? (Answer: "I feel optimistic.")

13 *Pointing out contradictions*—Wait a minute, you just told me you would like it to be less greasy and now you're telling me it works because it's greasy and oily—how do you explain it?

14 *Sentence completions and extensions*—The ideal ORS product is one that ... The best thing about this new product is ... It makes me feel ...

15 *Role playing*—Okay, now you're the Chairman of the Board, or the Mayor of this city. What would you do? (Or) I'm the Mayor, talk to me, tell me what you want.

16 *Best-of-all-possible-world scenarios*—Forget about reality for a minute. If you could design your own diaper that has everything you ever wanted in a diaper and more, what would it be like? Use your imagination. There are no limits. Don't worry about whether it's possible or not.

17 *Script writing*—If you were able to tell a story or write a movie about this company or city (or whatever), what would it be about? Who are the heroines and heroes? Does the movie have a message? Would you go see it? Who would?

Source: Debus, n.d., pp. 32–33. Used with permission.

extent to which original insights are generalizable or must be modified for specific populations.

Pretesting

Even with the very best formative research, the development of marketing strategy is still necessarily a creative process. Managers work from limited information and craft products and services, delivery systems, communications messages, training programs, and the like in attempts to achieve their behavior-change goals. But there is much that can go wrong in this planning process, both major and minor. Pretesting serves three basic functions:

- Evaluate alternative strategies and tactics.
- Make sure that the chosen strategies or tactics have no obvious major deficiencies.
- Fine-tune possible approaches so that they speak to target audiences in the most effective way.

In the very best marketing organizations, the planning stage involves the preparation of a number of alternate strategies, only one of which will be used. The pretesting phase is then used to sort out the competing executions. This is sometimes a time-consuming and costly process but it avoids the fallacy of the one-best-strategy approach many organizations adopt. The latter organizations think hard about what to do, choose the action that looks best, and test it alone (or, worse still, implement it and wait for the monitoring stage—or the final evaluation—to see if it was a good choice). Preparation and testing of multiple executions makes it much more likely that seriously wrong choices—and the costs associated with them—will be avoided.

Pretesting requires that good social marketing managers once again *listen to their customers*. As before, this can be done on a one-on-one basis, in central location intercepts, depth interviews, or self-administered questionnaires. It can also be done in focus groups. In all cases, it is important to choose research subjects who represent the real target audience (which is unlikely to consist of the researcher's friends, secretaries, and passing colleagues). It is particularly important to test all the major audience segments and to test not only for positive reactions but also for negative reactions. Here, researchers are looking not only for things that might go well but also for things that might go wrong. They look for assertions that do not "ring true" for the target audience. They look for comments like "This spokesperson seems patronizing and insincere and isn't really very cool." Positive results can be comforting, but negative ones can be the most useful because they lead directly to program revisions.

As with formative research, pretests can be quantitative or qualitative. Organizations that do a lot of pretesting prefer to use at least some quantitative elements for their pretesting. They develop some type of rating system and then use it over and over again. Repeated use over time helps them develop benchmarks or norms for their tests. The desire for norms was one of the reasons that the National Cancer Institute developed the Health Message Testing Service in the late 1970s (National Cancer Institute, 1981). This service developed a specific protocol and tested a large number of social marketing ads over a period of time and developed appropriate norms and benchmarks. Each new proposed communication could then be tested against such norms and benchmarks. Marketers could then say, for example: If it does not exceed the norms by at least 20 percent on day-after recall, it is not worth spending our money on. Unfortunately, although the Health Message Testing Service was a great way of screening ads on a relatively scientific basis at relatively low cost while it lasted, it is no longer in operation. Researchers must now develop their own norms or try to adapt norms from commercial agencies and settings.

When setting quantitative benchmarks for pretesting, it is important to have clear criteria, that is, objectives that the particular product, service, message, or promotional event is supposed to achieve. The HealthCom project mentioned in the Introduction uses the following criteria in evaluating its advertising messages (Rasmuson, Seidel, Smith, and Booth, 1988, p. 55):

- Attractiveness
- Understandability
- Acceptability
- Capacity for inclining the audience to identify with the topic
- Overall persuasiveness

In addition, commercial sector advertisers look at:

- Credibility
- Personal relevance
- Originality
- Intrusiveness
- Memorability
- Interest

Many advertising professionals pretest ads by using a relatively straightforward process called *the Communications Test*. They expose audiences to new commercials or advertisements and then conduct thirty to fifty individual interviews. The interviews begin by eliciting respondents' thoughts and feelings while looking at the ad or hearing the commercial. Afterward, they are asked to recall what the advertisement said or showed and what the main messages were. In some cases, they will be asked to fill in rating scales for comparison with other executions (DDB Needham Worldwide, 1989).

Of course, pretesting is not just for advertising. A great many other elements of an integrated marketing strategy can be exposed to target customers' reactions. Packages, such as for condoms or oral rehydration ingredients, are typically subject to careful pretesting, particularly since several versions are typically considered. Other programs have investigated:

- Alternative rewards to be given to home builders who plant or save more trees (Andreasen and Tyson, 1993)
- Alternative brochures explaining the benefits of breast self-examination to young women
- Alternative fund-raising events for supporting homeless shelters
- Alternative fees for health examinations

Pretests can differ in the extent to which they are disguised or not. In an undisguised format, consumers are shown the proposed product or advertisement, or a description of a new service. They are then asked to respond either with quantitative ratings or with qualitative responses. The problem here is that the approach is relatively intrusive and subject to biases from interviewer effects or from respondents' attempts to look good or please the researcher by giving the "right" answer. Disguised pretests, on the other hand, attempt to mask the true purpose of the study and collect responses in the context of some broader set of questions. Thus subjects may be asked to view a new television show or listen to a new radio show in which is buried some social marketing commercial. In the process of asking about the entire show, the interviewer slips in questions about the commercial. This typically produces more valid measures of such things as comprehension and recall. However, interviewers cannot delve very deeply without alerting the subject to the true purpose of the study.

An Example

A good example of the use of pretesting to develop strategy was the work by HealthCom and its collaborators in the Philippines in developing radio and television commercials for a campaign to influence the way mothers treated dehydration associated with diarrhea (Hernandez, de Guzman, Cabañero-Verzosa, and Seidel, 1993).

> The process involved six separate studies before the campaigns were put on the air:
>
> 1.   *A baseline formative survey.* This revealed that mothers did not perceive dehydration to be a problem at all. There was no word in Tagalog or local dialects for dehydration. However, mothers were concerned about loose stools and did recognize behavioral signs of a weakened condition in their child. They tended to treat diarrhea very often with medication. This information led the strategists to decide to create a new "disease," dehydration, and to promote the use of an oral rehydration product, Oresol, as a medicine for its alleviation. They decided that a way had to be found to illustrate the concept graphically to the mothers.
>
> 2.   *A graphics test.* Artists developed a sequence of pictures showing successive images of child sitting on a chamber pot being drained of water and becoming weak and then being rehydrated and growing strong. The word "dehydration" was superimposed over the panel with the child in his worst stage. This

graphic was tested with three focus groups totaling twenty-eight mothers. The moderator asked mothers what the pictures showed and whether it seemed to them to be a true story. The mothers clearly could understand the concept of dehydration (and the English word) and the link to diarrhea.

3.   *A preliminary campaign plan*. It was then decided to give the two concepts of diarrhea and dehydration distinct personalities and to show their relationship to each other in radio and television commercials. The radio commercials featured two evil voices introduced as Diarrhea, a pest, and Dehydration, a traitor. They are coconspirators in attacking a baby. The announcer then explains how the water level in the baby goes down and it is weakened (as in the earlier graphic panels). Mothers are told to watch out for dehydration because it can kill. The commercial ends with the child rehydrated and a happy mother and cooing baby. A draft version of this commercial was tested with a hundred mothers intercepted for one-on-one interviews at eight locations in greater Manila. Respondents indicated how they now treated diarrhea and then listened to the new commercial three times. They were then asked open-ended questions about what the commercial was about and whether they thought it was informative, entertaining—or disgusting. The commercial was found to be believable, entertaining, and unique. It spoke to them personally, a key objective of social marketing. Comments were made about the voices and the conversations in the commercials that led to revisions. After the commercials, fewer women were planning to use antidiarrheal medicines and more were planning to use oral rehydration solutions.

4.   *An enhanced campaign plan*. The development team decided to use animation to bring the radio script to life in the television commercials. Three freelance artists produced sketches of twenty pairs of obnoxious characters. These were narrowed to three of each and shown to fifty mothers of lower socioeconomic status who had at least one child five years old or younger. Criteria to be used were apparent meanness, uniqueness, and the extent to which the characters adhered to the women's own concepts of diarrhea and dehydration. As the researchers noted, "It was important that the selected characters be memorable and distinct from one another, that they both seem dangerous, but that Dehydration seem to be the more threatening of the two.

On the other hand, neither character could seem so repulsive that a mother would not want to see it on television" (p. 73).

5.   *A refined plan.* The two winning characters were then tested informally at a Metro Manila Health Center with a group of twenty mothers who were seeking treatment for their children with diarrhea. The major objective of this test was to make sure that the Dehydration character was, in fact, meaner than the Diarrhea character—which it was.

6.   *The final ad.* The final draft of the public service ad was then tested with a hundred mothers from the target audience in one-on-one central location intercept interviews at twelve sites within greater Manila. The ads were shown twice and mothers were asked what they meant and what they liked and did not like about them. The research results led to further modifications of the ad to heighten the differences between the characters. Dehydration was given a more ominous voice and both characters had their names printed next to them. The commercial and its dialogue were also slowed to make them more comprehensible.

Cautions

It should be noted that, while pretesting is one of the most important hallmarks of modern social marketing, it is certainly not foolproof. As the National Cancer Institute noted in connection with their message testing service: "Pretesting is neither an absolute predictor nor a guarantee of success in terms of learning, persuasion, behavior change, or other measures of communication effectiveness. Pretesting in health communications is seldom designed to quantitatively measure small differences among large samples. . . . Pretesting is not a substitute for experienced judgment. Rather, it is a tool to provide direction from which sound decisions can be made" (National Cancer Institute, 1981, pp. 5–6).

They point out that pretesting of materials or concepts involving highly sensitive topics such as breast self-examination, gay sex, the use of condoms, or marital relations in particular may not yield valid or reliable results. As they note: "Respondents may become unusually rational when reacting to such pretest materials, and cover up their true concerns, feelings, and behavior. As a result,

the pretester must examine and interpret responses carefully"
(National Cancer Institute, 1981, p. 29).

Experimentation

In situations in which pretesting does not or—as in the case of sensitive topics—cannot provide the needed evaluations, marketers
can still resort to *real-world experimentation* as a device for testing
strategic approaches. This is not exactly a method of pretesting but
its function is essentially the same. Real-world experiments are different from laboratory experiments, in that the former are carried
out in natural settings where control is difficult, and the latter are
carried out in artificial settings where control is relatively easy—
but in either case experimentation is nothing more than trying
things out. It is what commercial sector marketers do when they
carry on test marketing or when they test one price in Des Moines
and another price in San Diego.

In social marketing programs, experimentation is most valuable when marketers need to know how a strategy or tactic will
work out in the complex real world. This reality check is not possible in the more artificial world of most pretesting systems. Real-
world experiments are of two kinds:

- Trials of tactics or strategies (test markets)
- Tests of alternative approaches (advertisement *A* versus advertisement *B*)

As I have noted elsewhere (Andreasen, 1988c, p. 120), experiments are relatively rare in social marketing. The principal reason, I believe, is that managers make up their minds and want to
get on with implementation. They do not want to wait for a pilot
test. Or they don't want to try something out that isn't what they
believe is their best strategy! So they just blunder ahead not knowing if they did the right thing.

Yet experimentation—particularly comparisons of alternative
strategies or tactics—is relatively quick and inexpensive. All that is
necessary is that, while the manager is planning to implement the
best approach with the bulk of the market, a separate group or
groups within it receive alternative, second-best treatments. Thus,

in developed countries, a social marketer may be planning to send out a mailer to areas known to have high gay populations with a message about a new confidential AIDS Hotline, an extremely effective service in this sensitive topic area (Helquist and Rosenbaum, 1993). The marketer has evaluated several message themes—even pretested some—and has chosen the one that looks best. However, the choice is not certain. For relatively little cost, the marketer could:

- Prepare a small set of alternative messages.
- Select a small random sample of addressees to receive the alternative message.
- Devise a way to learn which message each Hotline caller received (for example, using different Hotline numbers for each treatment).

With this approach, evaluation is a simple matter of sitting back and seeing which one works best. Such an experiment can yield extremely valuable strategic advice in a real-world setting. Think of the riches that a series of similar experiments would bring!

For further information on the intricacies of experimental research, see Campbell and Stanley, 1966, and Achenbaum, 1975.

Monitoring and Evaluation

The third stage of the strategy process during which marketers must listen to their customers is when they have begun implementation. Here, research can prove extremely valuable in finding out whether programs are on track and whether they are achieving their objectives. Monitoring and evaluation are two approaches to this task that are very similar. *Monitoring* denotes ongoing measurement of program outcomes: it is, in effect, continual evaluation. *Evaluation* typically refers to a single final assessment of a project or program, and may or may not involve comparisons to an earlier baseline study. In a sense, monitoring implies evaluation, although usually it is shallower than overall evaluations, which tend to look at multiple, global measures and relate these to levels of effort and so forth.

I will begin with what marketers are typically more interested in: monitoring.

Monitoring

Commercial sector marketers crave data. They want to know how they are doing. They want to correct things before it is too late. Too many social marketing programs with which I am familiar only carry out studies at the beginning and end of a project. These evaluations allow one to learn whether the project as it was developed was successful. They do not allow managers to make mid-course corrections that would make that development much more effective. Commercial sector marketers rarely worry about final summative evaluations; instead, they carry out focus group studies, small-scale surveys, and the like along the way to permit up-to-date measures of program effectiveness and rapid adjustments of strategy and tactics in response to market dynamics.

The major use of monitoring data is for *control.* In its ideal form, control will be a cybernetic self-correcting system that constantly looks at what is happening, diagnoses why it is happening, and takes corrective action as needed. The frequency with which the marketer checks on performance is a function of two things: uncertainty about the correctness of the chosen courses of action, and market volatility.

The major point to emphasize here is that the monitoring system should be based on measures closely related to program goals. The tendency in many organizations is to measure what can be measured. Thus, social marketers may be tempted to keep track of how well they are doing by looking at the number of brochures distributed, the number of advertisements run, the number of people attending various events, or the extent of distribution of the products involved in the behavior. The difficulty with this approach is that the data may or may not bear any relation to the program's objectives and goals. For example, large numbers of distributed but unread brochures accumulated by illiterate audience members should not be taken as a sign that the program is on target. Nor should television advertisements run at late-night hours with little or no audience.

Given social marketing's bottom line, the best monitoring systems are those that measure actual behavior or some close approximation to it. A good example is product usage. In social marketing programs involving products such as condoms or ORS packets, there are many measures one could use, varying in the degree to which they reflect actual correct usage (the ultimate goal). Among the possibilities—ordered in increasing distance from actual usage—are:

1. *Direct observation of usage.* This is probably only possible in ethnographic studies, which are costly and difficult to quantify.
2. *Self-reports of usage.* This is likely to be subject to forgetting and attempts to give self-protective or self-aggrandizing answers.
3. *Actual sales in retail outlets plus free distribution in public programs.*
4. *Changes in inventories at the retail level* (Andreasen, 1988a).
5. *Retailer estimates of actual sales.*
6. *Shipments to retailers and public health clinics from central storage areas.*

Periodic self-reports would probably be the best measure here. However, this is costly—especially if the social marketer attempts to carry out a large, scientific survey. Given the need to conserve costs, a more sensible approach would be to develop a simple, although biased, methodology for checking out a population's behavior—and then repeat this biased measure regularly. For example, one could measure ORT or contraception use by going to the same ten health clinics once a month (on randomly assigned days) and interviewing every third mother in the waiting room about her ORT or contraception practices. Although each monthly survey has a bias, it is reasonable to assume that the bias will stay constant from month to month and one will thus observe real changes. Good practical researchers know that bias isn't always bad!

Customer Satisfaction Measures

Customer satisfaction surveys are a particularly valuable monitoring approach for social marketing programs involving services (Andreasen, 1982). These are formal or informal interviews with people who have used a program service. Customers can be asked such questions as: How satisfied were you with the service? Did it meet your expectations? In what ways could it be better? Such questions could be asked for the program overall and for specific program elements. Attempts should be made to secure honest answers to these questions by asking questions away from any facilities or staff people and, if possible, having an independent research group (such as college students) do the interviews.

Satisfactions data can be very valuable in several ways:

• *They can provide early warning if things are going wrong in some aspect of a program.* For example, suppose a particular weight-loss or smoking clinic has hired some staff who are not very customer centered. If no interim satisfaction measures are obtained, management would only discover the problem when the drop-out rate increases for the problem clinic. The problem might show up in a decline in the number of new enrollees. However, a program can coast for a time on past successes and general reputation before the word about a particular bad unit gets around. The virtue of satisfactions data is that they alert management to the problem right away so that corrective action can be taken before the problem becomes really serious.

• *They can provide a basis for comparison.* It can be very useful to see how various delivery sites (clinics or whatever) stack up against each other, or to track the relative effectiveness of various aspects of a particular delivery site (for example, the reception staff versus the trainers).

• *They can see whether customers know what to expect from the service.* Expectations questions can alert management to a problem of raising expectations too high, as well as showing areas where realistic expectations are not being met.

• *They can reveal trends.* If carried out over time, data on consumer expectations and satisfactions can alert management to changes in the market, in competition, or in clientele. For example, management would have clear indications of the need for program changes if people begin to say:

"This program is not as good as your new competitor my friends went to."

"People who have been here before said that they were pleased at the group sessions, but I want individual treatment and you are not very good at that."

"You don't seem to have many Hispanics like me here. Many of my friends would like to come to such a place."

• *A mechanism can be established for correcting specific problems if that is appropriate.* For example, if an independent surveyor had a smoking clinic participant complain about the lack of individual attention, with permission, the participant's name could be passed to management who could offer the individual free entry into a program at another site with more individualized attention. (Remember that a clearly voiced concern about meeting the customer's needs will always pay off. Just think of how many of her friends the smoker will tell of the extraordinary interest of the clinic management in meeting customer needs. The payoff in favorable word-of-mouth advertising and potential future enrollees is worth any short-term losses.)

Despite their advantages, raw satisfactions data need careful analysis. In particular, the marketing manager needs to remember that customers tend to underreport problems where customers they think they are partly to blame. Self-attributions of blame can be a particular problem in cultures or in programs where staff members are higher status than their clients. In such cases, surly staff members may also excel at making clients feel that any problems are their fault. Status problems can be overcome to some extent by training peers of respondents as interviewers. Problems with respondents censoring episodes for which they might be to blame can also be overcome by simply asking for reports of experiences that were unsatisfactory for whatever reason.

One useful approach is to ask consumers how the organization performed on key consequences and how important these consequences were to them. A simple 1 (very dissatisfied) to 10 (very satisfied) scale is generally easy for both customers and staff to relate to. The resulting scaled ratings allow management to compare program elements and make judgments about what needs to be done—the central role of feedback. Table 3.1 reports the ratings received by a hypothetical weight-loss program.

The next step is to take these data and plot them in a two-dimensional graph like Figure 3.1. Here we see that there are four quadrants, each with its own implications for different managerial action.

The four quadrants are as follows:

Quadrant A: Concentrate here. These are cases where conse-

Table 3.1. Performance and Importance Ratings for a Hypothetical Weight-Loss Program.

Consequence	Performance rating	Importance rating
Staff is friendly	8.44	9.41
Other participants are like me	4.29	8.87
I get a lot of individual attention	4.16	7.26
I am not embarrassed	5.78	8.47
I can hear other people's problems	8.56	3.19
The results are fast in coming	4.39	4.30
I learn a lot about my problem	6.69	4.26
I get to practice cooking healthy food	3.93	6.77
Getting to meetings takes little time and effort	2.44	6.32
My family gets help also	1.52	3.38

quences are important to customers but where program performance is below average. In Table 3.1, participants are dissatisfied with four consequences each suggesting program implications. Management should consider:

- Making groups more homogeneous (more "participants are like me")
- Increasing the amount of individual attention
- Increasing the training in food preparation skills
- Holding programs in more locations nearer to customers

Quadrant B: Keep up the good work. These are cases where consequences are important to customers and where program performance is above average. These are clearly features about which the program can brag. In the example, they can brag about the friendliness of the staff and the fact that efforts are made not to embarrass the individual.

Quadrant C: Low priority. These are cases of consequences that are not important to customers but where program performance is below average. In these cases, managers must resist the tempta-

Figure 3.1. Performance/Importance Matrix.

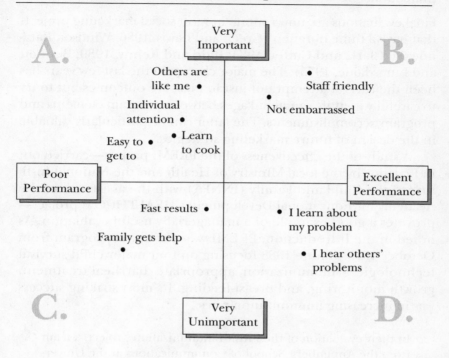

tion to put resources into these consequences because the manager notices a deficiency. The example suggests that, although the manager may be concerned that the weight program takes too long and does not involve family members (who may be part of the problem), these features are apparently not important to customers.

Quadrant D: Possible overkill. These are cases of consequences that are not important to customers but where program performance is above average. These may be aspects of the program that can be deemphasized with a possible saving in program costs. The participants represented in Table 3.1 are saying that they do not particularly appreciate the efforts the program makes to help them understand their own problems or to hear the problems of others. They may well be saying that they need to know more about what to do and not so much about why to do it.

Evaluations

Final evaluations are now routine in most social marketing projects that have a finite duration (Green and Lewis, 1986; Windsor, Baranowski, Clark, and Cutter, 1984; Judd and Kenny, 1980; Bennett and Lumsdaine, 1975). The major change in the last few years has been the careful attempt not just to measure outcomes but to try to carefully identify causal linkages between program elements and program accomplishments. The latter can be particularly valuable in the design of future marketing strategies.

A study of the effectiveness of the PREMI project—carried out in Ecuador by the local Ministry of Health and the National Institute of the Child and Family (INNFA) with the assistance of the Academy for Educational Development's HEALTHCOM project— provides a good example of a managerially useful evaluation. As noted in the Introduction, PREMI was a national program from October 1985 to June 1988 focusing on four major child survival technologies—immunization, appropriate diarrheal treatment, growth monitoring, and breast-feeding. Its most striking success was in increasing immunization rates.

In their evaluation of the PREMI immunization project, a team from the Annenberg School of Communications at the University of Pennsylvania (Hornik and others, 1991) sought answers to three questions:

- Did the PREMI program affect immunization rates?
- Were the effects equitably distributed across the socioeconomic spectrum?
- What was the process through which PREMI's communication activities affected vaccination behavior?

The major source of data for these evaluations was a series of KAP (knowledge, attitudes, practices) studies carried out before and during the latter stages of the project. The answer to the first question was clearly yes. The dramatic increases in immunization rates have been described in detail in the Introduction; here, it is sufficient to say that overall immunization rates for children over the age of twenty-seven months came close to 90 percent by the end of the program.

The approach to assessing cause-and-effect relationships was much more difficult since the project was not designed with careful controls and random assignment of population groups to different treatments. As a result, the researchers proceeded by specifying what they thought would be true if certain causal relations did exist, and then seeing if the evidence was consistent with these specifications. Two hypotheses were explored consistent with the development in this book:

• *The individual change hypothesis.* Here, the expectation was that program communications would inform community members of the benefits of vaccinations, explain to them at what age they should be completed, and show them where to go to get them.

• *The community effects hypothesis.* Here, there were two possibilities. One was a two-step flow hypothesis that proposes that a small number of members of the community were the primary sources of information for others not exposed to the PREMI program. The other was that there was a demonstration effect. That is, some members of the community changed their vaccination behavior, and others observed this behavior and copied it either because they wanted to be like the earlier adopters or because they now felt that there was social pressure to do so.

To test the first hypothesis, the evaluation team looked at three questions:

• Was there substantial exposure to PREMI's marketing communications?
• Did this exposure lead to knowledge about proper vaccination behavior?
• Did this knowledge lead to individual vaccination practice?

The answer to all three questions appeared to be yes. First, there was clearly exposure to the PREMI program. As discussed in the Introduction, PREMI focused its marketing activities primarily on seven sets of vaccination days or *jornadas*. After the first jornada, awareness of PREMI was about 30 percent. After two more jornadas, awareness was at 65 percent. Radio and television were the primary sources of knowledge about the program. Second, knowledge of when to begin vaccinations clearly increased over the course of the program (although there was little change in ability to name some needed type of vaccination). Further, cross-sectional analyses showed clear (bi-variate) associations between exposure to radio or television health messages and vaccination knowledge (on a seventeen-item index), even when education, wealth, and general media exposure was controlled. That is, the higher the radio or television exposure, the higher the vaccination knowledge. Finally, a somewhat more sophisticated analytic approach called path analysis of cross-sectional data showed a clear link between exposure to messages and to vaccination practice operating through vaccination knowledge. However, the overall level of explanation was relatively low (8 percent of the variance in age-adjusted vaccination level measures).

The evaluation of the hypothesis about community-level effects required stronger inferences from cross-sectional data but, again, suggested that a relationship may be present. The researchers found that among those who had low personal knowledge of vaccinations, living in a community where others had high knowledge levels increased practice rates. For people with high personal knowledge, no effect was shown. A path analysis that added community knowledge to the previously mentioned individual analysis added substantially to the model's predictive power. In addition, community vaccination level was the single strongest predictor in the model. Unfortunately, the researchers could not detect from the data any relationships between PREMI program activities and community behavior.

This level of evaluation contributes to proving the effectiveness of social marketing programs and demonstrating how they appear to work so that other social marketers can build on this experience in future. Unfortunately, many summative evaluations are carried out and reported long after they can be of any use to program officers.

Quality of Completed Research

Research results are always subject to a variety of interpretations. Throughout the social marketing process, whenever management is faced with completed research to be used for strategic purposes, careful assessment of the soundness of the assumptions and conclusions in the data is critical. Managers need to ask the following questions:

1. *How valid are the measures used in the study?* Did specific questions capture the traits to be used for strategic purposes? Is the relationship found in the study to be relied upon?

2. *How reliable are the measures?* Would one get the same results if the same procedure was used over and over again? For example, was the sampling procedure objective? Were interviewers allowed to pick respondents who were easy to interview? If the latter was the case, is it not reasonable to assume that a new group of interviewers would generate a different set of results?

3. *How generalizable are the measures?* Can results for population X (say, four cities and five villages regarded as "typical") be projected to other cities and villages, or to farm residents?

4. *If the study is supposed to offer explanations, what is the level of explanation achieved?* There are three possibilities:

- *Association.* The study shows that trait A is associated with response trait R or media behavior Y. For example, an association study could reveal that women with no children rarely have been to a health clinic for a personal health checkup while women with one or more children frequently have. One might be tempted to conclude that having children leads to personal clinic use. But these data do not prove this. It might be that women with children are just older and need more personal care, so that age rather than presence of children is the "cause."

- *Causation.* The study shows that trait A leads to response R. For example, the causal study could reveal that women reported that their first visit for their own health care at the clinic was almost always soon after the birth of their first child and seldom before. One could conclude that the birth of a child leads to clinic visits. However, one still does not know why this happens.

- *Explanation.* The study shows that trait A leads to response R for Q reasons. Here, for example, an explanatory study could reveal that new mothers very often reported that they went for a personal checkup because prenatal visits convinced them that the staff was competent and caring.

It is too often the case that managers overvalue the level of explanation in secondary (and primary) sources. They may believe that they have insight into causation and explanation where really all they have is an indication of association. This associational information may be adequate for such decisions as to whether to allocate more resources to one village or another. It is usually not adequate for a determination of different message strategies for the two villages.

Associational results are problematic for a second reason. It is often the case that strong associations merely mask another and more central causative relationship. For example, when evaluating the PREMI program in Ecuador, Hornik and his colleagues (Hornik and others, 1991) found community to be strongly associated with vaccination behavior. But when they attempted to explain this finding, they were forced to conclude: "The appropriate inference was that there existed communities that are more or less advantaged in many ways—in wealth and education, but also in access to mass media (and the messages broadcast on those media) and in knowledge of vaccinations. . . . There appeared to be substantial evidence that community influences on individual behavior were powerful, more powerful than any individual influence. However, we were unable to sort out the influences on the overall community behavior" (Hornik and others, 1991, p. 58).

In a similar example, McDivitt and McDowell (1991, p. 39) found that the age of a child was negatively related to Vitamin A coverage. However, they speculated that this is because health posts were the major source for Vitamin A, and health posts "function primarily as weighing and immunization posts for children under two years old." Older children appeared not to get Vitamin A because they did not go to clinics.

Similarly, in many studies, it is very difficult to understand the effects of media exposure on response behavior because of possible confounding with wealth. For example, Hornik and others (1991, p.47) found that television watching was a function of wealth and the ability to acquire a TV set, while radio listenership was not.

There is also the possibility that causal relationships may have their causation reversed. Again, Hornik and his colleagues note that, although they attempted to infer that exposure to health messages affected behavior, they must ask: "Is it possible that people who know more about vaccination are more likely to remember having heard health messages on radio and television rather than actually having a higher level of exposure to those messages?" (Hornik and others, 1991, p. 45).

Summary

Customer-driven strategies are the hallmark of good social marketing. Attention to customers, in turn, means being able to collect information about them before, during, and after the development of social marketing campaigns. Social marketing research is basically of three types: formative research (done to assist the preliminary design of programs and campaigns), pretesting, and monitoring and evaluation. In each case, social marketers are very careful to minimize research costs and, above all, to make the research useful.

Useful research means, first of all, research that helps managers make decisions. Research that merely satiates curiosity, discovers something interesting but not action oriented, is biased, is carried out to protect managers politically, or is unlikely to change a preordained decision is wasteful of the social marketer's extremely limited resources. Designing research projects backward from the decisions that have to be made is a good way to ensure that research outcomes are useful.

Formative research is of two broad types, quantitative and qualitative. Quantitative research helps managers make decisions about targeting, behavior-change strategies, and resource allocation. Because they are quantitative and typically follow accepted sampling procedures, such studies can provide projectable results whose sampling errors can be stated. Quantitative data can also be subjected to a number of statistical tests that allow one to assess associations and apparent causation. Quantitative research studies, however, can be very expensive. When expense becomes prohibitive, social marketers can save costs by reducing the quantity or quality of the data or by using secondary sources.

Although useful for many purposes, quantitative research is often relatively shallow and artificial. A richer understanding of target customers is often possible with qualitative research, which involves getting "up close and personal" with them. Among the most common qualitative techniques are ethnography, depth studies, and focus groups.

Pretesting research is very valuable in helping marketers choose among alternative executions of various strategy elements (packages, advertisements, brochures, prices) and in picking up potential problems with chosen executions. Pretesting also can be both quantitative and qualitative. One approach that combines both pretesting and monitoring is experimentation. In experimental designs, different sets of target audience members are exposed to different executions and some response measure helps managers choose among them.

Social programs often wait and conduct final evaluations of projects, but social marketers rely much more on ongoing monitoring research to get early warnings about successes and failures. Monitoring tells managers what is going right, so it can be built upon—and what is going wrong, while there is time to stop or change it. The best monitoring systems measure actual behavioral outcomes. Other indirect approaches look at such things as consumer satisfaction. Consumer satisfaction data can be analyzed along with data on the importance to consumers of various outcomes in ways that can help managers decide which approaches to keep up, change, ignore, or reduce.

Post-project evaluations are often much more detailed than monitoring studies. They can be designed to yield careful explanations of cause-and-effect relationships that are impossible to study with briefer on-the-run monitoring studies. Such evaluations can help deepen marketers' knowledge for their next interventions.

Chapter Four

Understanding How Customer Behavior Changes

Behavior change is the bottom line for social marketing programs—this cannot be said too often. It follows that target consumers hold the key to success for any social marketing program or campaign—they are the only ones who can actually change their behavior. Whether the target consumer is a mother with a sickly child, an obstructionist health care worker, an important government official, or a major media figure, the social marketer must understand where the target consumer is coming from and what can and should be done to bring about desired change. In simple cases, this may mean understanding the consumers' mood or preoccupations. In more complex cases, it will mean understanding their perceptions, knowledge, attitudes, and predispositions. In still other cases, it may involve understanding how environments affect their behavior.

The very best social marketers appreciate the crucial importance of understanding consumers. As a consequence, they develop over their careers serviceable frameworks—or *models*—for understanding consumer behavior (see for example, Fisher and Fisher, 1992; Maibach and Cotton, 1995). These models are a combination of their personal experiences and things they have learned more formally from seminars, from consultants, or from the popular and academic research literature. The more experienced the marketer, the more sophisticated and complex the framework.

The purpose of this chapter is to jump-start the development process for beginning social marketers by presenting a framework for understanding consumers that has served well in a wide range of settings. The framework is heavily influenced by a wide reading of the behavior-change literature in marketing, anthropology, psychology, and economics. Scholars and others who have studied consumers in social marketing settings will recognize contributions from leading social scientists like Martin Fishbein, Itzak Ajzen, Everett Rogers, William McGuire, Albert Bandura, Irwin Rosenstock, and James Prochaska—among many others. The framework is also based on considerable field experience, talking "up close and personal" with target consumers, and with a wide range of social marketing experts whose opinions and perspectives I value. The interplay between scholarship and field experience is reflected throughout. (For related approaches, see Maibach and Cotton, 1995; Baranowski, 1992–93; Baranowski and Jenkins, 1989–90.)

I begin by putting some limits on the type of behavior we will be considering.

High- and Low-Involvement Decisions

Private sector marketers make a distinction between consumer decisions that are high and low involvement (Celsi and Olson, 1988; Laurent and Kapferer, 1985). Low-involvement decisions are those that are not very important. Consumers do not think about them very much. They do not consider very many alternatives, often only one. They do not gather much information before making their choices. And they have few regrets (or even thoughts) after they have chosen. Examples of low-involvement decisions would be choices of most convenience items, fast food restaurants, movies, and what pair of socks to wear today. Petty, Cacioppo, and Schumann (1983) have noted that low-involvement decisions are evaluated without central cognitive processing and, as a consequence, very often can be influenced by relatively minor environmental factors such as package design, commercial jingles, availability, or chance comments by friends.

The behavior that social marketers typically must influence involves choices that are just the opposite, what marketers refer to as high-involvement decisions (Celsi and Olson, 1988). High-involvement decisions are those that are very important. Consumers collect a good deal of information, think about the decision at some length, and are often emotionally involved in the choice. The decision process goes by what Petty, Cacioppo, and Schumann call the *central route* and is often complex and time-consuming. In the private sector, high-involvement decisions include decisions to buy a car, take a vacation, or choose furniture. In social marketing, they would include behaviors such as practicing safe sex or birth control, getting a child vaccinated, influencing a friend or child to stop using drugs, or volunteering time to an important cause. As might be expected, bringing about changes in these behaviors can be very difficult and time-consuming. In this chapter, we will only be considering high-involvement consumer behaviors.

Overview of the Model

As I suggested in the previous chapter, one of the best ways for social marketers to get an insight into the behavior they are trying to influence is to venture into the field and listen to consumers talk about the proposed behavior. A number of such discussions will inevitably reveal six important insights. These insights form the core of the framework for understanding—or model—presented in this chapter. The insights are:

- *Stages.* Consumers do not undertake high-involvement behaviors rapidly and in one step. They move toward the desired outcome in definable stages.
- *Consequences.* People make decisions on the basis of the consequences they believe will follow from their choices.
- *Tradeoffs.* Consequences are both positive and negative and so consumers are faced with tradeoffs between expected costs and expected benefits.
- *Other Influences.* Besides perceived consequences, behaviors are also affected by:
    Customer belief about what they think significant others want them to do
    Customer confidence in their ability to actually carry out the behavior
- *Segmentation.* Consumers vary greatly in their beliefs about

costs and benefits and in the importance of those beliefs to them—as well as in the influence that significant others and self-efficacy play in their decisions. However, consumers usually can be grouped in managerially useful ways.

* *Competition.* Competition as it is perceived by the consumer is not always what the social marketer thinks it is.

I will discuss each of these insights in succeeding sections and in the next chapter.

Behavior Comes About in Stages

The first feature to understand about high-involvement behaviors is that consumers typically do not undertake them instantaneously. They work their way up to them gradually, often going through some clearly definable stages (Maibach and Cotton, 1995). This insight has been around in private sector marketing for a very long time. In 1978, William McGuire proposed a stage concept to explain the challenges advertising faced in trying to get someone to prefer a product or brand. He suggested that consumers go through six stages: exposure to a message, attention, understanding, persuasion, retention, and behavior (McGuire, 1976). Others inside and outside the field of communications (such as Lavidge and Steiner, 1961) have proposed similar models with similar stages. However, the hierarchy notion was mainly limited to communications effects, the ways a message led to a behavior. Such a focus is too narrow for marketing, where the range of tools is much broader than communication.

A second stage model frequently used in marketing is Everett Rogers' innovation adoption process model. As adapted by Wilkie (1990, pp. 360–361), the model proposes seven stages: unawareness, awareness, knowledge, liking, trial, use evaluation, adoption. In recent writings, Rogers would add an eighth stage: maintenance.

The most useful model for social marketing applications is a stage conceptualization developed by Prochaska and DiClemente. Beginning in 1983, Prochaska and DiClemente laid out an approach they labeled a Transtheoretical Model as an "integrative and comprehensive model of behavior change" (Prochaska and DiClemente, 1983, 1984a, 1984b, 1985, 1986). Prochaska and Di-

Clemente suggest that consumers move through five stages as they go from ignorance or indifference toward some important behavior to becoming committed to it. They label their five stages as follows (see Table 4.1, Column 1):

- *Precontemplation:* Consumers really are not thinking about the behavior as being appropriate for them at this point in their lives.
- *Contemplation:* Consumers are actually thinking about and evaluating recommended behaviors.
- *Preparation:* Consumers have decided to act and are trying to put in place whatever is needed to carry out the behavior.
- *Action:* Consumers are doing the behavior for the first time— or first several times.
- *Confirmation:* Consumers are committed to the behavior and have no desire or intention to return to earlier behavior.

There are three features of this model that are significant from a social marketing standpoint. First, Prochaska and DiClemente were able to show that it is possible to separate target consumers into these five stages by asking them a relatively few simple questions. Second, they found that the appropriate type of intervention strategy for each consumer depended on the stage where the individual was at the time. For example, they found that it was important to emphasize benefits in early stages and emphasize costs in later stages—a point we shall return to shortly. Finally, they emphasized that a social marketer's goal with respect to a given consumer should not be to get all the way to the Confirmation Stage in one step. Rather, a marketer's goal should be to move the consumer to the next stage. Only through a series of steps will any consumer reach the social marketer's goal of permanent behavior change.

The Transtheoretical Model has undergone considerable field testing. Since 1983, Prochaska and his colleagues have validated the model as useful for changing twelve types of behavior, all of which are relevant to social marketers:

Quitting smoking
Quitting cocaine

Controlling weight

Reducing fat in the diet

Reducing adolescent delinquent behavior

Practicing safer sex

Choosing condoms

Reducing sun exposure

Reducing radon exposure

Increasing activity and exercise by sedentary individuals

Increasing mammography screening

Increasing physicians' antismoking activities

Prochaska and DiClemente's intervention studies were carried out on a wide range of populations including smokers, students, women over forty, delinquent adolescents, work site employees, and family practice physicians. Their results were remarkably consistent, especially given the degree to which the behaviors they tracked differed on six dimensions of importance to social marketers:

- Acquisition versus cessation (that is behaviors requiring starting something and those requiring stopping something)
- Addictive versus nonaddictive
- Frequent versus infrequent
- Legal versus illegal
- Public versus private
- Socially acceptable versus socially unacceptable

Other researchers and scholars interested in social marketing have proposed more elaborate stage models. For example, in the 1980s, I suggested eleven stages through which a target consumer for a family planning program might go from complete ignorance about reproduction through to the point where he or she is practicing family planning correctly on a routine basis (Kotler and Andreasen, 1991, pp. 551–552). These eleven steps can be grouped into five broad categories in terms of the marketing tasks that face a behavior-change specialist who needs to secure progress toward the final stage (see Table 4.1, Column 2):

- *Creating awareness and interest.* The target consumer has to be aware that there is some desirable new behavior to be undertaken and that may be appropriate to the current situation.
- *Changing values.* For behaviors that involve important changes in customs and community norms, target consumers have to come to believe that the proposed behavior is acceptable to people like them.
- *Persuading.* Once the consumer perceives that it is OK to carry out the behavior, he or she has to be convinced that it is personally desirable to do so.
- *Creating action.* It is one thing to convince a consumer to believe that a behavior is a good thing. It is another to get action. The latter may be more a matter of making the behavior easy to undertake.
- *Maintaining change.* Many behaviors that social marketers want to influence are for a lifetime. Social marketing does not stop when consumers make the first necessary step.

These five tasks can be cross-referenced to the five stages of Prochaska and DiClemente's model. Consumers who are in Prochaska and DiClemente's Precontemplation Stage are those for whom social marketers must undertake education and value change to get the process started. Consumers in the Contemplation Stage require persuasion and motivation if they are to progress. Consumers in the Preparation Stage need help with logistics of action and possibly support for their sense of behavioral control. Finally, those in the Action Stage (who have undertaken the desired behavior for the first few times) must have their changed behavior confirmed through training and reinforcement so that they will move to the final Confirmation Stage. And for each of these marketing tasks, different technologies will be paramount.

It is clear from Table 4.1 that the marketing tasks facing those who wish to bring about changes in behavior differ for each of the five broad stage categories of the Prochaska and DiClemente model. Second, the principal behavior-change technologies that one uses will also change. In order to simplify the exposition in this and succeeding chapters, I will simplify the stage structure. In effect, I have collapsed the third and fourth stages of the Prochaska and DiClemente model (Preparation and Action) into one stage.

Table 4.1. Stages in Behavior Change.

Prochaska and DiClemente's Stages	Marketing Task	Andreasen's Modified Stages
Precontemplation	Create awareness and interest	Precontemplation
	Change values	
Contemplation	Persuade; motivate	Contemplation
Preparation	Create action	Action
Action		
Confirmation	Maintain change	Maintenance

This is to align this stage more clearly with its marketing task (creating action). I have also relabeled the stages to more closely conform to the marketing tasks. The resulting four stages as seen from the consumer's perspective (as always) are:

- Precontemplation
- Contemplation
- Action
- Maintenance

These stages are outlined in the third column of Table 4.1. In a subsequent section, I will modify this framework once more to subdivide the Contemplation Stage into Early and Late stages. This is because it will be argued that the consumer's thinking differs in important ways later in the Contemplation Stage from what it was at the beginning, and that this distinction has important implications for social marketers.

Precontemplation Stage

During the Precontemplation Stage, the social marketing challenges are to make the target population aware of the new behavioral possibility and to show them that proposed behaviors are not antithetical to the values of the consumers' society and that they may improve individual audience members' own lives. Here, the appropriate technologies are the tools of education and propaganda. Major players that social marketers will need to bring to bear here will be educators, popular communications media, and various public agencies and figures. However, it should be noted that the social marketer's approach to the education and propaganda task is not always the same as that of those trained in education, propaganda, or media advocacy (Wallack, Dorfman, Jernigan, and Themba, 1993)—even health educators. There are two important differences.

Educators, propagandists, and media advocates are apt to be organization centered, while social marketers are customer centered. Educators and other communications specialists tell customers what they want them to hear. They often inundate target audiences with information that the source thinks is important and thinks audiences ought to know. By contrast, social marketers start by listening to consumers. As a consequence, they adjust their messages to what is important to the audience, in language the audience can comprehend, and through vehicles to which the audience pays attention. They do not force messages on audiences. They seek natural opportunities that fit with the audience's lifestyles. They do not overwhelm. They take account of audience misperceptions and prejudices and fears. They tell audiences what audiences want to hear.

Educators, propagandists, and media advocates tend to regard getting out the message as the important part of their job, while social marketers concentrate on changing behavior. Thus, social marketers' interest is not in telling customers everything that they could tell them or trying to change every value that could be changed. They focus on those educational and propaganda elements that are likely to influence behavior—or to move potential customers on to the next stage in the behavior-change process.

Thus, social marketers have important roles to play during the Precontemplation Stage in making sure that the necessary education and value change takes place. This will be critical in cultures where a new behavior is being introduced for the first time. It is also critical in many cultures where some segments have moved on to the Contemplation and Action Stages, but where there are important segments that are still in Precontemplation and must be addressed by a social marketing campaign with basic educational and propaganda messages to get them over that first hurdle. Throughout, social marketers have a very important role to play in bringing their customer-centered, bottom-line perspective to bear on the education and propaganda process.

Clearly, for markets at the Precontemplation Stage, the success measures that social marketers will use to monitor progress toward ultimate behavior change are measures of mental states such as knowledge, values, and attitudes. These are difficult to calibrate. However, this should not cause marketers to fall back on measures of activity (such as brochures printed, meetings held, or ads run) as proxies for their real objectives. Further, where knowledge, values, and attitudes are measured, there should be careful attention to pinpointing those mental states that are likely to lead to movement to the next stage of the process, rather than those that are only vaguely relevant and interesting.

Contemplation Stage

Although social marketers will often target consumers at the Precontemplation Stage with carefully tailored education and propaganda, their major strength is in the next two stages, Contemplation and Action. Because of their particular mindset, social marketers are especially adept at understanding how consumers make highly complex decisions and how they can be influenced to make the preferred decision and motivated to undertake the desired action. For this reason, the remainder of this book is primarily devoted to these two stages.

To be effective in these two stages, it is critical that we have a useful way of thinking about how consumers go about contemplating and taking action on highly involving behavioral choices. There are a great many models of this process in the marketing and social psychology literatures from which we could draw. Among the work that has been most influential in my own thinking on this matter have been Fishbein and Ajzen's Theory of Reasoned Action (1975; restated in Ajzen and Fishbein, 1980), Ajzen's Theory of Planned Behavior (1991), Bagozzi and Warshaw's Theory of Trying (1990), and, in the health care field, the Health Beliefs Model (Rosenstock, 1966).

A core element in all of these models is the proposition that individuals act on the basis of beliefs. Beliefs about social problems can be at the macro or micro level—for example, beliefs about the desirability of legal restriction or protection of abortion rights contrasted with beliefs leading to a personal decision about a specific pregnancy. However, a good deal of past research makes it clear that the relevant beliefs are those at the micro level that relate to the specific behavior—and the reader's own self-reflection will almost certainly confirm this. Four important sets of beliefs are important here—beliefs about the positive consequences of the behavior, about the negative consequences of the behavior, about what others expect, and about ability to carry out the action. The importance of each of these behavioral determinants will depend on the culture, the type of behavior, and the behavioral context.

Beliefs About Consequences

In a great many situations, people make decisions in large part based on how they think the behavior will turn out. To intuitively sense the reality of this, the reader need merely imagine a male friend calling with an invitation to go out for dinner and a movie on a particular Friday night. The caller is, in effect, a marketer attempting to influence your behavior.

Put yourself in this situation. What are you thinking about?

If you are typical of a great many others to whom I have posed the same hypothetical situation in the past, what is likely to go through your head are thoughts like these: It will be the end of the week, and I may be too tired to enjoy going out. . . . My friend is such a bore—but then his wife is not and she just returned from Paris and probably has great stories to tell. . . . I'm trying to diet and they always want to go to an Italian restaurant. . . . I've heard that the movie he mentioned is really good and I could use the relaxation. . . . I turned down his invitation three weeks ago, and I am reluctant to cause any hard feelings by doing it again. . . . And so on, through a whole range of self-centered cost-benefit calculations.

The important feature of this internal dialogue is that you (the target audience) are thinking through the consequences of going ahead with the proposed behavior. There is nothing unique about this. It is the way that a rural mother makes decisions about whether to follow up the suggestions of a community outreach worker that she go to the public health clinic to get her child vaccinated. She thinks to herself, if I go: It will help my child be healthier. . . . I'll have to walk five miles each way and probably wait several hours for an appointment. This will be very arduous given my poor health. . . . If I go, I will have to leave my other children behind with someone and I will not be home in time to cook dinner for my husband when he wants it. . . . I will not be able to take care of the garden in back of our living area and do the wash I do every day. . . . And so on through a series of calculations that will be instantly recognizable in form, though the specifics change according to the mother's lifestyle.

The same internal dialogue, so to speak, occurs with smokers thinking of quitting, college students contemplating using condoms in future sexual encounters, gang members considering giving up drugs, and media directors thinking about covering a public relations event. In each case, the set of factors considered—positive and negative—depends in part on the target consumer's needs and wants. Marketers know that positive and negative consequences are tied closely to deeper needs and wants—and these, in turn, are tied to still deeper values (Bush, Ortinau, and Bush, 1994; Homer and Kahle, 1988). Thus, a mother who says "It will help my child be healthier" may be reflecting an underlying need to be a good mother. This, in turn, may be linked to other needs and wants, perhaps to impress her mother-in-law, and (at a level more fundamental to basic values) to live up to an internalized principle that "the first priority for a married woman with children is to be a good mother."

Competition

But choices do not occur in a vacuum. An important point that occurs naturally to marketers—and to anyone who has taken the trouble to listen to target audiences carefully—is that decisions about behavior always have alternatives. In the private sector, these alternatives are other brands or other products and services vying for the consumer's pocketbook. In social marketing, the competition most often comes from past habits or from inertia. A marketer considering trying to persuade a teenage drug user to enter a treatment program or otherwise give up drugs must explicitly recognize that the drugs and the lifestyle that goes with them are vigorous competitors for the new alternative. The present use of drugs undoubtedly meets all sorts of personal and social needs of the target audience members.

To proceed to develop a strategy that is simply concerned with the benefits and costs of the new behavior denies the mental reality of the consumer's contemplation. In the case of drug-using teenagers, their contemplation involves both the new and the old behavior. And for the mother asked to get her child immunized, contemplation will be include alternatives such as doing chores around the house, taking care of other siblings, or meeting her husband's needs.

Social marketers need to be careful in identifying competition. In my experience, it is very often the case that marketers have read the competition all wrong. As a result, they wind up competing at one level while the target consumers are competing at another level entirely. For example, in promoting the use of condoms to the gay community, the marketer may think that the consumer sees the choice as between the pleasure and spontaneity of unprotected sex and lesser pleasure and spontaneity but greater safety of the condom (service form competition). But the target audience may see the choice as between having an active social life (without ruining encounters or relationships by mentioning condom use) and not having an active social life (generic competition). Clearly, the type of marketing that is needed in the latter case is very different from that needed in the former.

In sum, marketing a new behavior inevitably means demarketing an old one (Kotler and Levy, 1971).

Positive and Negative Consequences

Analysis of the kinds of consequences people think about divides them naturally into positive and negative. Thus, one can think of the dilemma facing consumers in high-involvement social marketing situations as having to make trade-offs between good outcomes (benefits) and not-so-good (or bad) outcomes (costs). Decisions to act then come about (other things equal—which is rare) when the customer believes—presumably, as a result of strategies and tactics the marketer has employed—that the benefits exceed the costs.

Another way to look at this phenomenon is as an exchange. This is, in fact, what many scholars see as the central paradigm of marketing (see Bagozzi, 1978). The consumer, in effect, is saying: I am going to have to give up some things (endure negative outcomes such as lost time, lost money, a decline in peace of mind) in order to get some things I value (enjoy positive outcomes such as a better life for my child, less worry for me, praise from my neighbors). This is a framework with which marketers feel quite comfortable since it applies equally well to transactions involving the exchange of money for Big Macs or Buick Regals.

Bundles of Cost-Benefit Beliefs

Private sector marketers have a further contribution to make. They suggest that what is really being exchanged is bundles of benefits for bundles of costs. In the Big Mac analogy, this means that a consumer contemplating going to McDonald's for a Big Mac instead of staying home is considering the trade-off between the following bundles of costs and benefits:

Benefits	Costs
Getting good basic nutrition	Spending $1.89
Being served quickly	Having to drive a long time
Experiencing good tastes	Feeling guilty about eating high-fat food
Having a variety of options to choose from	Having to eat off paper wrappers with plastic utensils
Having a pleasant encounter with staff	Having to get dressed

Marketers would then say that, in general, they will get more sales (that is, more behavior) if they can improve the ratio of benefits to costs in comparison to alternatives (eating at home, eating at Burger King, or eating at Chez Pierre). There are basically four ways to do this:

• *Increase the extent to which people believe they will get the benefits that they want* (for example, increase the number of dessert options)

- *Decrease the extent to which people believe they will get the costs that they would like to avoid* (for example, decrease the price or the fat content of the food)
- *Add new benefits* (such as a chance to win a prize)
- *Decrease the perceived benefits and increase the perceived costs of the likely alternative* (such as eating at home or eating at some unknown new restaurant)

Importances

So far, we have assumed that all costs and benefits are equally important. But private sector marketers will point out that this is rarely the case. That is, some benefits may be really important to some consumers, and a small improvement may make a big difference in their eventual behavior. On the other hand, creating a really big improvement in a consequence they do not care about may have little or no payoff in behavior change. A mother with a domineering husband may weight the costs of not being able to cook her husband's meal as much more important to her than the benefits of getting her child better health. For this mother, a social marketing program that emphasizes the benefits of the vaccination to the child—and perhaps even offers an extra incentive like a free meal at the clinic—will be missing the point. Unless something is done about the cost of missing the husband's meal, nothing will happen! The marketer will have to find some way of feeding the husband—or getting the mother to and from the clinic in less time so she can still prepare the meal—in order to have any hope of success. These crucial costs and benefits are often referred to as *determinative*.

If we grant that benefits and costs differ in their importance to target consumers, we may ask whether the importance of the overall bundles varies over the Contemplation Stage. The research of Prochaska and DiClemente again suggests that the answer is yes. Adapting Janis and Mann's concept of the Decision Balance Sheet (Janis and Mann, 1977), Prochaska and DiClemente found that, across the twelve social behaviors they studied, the benefits of adopting the behaviors were perceived to be higher in the Contemplation Stage than in the Precontemplation Stage, which is certainly reasonable. In the Precontemplation Stage, consumers presumably see few benefits of the behavior and (again presumably) many costs.

Prochaska and DiClemente also found that in nine of the twelve behavior-change programs, the costs of the proposed behavior were perceived to be lower in the Action Stage than in the Contemplation Stage. The authors suggest that moving consumers toward action may be largely a matter of reducing costs, rather than promoting benefits. This presumably would apply to consumers in the later portion of the Contemplation Stage and, almost certainly, to consumers in what I call the Action Stage. My own experience from interviewing the targets of social marketing programs, particularly in the arts, supports the Prochaska-DiClemente findings.

This distinction has important implications for social marketers. Take, for example, the following case. Suppose a mother in a developing country is currently treating childhood diarrhea ineffectively with traditional herbs and teas. She is contemplating using oral rehydration therapy but knows little about it. Before she is likely to move on in the Contemplation Stage, she will need to be shown its benefits. The social marketer's challenge at this stage will be explaining what ORT does and how to use it and touting the great advantages it has over other alternatives—while, of course, being sensitive not to attack traditional cultural values. Once the target mother sees the potential benefits of the new behavior, existing experience suggests that her thinking will then focus on all the reasons why she can't carry the behavior out. She may think about how she cannot find uncontaminated water or how she could not find the time and patience to feed the child the amount of ORS that is desirable. It is at this point that the marketer needs to stop emphasizing benefits and focus on minimizing or eliminating the costs that now loom large in the consumer's mind.

This scenario leads us to propose separating the Contemplation Stage into two substages: Early Contemplation and Late Contemplation.

Implications

The discussion to this point suggests the following implications for a social marketer thinking of undertaking a major intervention in a new marketplace where consumers are in the Contemplation Stage:

- *Formative research.* The project should begin with formative research with the target audience to determine the nature of the benefits and costs this audience contemplates when considering undertaking the proposed behavior. Then, for each benefit and each cost, the research needs to find out how likely the audience thinks it is that the consequence will occur, and how important each benefit and cost is to them. In addition, the research needs to find out what competition the marketer faces.

- *Strategic planning.* Given the results of the formative research, the marketer should consider ways to increase the total weighted value of the benefit bundle as compared to the cost bundle. *Benefit-enhancing strategies* include increasing the number of benefits, increasing the perceived likelihood that each major benefit will occur (especially those that are determinative), and increasing the importance of major benefits perceived to be very likely to occur. *Cost-reduction strategies* include decreasing the perceived likelihood that each major cost will occur (especially those that are determinative), and decreasing the importance of major costs perceived to be very likely to occur.

- *Demarketing.* If necessary and desirable, increase the perceived costs and decrease the perceived benefits of the most common alternatives that compete with the proposed behavior.

- *Tailored messages.* Emphasize benefit-enhancing strategies for consumers early in the Contemplation Stage and emphasize cost-reduction strategies for those late in the Contemplation Stage.

The strategic and tactical approach that social marketers can use to implement these alternatives will be discussed in later chapters.

Role of Significant Others

Research and common sense also make clear that beliefs about consequences are not the only things that consumers contemplate for highly involving decisions. These beliefs only consider personal consequences, that is, the benefits and costs to the individual of taking on the new behavior. Consumers, of course, do not make decisions in a social vacuum. They are part of couples or families or villages or societies. Other members of these various groups can have very important roles to play in influencing what consumers do. They can participate in the decision—and sometimes in the behavior, as with condom use. Or they can act as facilitators (such as acquiring ORS for family use). But they also serve as sources of information and sources of social pressure.

Sources of Information

Family members, peers, neighbors, co-workers, and even media personalities and movie stars can pass along facts and opinions to individual consumers that can have direct influence on the consumer's own perceptions of specific consequences and the importance attached to them. A neighbor can describe the long wait she had at the health clinic and how poorly she was treated. A relative can offer an opinion about the health effects of immunization on her children. A village leader can report an increase in hours during which the clinic in the next village is open.

It has long been known that many marketing communications campaigns work in a two-step fashion. The campaigns first communicate their messages to key individuals in communities called *opinion leaders,* and these individuals then pass on this information to target consumers through word of mouth. It is often how doctors learn about new drugs and how villagers learn about new health practices (Rogers, 1983).

Besides providing factual information, other individuals can also have major effects on the importance weightings that individuals give to various consequences. These influences can occur over very long periods of time and in very subtle ways. Consumers acquire basic values as they are socialized into a culture and then more particularized values from their mothers and fathers. These values are then changed as cultures change and as the individual becomes part of other social organizations, families, work forces, neighborhoods, and villages. Thus whether a mother places greater importance on having a healthy child or on having a happy husband will depend, at least in part, on what part of the world she is in, what her parents told her, and what the neighboring women think is important.

Finally, other individuals can serve as silent sources of information simply by providing models for the desired behavior. Marketers have long noted the role that reference groups can play in influencing behavior (Bearden and Etzel, 1982; Witt and Bruce, 1972). These references can comprise others in membership groups ("people like me"), aspirations groups ("people I would like to be like"), and negative reference groups ("people I want to be the opposite of"). Reference individuals can be particularly important when the social marketing behaviors are public and target customers can watch closely what other people do. In many situations, celebrities can play an important role in modeling desired behaviors for others.

I will return to the role of others in modeling behavior later in this chapter.

Sources of Social Pressure

Everyone at one time or another has had the experience of doing something they did not really want to do. There is the time you were too tired to go out, but your wife insisted. Or the time you did not want to give money to the homeless person, but the person with you did and shamed you into it. This social pressure is independent of the role of others in affecting consumers' perceptions of consequences. Social pressure is a particularly important part of the Fishbein and Ajzen Theory of Reasoned Action, which they refer to as the *Normative* component of their model. They argue that in order to predict individuals' intentions to take a particular action, one must understand not only their perceptions of personal consequences but also their perceptions of what they think others want them to do and how likely they are to be influenced by these others. In social marketing settings, professionals such as health care workers and physicians can be very important sources of this kind of social pressure.

When social influences are added to personal consequences in the Theory of Reasoned Action (TRA), the model is particularly powerful in explaining individual intentions to take a particular action, which, in turn, are found to be good predictors of actual behavior. Much of the research validating the model has been with respect to behaviors of interest to social marketers. For example, Baker (1988) found that the TRA accounted for 38 percent of the variance in intentions to use condoms with steady partners. Jaccard and Davidson found the model to account for 79 percent of the variance in intentions to use birth control pills among college students (Jaccard and Davidson, 1972) and 74 percent of the variation among married women (Davidson and Jaccard, 1975).

In another important line of research on social pressure, Hornik has argued that results from the HEALTHCOM project suggest that community norms may play a more important role than individual attitudes in communities where more than half the population has already adopted a target behavior (Hornik, 1992). This finding has interesting implications for the stage model. If one can assume that in communities with 50 percent adoption, most target consumers who have not adopted the new behavior will be at the Late Contemplation Stage, then Hornik's research would suggest that movement from the Late Contemplation Stage to Action may be brought about by applications of social pressure in addition to (or instead of) reductions in perceived costs.

Implications

The significant role others play in the Contemplation Stage suggests several implications for social marketers.

•   *Formative research.* In addition to the questions about individual reactions, include questions in formative research about significant groups of others asking what groups the individual pays attention to. For each group, find out what action the individual believes the group wants, and how likely the individual is to accede to the perceived wishes of the group.

•   *Strategic planning.* Consider using opinion leaders in each community as conveyors of information to others, role models for targeted behaviors (especially if it is a public behavior), and sources of social pressure. Workplace sites where there are clear leadership hierarchies may be particularly good locations in which to make use of interpersonal influence as a vehicle for change.

•   *Tailored messages.* For those consumers in the Late Contemplation Stage, consider applying social pressure extensively using reference groups identified by target consumers as being influential.

Action Stage

For an individual to move from concluding that a behavior is a good idea—either because it is personally rewarding or because social pressures make the action imperative—to actually taking an action, he or she must hold one additional important belief. This is the belief that the behavior *can actually be accomplished.* Both Bandura (1977a) and Ajzen have placed considerable emphasis on this behavioral determinant. Bandura called it "perceived self-efficacy" while Ajzen uses the broader term "perceived behavioral control" (Ajzen, 1985, 1991). Ajzen defines this component as "the person's belief as to how easy or difficult performance of the behavior is likely to be."

Ajzen's concept of behavioral control has two parts, a distinction also made earlier by Balch (1974). One component is the individual's perception that he or she has the knowledge, skills, and so forth to carry out the behavior personally. This component, which Balch calls "internal efficacy," is equivalent to Bandura's concept of self-efficacy. The second component is the individual's perception that environmental factors will permit the behavior to occur. Balch calls this "external efficacy." Environmental factors that might interfere with behavior would be the unavailability of needed products or services or the unwillingness of another person to cooperate (as in practicing safe sex). The model has considerable support in areas where volitional control is substantial, such as voting (Balch, 1974), weight loss (Netemeyer, Burton, and Johnston, 1991), problem drinking, and exercising (Ajzen, 1991), and in behavioral areas where volition is less because others are involved, such as condom use and limiting infants' sugar intake (Ajzen, 1991).

In other recent work, Bagozzi and Warshaw (1990) suggest that *self-efficacy* confuses two notions of efficacy. One is the consumer's judgment that he or she has the necessary wherewithal to perform the act. The other is the consumer's estimate of whether the action will achieve the individual's behavioral goal. In this chapter, the latter notion of *action efficacy* is included in the perception of positive consequences. That is, it is argued that asking a target consumer how likely it is that a particular action will lead to a particular consequence is equivalent to asking about action efficacy.

Constructive Blame

In the model proposed here, I will adopt Ajzen's two-factor component in part because it points relatively unambiguously to steps social marketers need to take in order to get target consumers to undertake needed behavioral change. The steps needed depend on where consumers attribute the blame for their perceived inability to carry out a proposed action. There are two possibilities here: blame can be attributed to themselves or to others or to the general environment (Mizerski, Golden, and Kernan, 1979; Kelley, 1973).

When consumers attribute blame to themselves, the marketer's challenge is to increase the consumer's perceived self-efficacy, for example teaching them new skills. For example, smokers must learn how to quit, what to do when they are nervous, how to fend off friends (or spouses) who offer cigarettes, and so on. Sex workers need to learn how to negotiate with customers in order to get them to agree to wear a condom and then learn how to put them on their customers (Ramah and Cassidy, 1992). Mothers with kids who get diarrhea need to know how to mix oral rehydration solutions, dieters need to learn new eating (and cooking) habits, sedentary individuals must learn how to exercise safely and productively, and individuals with high blood pressure need to learn how to detect harmful foods and what to substitute for them.

The likelihood that people will intend to carry out any of these activities, therefore, is in large measure a function of whether they think they can actually carry it off themselves. As we shall see in subsequent chapters, one of the most effective methods for increasing this sense of self-efficacy is with a technique called *behavioral modeling*. The approach, originally developed by Bandura, was used successfully in the California three-city Heart Health Study to reduce smoking (Maccoby and Farquar, 1975).

Where consumers attribute blame to other people, the marketer's challenge is more difficult. If consumers' attributions are wrong—for example, if they incorrectly believe that others will not cooperate with a desired behavior—then the solution lies in changing what consumers perceive to be the likely behavior. It has been suggested that many teen and college-age students do not use condoms because they incorrectly believe that this is not what their partners want. Clearly, a marketing strategy here would be to get partners talking to each other (to learn the truth) and to get out the word through advertisements, press releases, and magazine articles that many more young people support the use of condoms than is routinely thought. On the other hand, if typical behavior is not supportive (and consumers perceive things correctly), then the challenge is to change that behavior—which, of course, is the basic problem we began with!

Finally, if consumers attribute a lack of behavioral control to the "system" and that system is under the marketer's control, then solutions are relatively straightforward. Again, if perceptions are wrong, the marketer must teach consumers the facts—for example, that condoms are available everywhere; that ORS comes in many flavors, one of which will please your baby; that health workers will never "tell" if you get birth control products at the clinic; and so on. On the other hand, if the customer's perception of reality is correct, then the marketer has to get the condoms widely distributed, make ORS in more flavors, and ensure that health clinic personnel do not ever reveal confidential information.

Implications

This section makes clear the need for social marketers to adapt their projects still further.

- *Formative research.* Include questions about perceived behavioral control in any future formative field research studies.
- *Strategic planning.* Plan on including skill training and confidence building in any social marketing program where new abilities are required. In addition—and perhaps more important—make sure that no aspect of the marketing system is at fault in holding back consumers from carrying out the desired activities.
- *In-flight adjustments.* Include questions about perceived behavioral control in monitoring activities in the Contemplation Stage. Where perceptions of blame do not square with reality, change the perception. Otherwise, change the reality!

Maintenance Stage

In a relatively small number of cases, social marketers are only concerned with a single act. Thus, if a man has a vasectomy or a woman has a tubal ligation, the social marketing task is essentially over (although the social marketer would want the target customer to continue to spread positive messages to others who can be influenced). In the majority of cases, however, the marketer is interested in continuous behavior as well as in correct behavior. In some cases, such as in mixing and administering an oral rehydration solution, correct behavior means doing something properly. In other cases, such as in the use of condoms to prevent AIDS and other STDs, it means doing the proper behavior every time.

Initial behaviors are sometimes really trials in the consumer's mind, with subsequent behaviors following only upon a positive evaluation of the actual consequences. In other cases, the consumer may have moved beyond trial and be committed to the new behavior, but there is still always a very real risk that the consumer will drop out. The latter is a serious problem for certain kinds of socially desirable behaviors. Recidivism rates for quitting smokers and dieters are over 70 and 80 percent. Thus, marketers cannot let down their guard once the first action is completed.

There are two consumer behavior constructs that are valuable in the Maintenance Stage. One is cognitive dissonance; the other is behavior modification. In the former case, it has been relatively well documented that, after a high-involvement decision in which the choice was a difficult one, consumers will go through a period in which they will experience high *cognitive dissonance* (Brehm and Cohen, 1962; Engel, 1963). In this condition, consumers realize that they have declared a preference where only minutes before the choices were relatively close. At this point, two cognitions that are in conflict (*the choices were close* and *I committed to one of them*) produce a state of anxiety or dissonance. This dissonance leads consumers—among other steps—to eagerly seek out confirmation that they did the right thing. (The reader undoubtedly will recall this process taking hold after a major decision. After buying a new car, for example, almost everyone starts noticing more of the same models on the road, reading more ads for the chosen car, and becoming aware of many nice features of the vehicle that were never noticed before. This is cognitive dissonance at work!)

The implication for social marketers here is that, after the first action step, a good deal can be done to help the consumer come to a conclusion that the choice was correct, that is, to help reduce the cognitive dissonance resulting from the choice. Thus, a mother who just had a baby vaccinated for the first time should not be simply dismissed to go home. Where possible, time should be taken to remind her of the benefits she has obtained from her action and how the baby will now have a much better chance for a healthy life. Materials should be given to her to take home so that she can keep convincing herself that she did the right thing—otherwise she may regret the behavior change and revert to her former behavior, skipping follow-up vaccinations. This is obviously relatively easy to do—certainly easier than returning an unsatisfactory car.

This is a cognitive-persuasive approach to securing repeat behavior. An alternative—often complementary—approach is to use principles from behavior modification theory. Behavior modification theory argues that much of behavior is influenced by environmental factors that appear both before and after the desired behavior. *Preceding* factors would be cues that trigger the event, such as posters or urgings by neighborhood opinion leaders to secure a vaccination or a supply of Vitamin A for the child. These cues can be important determinants of behavior. The Academy for Educational Development found that offering a chance at a lottery provided the cues that got many women in The Gambia to come to sessions to learn oral rehydration mixing skills (Rasmuson, Seidel, Smith, and Booth, 1988).

The other important contribution of behavior modification theory is its emphasis on the role of postpurchase contingencies in *reinforcing* desired behavior. In a modern adaption of B. F. Skinner's early experiments on pigeons, behavioral theorists urge social marketers to pay close attention to the rewards that can follow behavior. They point to the simple fact that, other things equal, people tend to repeat behaviors they find rewarding. As Graeff, Elder, and Booth (1993) point out, a great many social marketing behaviors are not intrinsically rewarding. When a child is immunized, the mother does not automatically feel good about it. Indeed, the contacts with health clinic staff and the wails of the child may have made the whole occasion rather unpleasant. Social marketers are therefore admonished to make sure that the behavioral event has as many positive contingencies as possible and that extrinsic rewards be employed wherever possible. Thus, to increase recycling, contests can be held among participating households for tickets to sporting events. And brightly colored containers can be offered free so that, when individuals put out their recyclable trash, they can imagine that neighbors will easily observe—and presumably praise—their admirable behavior.

However, behavior modification may not work in all cases. As Kotler and Andreasen (1991, p. 535) note, three conditions must be present:

- *The desired behavior must be under the individual's control.* Thus, behavior modification is not particularly effective with physical drug dependency.
- A *clear link can be established between the behavior and the reinforcement,* although this need not always be apparent to the subject. The closer the reward is to the time of the behavior, the greater the effect—praising someone two days after a desired behavior (for example, cutting down on smoking on certain occasions) is less effective than immediate praise.
- *The reinforcer must constitute a meaningful reward to the individual.* Praise from someone the individual fears would be less rewarding than praise from a respected person such as a doctor, or praise from a close friend.

Operationalizing the Approach

There is a key set of information that a social marketer needs to know about consumers in order to bring about behavioral change. To put this in specific terms, consider the behavior of a hypothetical target village mother of a one-year-old boy needing immunization. In one-on-one situations, health workers can learn much of this information in simple conversations. And then social marketers must turn this information into effective interventions to move the mother on to the next stage of the behavior stage continuum, that is, from Precontemplation to Action and Maintenance.

- *Is the mother at least at the stage where she is contemplating taking her child to the health clinic for his first immunization shots?* Does she know what immunization is and why it might benefit her son? Does she have any religious or cultural reservations about immunizations?
- *What are the major alternatives she is considering?*
- *What does she see as the costs and benefits of going for the first time to*

get the first immunization shots? For each cost and each benefit, (a) how likely is it to occur? (b) how important is it to her?
- *What does she think others who are important to her want her to do?*
- *Does she think that she can actually take the child for immunization* at the next opportunity (that is, does she know where and when to go)?
- *If she has undertaken the behavior before, how did it turn out?* What did she find particularly rewarding about it? What was negative about it?
- *What is the probability she will undertake the behavior again?* What could increase this probability?

The answers to these questions should give the social marketer a very good sense of what to do at the next step in the social marketing process.

Summary

In order to understand target consumers and develop strategies that respond to them, social marketers must have a way of both researching those consumers and then understanding what they learn about them. This requires a framework for understanding. The framework presented in this chapter is based on a number of insights from the social science literature about the kinds of high-involvement decisions social marketers try to influence. These insights show that consumers do not undertake high-involvement behaviors rapidly and in one step. They move toward the desired outcomes in stages. So, at any point in time, the social marketer's challenge is to move the consumers to the next stage of the process.

Decisions to take action along this process are made on the basis of the consequences perceived to follow from the choices. These consequences are both positive and negative, so consumers face tradeoffs between expected costs and expected benefits. The insight that behavior comes about in stages provides the spine of the consumer analysis framework used in this book. It turns out that the role and importance of the various behavioral influence factors varies by the stage of the process and therefore the challenge facing the social marketer also varies dramatically. For the purposes of this book, I have divided the process into four stages: Precontemplation, Contemplation, Action, and Maintenance. I have further divided the most important stage, Contemplation, into Early and Late substages because research has suggested that the relative importance of benefits versus costs shifts across this stage.

During the Precontemplation Stage, the social marketer's challenges are to make the target population aware of the new behavior as a possibly acceptable addition to their culture and their own lives. Here, the appropriate technologies for the social marketer are the tools of education and propaganda. Media advocacy can also play an important role here.

Social marketing comes into its own during the Contemplation Stage. This is where consumers are considering action. Previous research suggests that their contemplation primarily involves four things. First, they think about how the behavior will turn out. This includes both the good things that will happen (the benefits) and the bad things (the costs). Then, they think about what others want them to do. Finally, they think about whether they can actually make the behavior happen, a condition marketers call "behavioral control." Marketers must understand all of these potential influences if they expect to develop an effective program for a specific target market. And they must understand them not only for the behavior being contemplated but also for its most prominent rivals.

During the Contemplation Stage, costs and benefits are probably the most important cognitive elements influencing movement to the next stage, Action. Early in the Contemplation Stage, benefits are more important—consumers must know that the behavior has many positive features or they are not going to think about it further. But as they get closer and closer to action, costs loom larger and more daunting. It is during the latter substage that marketers must focus primarily on reducing these perceived costs.

Other people play an important role in the Contemplation Stage. They can provide information and serve as role models, and they can bring direct social pressure to bear. Sometimes people will act in a desired way even though they personally think the benefit-cost trade-off is unsatisfactory, because they believe their relationships, reputation, or social position will suffer if they refuse.

At the Action Stage, the most important factor is perceived behavioral control. This factor is made up of two parts: (a) the perception that the customers can actually bring the action about— that is, that they have the necessary skills; and (b) the perception that the environment (that is, physical factors and other people who must cooperate) will permit the behavior.

Most social marketing programs require permanent behavior change—people must stay on diets or off drugs or keep on recycling. This is why the Maintenance Stage is so important. Here, many of the principles of learning theory are especially relevant. Individuals need to be rewarded for what they do—their behavior must be reinforced. Further, they need to be helped to resolve the cognitive dissonance they go through when they undertake something that they once were not sure was a good idea. Social marketers must work effectively on both mechanisms if their programs are to have permanent influence.

Part Two

Doing Social Marketing

Chapter Five

Targeting Your Customer Through Market Segmentation Strategies

In the preceding chapter, I outlined a framework for understanding how target consumers go about making decisions to undertake behavior advocated by a social marketing program. This framework provides a basis for carrying out the first two stages of the strategic planning process outlined in Chapter Two. These stages were:

1. *Listening.* Conducting extensive background analysis, including listening intently to target customers.
2. *Planning.* Setting the marketing mission, objectives, and goals, and defining the core marketing strategy.

In this chapter, I will assume that Stage 1 has been completed and the social marketing manager must turn attention to Stage 2. I will also assume that the marketing mission has also been established (as something along the lines of reducing infant mortality or cutting down on the number of smokers) and that this mission has been turned into specific objectives (such as reducing the number of childhood deaths from polio or measles or increasing the number of children who never start smoking) and quantified goals (like reducing deaths from polio from 20 to 10 per 100,000 or increasing the rate of nonsmoking among teenagers from 60 to 80 percent). The challenge on which I will now focus is devising the *core marketing strategy*.

The core marketing strategy has two major components: the target market and the strategy designed to influence the target market to undertake the desired behavior. In this chapter, we shall be concerned with selecting target markets. This neat separation into components, of course, does not reflect reality. As we shall see below, decisions about segmentation inevitably require that marketers think through—at least to some extent—how they might market to individual segments (Slater, 1995). Further, it is also inevitably the case that as marketers get deeper and deeper into their understanding of target markets in order to develop the detailed strategies I will discuss in the next chapters, they will think of new and better ways to segment the market (or, in some cases, not segment the market). Core strategy formulation is not a linear process. It is interactive and cyclical like much of social marketing planning in general.

Targeted Marketing

Social marketing programs have extremely ambitious goals. Typically, these goals involve targeting a very large, relatively undifferentiated population such as "all children under age five" or "all adults who drink alcoholic beverages." As a result, many programs end up employing what commercial sector marketers call *undifferentiated target marketing*. In such strategies (which resemble the one used by Wrigley's chewing gum, for example), they consider the target audience to be a relatively homogeneous mass—at least with respect to the product offered (equivalent to anyone with teeth!)—and develop one best strategy to address all of them.

However, it is a blunt fact that virtually all social marketing programs must operate with very limited resources. This reality puts great pressure on program managers to become more efficient and effective in their use of the resources entrusted to them. In the commercial sector, such pressures lead managers to think seriously of rejecting undifferentiated marketing in favor of *market segmentation* (Frank, Massy, and Wind, 1972; Dickson, 1982). Market segmentation can be extremely helpful for increasing both efficiency and effectiveness.

In concept, the idea of segmentation is very straightforward. It involves the partitioning of target populations (individuals, households, villages, health workers, businesses, and the like) into subsets. In theory, these subsets are mutually exclusive, though this is sometimes difficult. The marketer then treats some or all of these subsets—or segments—differently with respect to the amount of resources committed to marketing to them and the way in which these resources are used to influence target customer behavior.

In the commercial sector, segmentation allows marketers to carry out one of two types of strategy:

Segmented marketing. This involves developing different strategies for different segments.

Concentrated marketing. This involves selecting only a few of all possible segments and targeting them (possibly with different strategies for each of the few segments chosen).

Segmentation is, of course, already practiced in most existing social marketing programs. Men are treated differently from women, children differently from adults, nurses differently from doctors. However, such approaches employ relatively obvious variations among customers, usually based on gross or unavoidable distinctions. The segments rarely emerge from any systematic evaluation of alternative possibilities, nor do marketers often carry out segmentation as extensively as careful analysis would recommend. Thus, for example, an inexperienced social marketer might prepare campaign materials in two languages for two different market segments, yet keep the content identical for the two segments (ignoring important differences in perceptions and motivations) and distribute the materials in equal amounts to the two markets (ignoring differences in likely responsiveness).

The lack of systematic attention to segmentation possibilities in social marketing programs to date can be attributed to one or more of several barriers:

- A belief that the sponsors of a program or the government that has authority over it will forbid any segmentation of markets.
- A lack of appreciation of the potential of segmentation to significantly increase program impact while reducing program costs.
- A mistaken devotion to program uniformity, based on the belief that this is essential in order to keep costs down through

economies of scale and assure that messages are always
consistent.

- A lack of understanding of just how to go about extensive
  segmenting markets and when to do so.
- A lack of available data on which to base a sound segmentation strategy.
- An unwillingness to collect new segmentation data—either
  because marketers do not know what data to collect or how to
  collect it or because they believe that such research efforts will
  never be cost-effective.

But none of these barriers should apply! Segmentation is one
of the most powerful contributions that commercial sector marketing has to make to the solution of social problems. It may be
that a program will consciously decide not to segment its markets
for resource allocation purposes. Many thoughtful scholars and
practitioners argue that, in some circumstances, it would be unethical to segment a market and devote more resources to some segments than to others (Bloom and Novelli, 1981). Further, in
publicly funded programs, any signs of partiality may be politically
dangerous—unless, perhaps, the favored segment is the most
needy. However, the fact that one chooses not to allocate resources
differently across segments does not mean that segmentation concepts cannot be useful for developing differentiated strategies.

For the aspiring social marketer to use these techniques, four
issues need to be addressed:

- When should a market be segmented?
- What are the possible ways that markets could be segmented?
- How does one choose among the various bases?
- How does one implement a segmentation approach?

Readers interested in further reading on segmentation are
referred to Wind and Massy (1994); Frank, Massy, and Wind
(1972); Fine (1980); Dickson (1982); Kotler and Andreasen (1991,
Chapter Five); Lovelock (1975); Sheth (1990); and Simon (1968).
Readers interested in further reading on the related, but not central, topic of carrying out segmentation field research under limited budget restrictions are referred to Andreasen (1988c).

When Should a Market Be Segmented?

Segmentation can help managers achieve both efficiency and effectiveness. Greater efficiency is achieved when managers allocate resources to target customers in proportion to likely payoffs. This can be achieved by minimizing allocations to unproductive or undesirable market segments and reallocating resources to more productive uses. Greater effectiveness can be achieved by helping managers develop a set of marketing strategies and tactics that would meet the needs, wants, and perceptions of specific subpopulations rather than approaching them all with one general strategy that does not quite speak to anyone particularly well.

Resource Allocation

The simplest approach to allocating resources in a social marketing program—the default strategy—is equally across all segments of the population. The question then is: under what circumstances would a marketer want to allocate disproportional resources to some segment? There are basically three reasons to do so:

- *Different Needs.* Some market segments may be more in need of a social marketing intervention than others. This difference can be a function of several factors:

    Size of the segment.

    Problem incidence. There may be higher rates of some problem behavior in some segments than others—for example, more polio cases per 100,000 in segments *A* and *B* than in segments *C* and *D*.

    Problem severity. For whatever reasons, a given incidence of a problem may be more severe in some segments than others.

    Population defenselessness. Some market segments may be less able to take care of their problems themselves than others.
- *Different General Responsiveness.* Some market segments may be more ready, willing, and able to respond to intervention than other segments.
- *Different Costs.* It may be harder to deliver effective marketing programs to some market segments than to others. This is

primarily a function of *reachability*. Some market segments may be harder to reach than others either because they are harder to find or because the vehicles one must use are more costly.

Strategy Differentiation

The default approach to differentiating strategies across segments is not to do so, that is, to develop one strategy for everyone. One would only do otherwise if the incremental costs were exceeded by the incremental benefits.

- *Incremental costs.* As one progresses from a single mass marketing strategy to one or more differentiated strategies, there are incremental costs for each segment added. These costs are both economic and human. More segments means more dollars spent, and also more managerial thought and staff attention.
- *Incremental benefits.* As one makes strategies more closely tuned to the needs and wants of individual segments, payoffs as measured in program effectiveness (things like vaccinations achieved, smokers quitting, and so forth) typically increase. This happy result depends on three major factors:
  Each segment has to be large enough to merit separate treatment.
  Segments differ in responsiveness to marketing mix elements. For instance, some segments might respond to mass media approaches featuring appeals to hope, some might respond to facts and effective distribution of services, still others might respond to personal contact and fear messages.
  The organization has the ability to create and deliver differentiated strategies. Even though an organization is aware of differences in responsiveness, it may not have the creative brilliance to develop the needed implementation and the human resources to carry it out. I will refer to this characteristic as *organizational feasibility*.

The assumption of differential responsiveness is crucial. Its centrality reflects both logic and the origins of much theorizing about segmentation that are found in the economic literature on price discrimination (Robinson, 1954).

In summary, then, there are nine factors to look at when deciding whether to segment a market:

1. Segment Size
2. Problem Incidence
3. Problem Severity
4. Defenselessness
5. Reachability
6. General Responsiveness
7. Incremental Costs
8. Responsiveness to Marketing Mix
9. Organizational Capability

Potential Segmentation Bases

The most important step in the segmentation process is choosing the basis for a segmented marketing strategy. There are a great many possible bases and the choice among them will depend a great deal both on what is possible and on what is desirable from the standpoint of program strategy. These factors, in turn, will depend on whether the segmentation objective is primarily resource allocation or primarily strategy differentiation. If one is merely interested in making resource allocation decisions, the data demands are smaller. However, if the goal is to develop tailored interventions that speak precisely to groups of customers, then very sophisticated may be chosen.

Alternative Dimensions

There a number of different dimensions one can use to array segmentation alternatives. Frank, Massy, and Wind (1972) distinguish between *a priori* and *self-selection* bases. *A priori* approaches require that the marketer determine in advance the characteristics to be used, generally things like sex, age, residential status, and so forth, and then develop an approach to each subsegment. *Self-selection* approaches allow segments to define themselves through their differing responses to specific marketing tactics. The self-selection approach is seldom satisfactory because it rarely indicates why a segment responded. It also tends to neglect segments that do not respond to the proffered strategy.

If a marketer chooses an *a priori* approach, there is a very wide range of traits that can be used. Frank, Massy, and Wind have suggested that the alternatives can generally be grouped along two dimensions:

- *Objective Versus Inferred.* Some traits, such as gender and residence, can be measured or observed objectively. Other traits, such as attitude or personality, can only be inferred (from responses to a paper-and-pencil test, for example) and not observed directly.
- *General Versus Behavior-Specific.* Some traits, such as gender and personality, are general and can apply to a wide range of behaviors a marketer may wish to influence. Other traits, such as past vaccination history or attitudes toward a health care clinic, are specific to the behavior to be influenced.

Table 5.1 presents a sampling of traits within the four cells defined by these dimensions. Detailed descriptions of many of these traits can be found in most marketing texts (such as Kotler and Andreasen, 1991, Chapter Five; McCarthy and Perrault, 1993, Chapter Three).

Each of the four segmentation bases has its advantages and disadvantages, but two are most interesting for the purposes of this book. *Objective general* segmentation bases have one considerable advantage going for them. In most markets, even relatively remote and underdeveloped ones, data on such characteristics are available from secondary sources. Thus, one can usually find out the size of various cities, the number of women in them, the education levels of the population, their racial and ethnic breakdowns, and so forth. And to the extent these data can be broken down by residential area, they can provide a basis for assessing reachability. In more developed countries, objective general data are often available for major magazines, newspapers, and radio and television stations as well, helping considerably with media allocation decisions. Overall, managers faced with resource allocation decisions often find objective general measures very attractive.

Table 5.1. Taxonomy of Household Segmentation Variables.

	General	Behavior Specific
Objective Measures	Age of adult	Contact with system
	Income	Past behaviors
	Sex of adult	Access to products
	Place of residence	Distance to sources
	Race, ethnic group	Behavior of relatives
	Language	Behavior of village
	Size of home	Hours watching TV
	Quality of home	Hours listening to radio
	Number of children	
	Education	
	Presence of husband	
	Age of children	
	Sex of children	
	Community wealth	
	SES index	
Inferred Measures	Personality	Self-efficacy
	Lifestyle	Perceived benefits
	Values	Perceived costs
	Risk preferences	Stage of behavior change
	Media preferences	Message recall
	Self-confidence	Relevant knowledge
	Perceived health	Social norms
	Discretionary time	Perceived risk
	Innovativeness	Perceived severity
	Attitude of community leader	Satisfaction with clinics

Objective general measures, however, have major disadvantages. Because they are general, they do not indicate cause-and-effect relationships that help social marketers create strategies. Thus, a marketer may know that residents of District X in Jakarta have higher vaccination levels and visit their local health clinic more frequently than residents of District B. He or she may also know that these residents have medium incomes, high school educations, small families, and one servant per household. Yet none of this explains why these households use the health system more. The marketer can only make informed speculations.

At the other end of the spectrum are *inferred specific* measures. Measures like these are very valuable for developing specific marketing strategies, messages, promotions, products, and so on. As I noted in Chapter Four, in order to develop effective marketing strategies, we need to get "inside the heads" of target audiences to learn where they stand with respect to the stages of the behavior-change process. This stage will determine such things as whether positive or negative consequences are more important, whether social pressure should be brought to bear, whether marketers need to help consumers with behavioral control. All of this information will allow the social marketer to fine-tune the strategy. And if these factors—which we infer from our research and other listening activities—differ across segments in important ways, then we must treat the affected segments differently!

It should, of course, be noted that a disadvantage of using inferred measures is that they require new, original research that often involves relatively sophisticated measuring instruments. On the other hand, as I noted in Chapter Three, these methods need not be all that sophisticated to provide management with very useful insights.

The Importance of Behavior-Change Stages

The single most valuable basis for segmenting markets for social marketing strategies is the target's stage in the behavior-change process. As I note throughout this volume, information about whether a target audience is in Precontemplation, Contemplation, Action, or Maintenance is the principal determinant of how one should approach people to move them toward desired objectives. It determines the types of messages one should use (Maibach and

Cotton, 1995) and the channels through which they should be placed, the relative importance of skills training, the need for social influence to be brought to bear, and so on. Learning the target's stage is relatively straightforward and will depend on the behavior or behaviors at issue. When developing major overall strategies, social marketers should profile the stages of their target audiences through large-scale formal surveys. However, even at the simplest level, naive queries (qualitative research) about a person's stage can be extremely helpful to interventionists making tactical choices on how best to move a specific target individual toward the next stage in his or her change process.

Implementing a Segmentation Approach

There are a number of steps involved in implementing a segmentation approach:

1. Specify a modest set of candidate segmentation bases for careful evaluation and determine specific subpopulations to investigate.
2. Assemble (or create) information on potential market segments.
3. Decide whether to allocate different levels of resources to different segments.
4. Decide whether to create different strategies for different segments.
5. Choose segments to address with different levels of resources or different strategies, or both.
6. Proceed to implement the segmentation plan (that is, with specific allocations and strategies).

Step 1 is straightforward. The social marketer merely lists a number of possible bases for segmentation and then divides the population into sensible subgroups. The bases and groupings could come from other projects or emerge as common sense. Ideally, however, they should emerge from the project's formative research. The candidate set should be relatively broad at the start—many options will drop out quickly—but not so broad that the task is overwhelming.

As an example of the procedure, let us follow a social marketer working for a private nonprofit that is developing strategies for an AIDS prevention project in the United States (similar to the one described in Smith and others, 1993). She has a limited budget and so can focus on only a limited number of sites and target populations. She knows that risk and knowledge of AIDS varies significantly by age, gender, and region of the country. Further, she believes that prevention programs will likely be more effective if they are targeted to specific racial or ethnic groups. Thus, she decides that the most promising bases for segmenting her audience are age, gender, region, and race. Because of her desire to focus her eventual program, she further decides up front to limit the regions she will consider to three that she believes have received relatively little attention to date: the Deep South (Mississippi, Louisiana, Alabama, and Georgia); the Mountain States (Montana, Idaho, Colorado, Wyoming, and Utah); and the Southwest (Arizona and New Mexico). The subgroups and possible combinations are set out in Table 5.2. (The three blocks marked with double asterisks (**) will be used in further discussion later in the chapter.)

The next step is to assemble information on each of the fifty-four potential market segments with respect to the nine segmentation factors outlined earlier in this chapter in the Strategy Differentiation section. The tricky problem is figuring out what the relevant measure for each factor should be. It is at this step that the marketer may go back into the field, recognizing that she does not have some important pieces of information.

Where possible, the marketer wants to use direct measures to derive information about each of the nine segmentation factors; in the absence of direct measures, she will look for a measure that could be a proxy for an inaccessible piece of information. The factors are further divided into two groups: those affecting allocation of resources, and those affecting strategy.

Resource Allocation Factors

Here are some specific measures that could be used to address resource allocation questions:

Size of the market. Factor 1, Segment Size, indicates whether there are enough people in a potential grouping to comprise a useful market.

Table 5.2. AIDS Project—Possible Segments.

Age	18–24		25–34		35+	
Gender	Male	Female	Male	Female	Male	Female
White	XXXX	XXXX	XXXX	XXXX	XXXX	XXXX
Deep South						
Mountain				**		
Southwest						
Black	XXXX	XXXX	XXXX	XXXX	XXXX	XXXX
Deep South		**				
Mountain						
Southwest						
Hispanic	XXXX	XXXX	XXXX	XXXX	XXXX	XXXX
Deep South						
Mountain						
Southwest	**					

- *Direct Measure:* Direct census count.
- *Proxy Measure:* Multiplication of total population times (percent in each age group) times (percent in each gender group) times (percent in each race group). For example: 17.312 million population x (50.7 percent female) x (9.77 percent age 18–24) x (28.8 percent black) = 247,968 black females between ages eighteen and twenty-four in the Deep South.

Prevalence of problem behavior. Factor 2, Problem Incidence, helps determine whether a potential segment offers sufficient scope for the marketer's program.

- *Direct Measure:* Rate of AIDS per 100,000 population.
- *Proxy Measure:* Frequency of sexual relations and intravenous drug use.

Severity of problem behavior. Factor 3, Problem Severity, also contributes to the picture of a potential segment's need for the program.

- *Direct Measure:* Rate of AIDS deaths per 100,000 population.
- *Proxy Measure:* Rate of deaths from any cause per 100,000 population.

Relative inability to cope with the problem. Factor 4, Defenselessness, provides an important indicator that the marketing program will be particularly useful to a potential segment.

- *Direct Measure:* Weakness of alternative programs aimed at target audience (on a scale of 1 for many strong programs to 100 for none).
- *Proxy Measure:* Percent unaware of AIDS and AIDS prevention behaviors.

Ease of access. Factor 5, Reachability, helps assess the likelihood of a given resource dollar reaching a potential segment.

- *Direct Measure:* Number of alternative media (TV and radio stations and newspapers) per 100,000 target population.
- *Proxy Measure:* Percent of households with TVs or radios.

Probable willingness to listen. Factor 6, General Responsiveness, also helps assess the amount of change the available resources are likely to generate.

- *Direct Measure:* Percent of individuals not now practicing safe sex or sharing needles who say they (a) know about AIDS and (b) are interested in learning more about how to prevent it. (Note: This index of responsiveness assumes target audience is in Contemplation Stage.)
- *Proxy Measure:* Measure of socioeconomic status.

Note that SES factors often prove good predictors of responsiveness to a proposed social marketing program. For example, evaluations of HealthCom programs have shown education to be positively associated with knowledge about vaccinations and proper mixing skills in Ecuador (Hornik and others, 1991), and knowledge of ORS and trial of Vitamin A in West Java (McDivitt, McDowell, and Zhou, 1991). Radio ownership was positively related to ORS knowledge in West Java (McDivitt, McDowell, and Zhou, 1991) and with measles knowledge and vaccination behavior in the Philippines (Hornik, Zimicki, and Less, 1991). Wealth and SES were associated with vaccination knowledge in Ecuador (Hornik and others, 1991).

There is also some evidence in the marketing literature that individuals who are undergoing status changes may be more willing to change behavior (Andreasen, 1984; O'Rand and Krecker, 1990). Thus, individuals who have just gotten divorced, just been married, or just moved to a new community may be particularly good targets for behavior-change programs.

Strategy Factors

Here are some specific measures for factors influencing strategy definition:

Segmentation expense. Factor 7, Incremental Costs, measures the additional costs required to address the group as a separate segment.

- *Direct Measure:* Average costs to produce additional promotional materials, such as posters, TV ads, radio ads, and so forth with different models, spokespersons, and copy.
- *Proxy Measure:* Number of advertising agencies in area catering to specific population.

Sensitivity to various tactics. Factor 8, Responsiveness to Marketing Mix, suggests the kind of strategy that may be effective with a potential segment.

- *Direct Measure:* Profile of typical target individual on each of the following characteristics:
  a. Perceived benefits of engaging in prevention behaviors
  b. Perceived costs of engaging in prevention behaviors

    c. Perceived social pressure to engage in prevention behaviors
    d. Perceived behavioral control over prevention behaviors
    e. Competitive behaviors
- *Proxy Measure:* For each of the characteristics:
    a. (Perceived benefits) Principal needs and wants with respect to health
    b. (Perceived costs) Perceived risk of HIV infection
    c. (Perceived social pressure) Estimates of group social cohesiveness
    d. (Perceived behavioral control) Interpersonal self-confidence
    e. (Competition) Percent single (for singles, there would be more concern to maximize the number of personal and sexual relationships)

Marketing organization scope. Factor 9, Organizational Capability, provides a reality check for the marketer's ability to design and implement a strategy aimed at a particular potential segment.

- *Direct Measure:* Availability of staff or outside resources with expert insight into the language and cultural norms of the potential segment.
- *Proxy Measure:* Number of segment members on organization's staff.

Using the Information

Table 5.3 presents hypothetical results of gathering information on the nine factors for three of the fifty-four potential AIDS segments outlined in Table 5.2. The results are separated according to d or direct measures and p or proxy measures. Note that many of the numbers may be estimates or projections from other segments or other data. For example, results may be derived from a national study and assumed to apply to each segment.

Allocating Resources to Segments

Once information like that reported in Table 5.3 has been gathered, the next task is to decide on resource allocation. To recall, the key criteria are:

Table 5.3. AIDS Project—Evaluation of Possible Segments.

		Black, 18–24, female, in Deep South	White, 25–34, female, in Mountains	Hispanic, 18–24, male, in Southwest
	Allocation Factors			
1 *d*	Number of individuals per census	248,000	559,000	62,000
1 *p*	Estimated group size	Same	Same	Same
2 *d*	AIDS rate per 100,000	34.2	25.8	28.8
2 *p*	Frequency of sexual relations per month	19	23	10
3 *d*	AIDS mortality per 100,000	11.0	3.7	8.5
3 *p*	General mortality per 100,000	833	970	1,211
4 *d*	Weakness of alternative programs	20	40	90
4 *p*	Percent aware of AIDS	32	41	50
5 *d*	Number of media per 100,000 population	31	18	44
5 *p*	Percent of households with TV	87	82	80
6 *d*	Percent wanting to know about AIDS	23	11	32
6 *p*	Percent of households above poverty	63	72	70
	Strategy Factors			
7 *d*	Costs of additional promotion	Low	Moderate	Moderate
7 *p*	Number of specialized advertising agencies	51	123	21
8 *d*	a. Perceived benefits	Fewer STDs	Longer life	No early death
8 *d*	b. Perceived costs	Angry boyfriends	Condom costs	Less pleasure
8 *d*	c. Perceived social pressures	Low	High	Medium
8 *d*	d. Perceived behavioral control	Low	Medium	High
8 *d*	e. Competitive behavior	Unprotected sex	Unprotected sex	Unprotected sex
8 *p*	a. Health needs and wants	Healthy motherhood	Health for work	Athletic
8 *p*	b. Perceived HIV risk	High	Very low	High
8 *p*	c. Group cohesiveness	Families/low Peers/high	Families/high Peers/low	Families/high Peers/low
8 *p*	d. Interpersonal self-confidence	Low	High	Medium
8 *p*	e. Percent single	88	31	70
9 *d*	Organization experience	Moderate	Low	Moderate
9 *p*	Number of segment members in organization	Very many	Very few	Few

- *Need for intervention,* which is a function of Segment Size (Factor 1), Problem Incidence (Factor 2), Problem Severity (Factor 3), and Defenselessness (Factor 4)
- *Reachability* (Factor 5)
- *General Responsiveness* (Factor 6)

In order to allocate resources across the segments, one must first determine the relative importance one is going to give to each of the six sets of factors. Some programs in some situations may give high weight to problem incidence and defenselessness and lower weight to responsiveness. Others may do the opposite. There is no magic formula that would fit all programs.

Segments to Ignore

Once some attention has been given to the weighting of the criteria, the next decision is: should one allocate zero resources to any segments? Given limited resources of most social marketing programs, the answer should often be yes. One may chose to ignore a segment for one of two basic reasons. First, the segment may be relatively well off with respect to the problem. It may be small, have low problem incidence, low severity, or high capacity to defend itself. Alternatively, the segment may be a really tough case because it is hard to reach or because it is not likely to respond to the sort of input that can be provided by available resources. Social marketers should eliminate such segments from further consideration, unless political pressures make such a judgment impossible. It simply wastes resources and increases the burden on management to bother with relatively well off or intractable segments.

Just such a situation was found to be the case in recent Health-Com work in West Java. There, McDivitt and McDowell (1991) concluded that "One quarter of the mothers can be considered the 'hard to reach' group: they did not listen to the radio more than three times a week and had not been to the health center or health post in the last two months. It is unlikely that this group would be reached by the channels used in this campaign" (p. 4).

The fact that a market segment is a tough case may argue against allocating resources to behavior-change programs at the individual level. However, as Wallack and others promoting media advocacy have argued (Wallack, Dorfman, Jernigan, and Themba, 1993), strategies aimed at the community level may be warranted so that the so-called tough cases can be brought to the point where a social marketing intervention is feasible and cost-effective. Thus, a crime- and drug-infested public housing project may not be a sensible site for a prenatal care program, even though one is desperately needed. Social marketers for the prenatal program, however, may wish to urge community organizers to do something about safety and crime in the area so that later the social marketers can intervene to deal with basic maternal health problems.

Dividing the Pie

The second step is to allocate resources across the remaining segments. The naive approach would be based simply on the size of the affected segment, with large segments getting proportionately more than small segments. But as suggested above, this figure should be adjusted for each of the other five factors in the first part of Table 5.3. One approach would be to use indexes for each of the other factors and then adjust the population figure by the index. (As a further refinement, each of the five factors making up the index can be given a weight depending on the social marketers' view of its relative importance.) One would proceed as follows:

1. For each of the five criteria, assign the value 1.0 to represent an "average" segment. Values above 1.0 should be assigned to segments that are "worse" in the case of incidence, severity, and defenselessness—or "better" in the case of reachability and responsiveness. (Thus, a value of 2.33 on severity would mean that the segment had a problem rate two and a third times the average for all the segments.) A value below 1.0 would have the opposite meaning.
2. Once values are assigned, average them and multiply them by the total population groups to get what might be called an *index-adjusted population* (IAP) score.
3. Add the IAP scores together to get a total IAP.
4. Convert each segment's IAP into a percentage of total IAP.

5. Use this percentage (other things equal) to represent the segment's share of the total resource budget.

To see how this would work, let us consider the three segments in Table 5.3. We will assume that they will receive all the resources and that none of them will get zero. How would we go about calculating their allocations? To further simplify the example, we shall focus only on the direct measures, not the proxies.

- *We would begin by computing indexes for each of the segments on each of the five criteria* based on the average results for each criterion assuming the overall averages given below, which translate into the resulting indexes for the three segments given in Table 5.4.
    a. Incidence: Average AIDS rate is 29.6 per 100,000.
    b. Severity: Average AIDS death rate is 7.7 per 100,000.
    c. Defenselessness: Average weakness score for programs aimed at target population is 50.
    d. Reachability: Average percentage who heard of AIDS in the past month is 31 percent.
    e. Responsiveness: Average percentage wanting to know about AIDS is 22 percent.
- *We then calculate the IAP for each segment* by multiplying the target population in the segment (Table 5.4, row 7) by the average of the five indexes (row 6). To simplify the example, it assumes that the indexes have equal weights. The results are recorded in row 8.

These steps result in an allocation of 35.9 percent of the resources to young black Southern women, 52 percent to twenty-five to thirty-four-year-old white women living in Mountain states and 12 percent to young Hispanic men living in Arizona and New Mexico. This means that the last group gets two-thirds more than its population alone would justify, while white Mountain women get proportionately less. This makes sense. Young Hispanic men are much more defenseless than the other two segments and, at the same time, are much more reachable and potentially responsive. Mountain women, on the other hand, are somewhat defenseless but are much harder to reach and are predicted to be significantly less responsive.

Table 5.4. AIDS Project—Allocation Calculations.

		Black, 18–24, female, in Deep South	White, 25–34, female, in Mountains	Hispanic, 18–24, male, in Southwest
1	Incidence	1.16	.87	.97
2	Severity	1.43	.48	1.10
3	Defenselessness	.4	.8	1.80
4	Reachability	1.00	.58	1.47
5	Responsiveness	1.05	.5	1.45
6	Average adjustment factor	1.01	.65	1.35
7	Population (percent of total)	248,000 (28.5)	559,000 (64.3)	62,000 (7.1)
8	Index Adjusted Population (IAP) (percent of total)	250,480 (35.9)	363,350 (52.0)	83,700 (12.0)

We should note three points here:

1. *Index calculations like these are in many cases subjective.* Managers should use the resulting quantitative calculations simply as a starting point for making judgments about allocations. At least the quantification process will force managers to set down their assumptions about the market, and this process alone can be very suggestive.

2. *The example put no weighting on the various indexes.* Management may look at the results in Table 5.3 and decide that not enough weight was given to, say, defenselessness, which would indicate that even more resources should be given to Hispanic males because there are few other AIDS programs targeting them.

3. *In many real-world situations, managers may decide to ignore a segment altogether if the IAP falls below a certain minimum cutoff.* Management may determine that the hassle of developing a separate treatment is excessive given the significance of the segment and its problems. In such cases, the strategy would be labeled a *concentrated* one. In the commercial sector, this is often called *niching*.

Differential Strategy Decisions

Given that resources will be allocated disproportionately across segments, one must next decide whether to spend these resources on
different strategies across segments. The principal determinants
of this choice will, of course, be the various factors identified in
Chapter Four to influence behavior, plus considerations of costs
and actionability. These decisions, however, cannot be quantified.
One must simply look carefully at the data and answer three
questions:

- Should we approach each segment in a different way?
- Can we afford to?
- Can we actually make it happen?

In the case of our hypothetical three AIDS segments, the answer
to the first two questions is clearly yes. Based on the data in Table
5.3, different approaches to each segment seem appropriate:

> *For the young black women in the Deep South:* Many in the audience
> will be in the Precontemplation Stage. Awareness of AIDS and
> AIDS risk is low. These women need to see that the risks are real
> and serious. However, with this group, the focus should be on
> sexually transmitted diseases, not just on AIDS alone. Ads and
> brochures should point out the risks of AIDS and STDs and the
> benefits of using condoms. The principal benefit to stress would
> be that having protected sex would increase the chances that the
> target audience would be able to be healthy mothers of many
> happy children. The campaign, however, must also help the
> women cope with angry boyfriends who will insist on not wear-
> ing condoms. Because of low literacy levels in this population,
> comic books might be used to portray interpersonal strategies
> for deflecting male anger. Broader efforts to empower these
> women generally may also increase their sense of behavioral con-
> trol. Because peer pressure is important, carefully chosen spokes-
> people who resemble them might be very effective in delivering
> messages and in modeling the desired behavior. Encouraging key
> young women in this segment to talk directly to their friends
> about the desired behavior may prove especially powerful.

> *For white twenty-five to thirty-four-year-old women in Mountain States:*
> This group is almost completely in the Precontemplation Stage.

Awareness of AIDS is moderate and perceived risk is low. In addition, interest in learning more is very low. (This is to be expected in that the hypothetical AIDS rate per 100,000 is lowest for this group. Further, because the region is so spread out, target audience members may not have known anyone with the disease.) While information on potential risks needs to be communicated, the consequences of not having protected sex should focus on the debilitating effect this would have not on the audience members themselves but on their families and the families' incomes. Two-thirds of this group is married and most work. Being sick from AIDS (and STDs) can mean they cannot provide for themselves or their families. Social pressures can be helpful in this part of the country, but the source of pressure will be family, not peers. Thus, spokespeople should be older individuals talking about risks and benefits. Finally, the campaign for this market should probably include free condom distribution—at least during initial stages. Condom costs are perceived to be an important barrier by this group.

For young Hispanic men in the Southwest: This group is primarily in the Contemplation Stage. They have relatively high rates of awareness of the AIDS problem and many of them want to know more about the disease and how to prevent it. They like life a lot, which means marketers have to emphasize the risks of death from AIDS, not just poorer health. But also because they like life, they think of condoms as inhibiting pleasure. Thus, the campaign needs to show them ways in which using condoms can enhance sexual pleasure, to reduce the impact of condom use as a negative factor. Spokespeople should be athletic individuals (Magic Johnson might be very powerful for this group). The group has high self-confidence, so the campaign does not need to worry extensively about behavioral control. Obviously, materials would need to be produced in Spanish. Use of *foto-novellas*—popular with this group—may be very effective.

As to cost, data in Table 5.3 would suggest that segmentation costs are reasonable. And specialized commercial sector advertising agencies are relatively abundant to help out with campaign development in each market (and to shore up any tactical weaknesses the social marketer may have). Some waste may be encountered in addressing Mountain States women due to the absence of targeted media.

Strategies seem actionable in the black Deep South market where the social marketer has a good deal of past experience. Assistance from outside agencies may be necessary in the Mountain States. A Hispanic advertising agency would also be helpful in the Southwest because of language and cultural idiosyncrasies of which the program should be aware.

Summary

Once the social marketer has carefully studied the intended market, the next step in the process is to begin planning specific strategies for influencing behavior. One of the most central elements of such strategies is a plan for segmenting the market. While it is possible to treat markets as undifferentiated masses, it is typically better to carry out *segmented marketing,* where different strategies are developed for different markets, or *concentrated marketing,* where the organization focuses on a few groups on whom it can have a major effect. Segmentation is one of the most powerful contributions that commercial sector marketing has to make to the solution of social problems.

There are two broad classes of decisions for which segmentation can be helpful: *resource allocation decisions,* deciding how much staff time, capital, and cash resources to devote to each target group, and *strategy decisions,* deciding what to say and do to each group, and where and through what medium to address it. In order to assign resources, marketers can always allocate proportional to population. But for most social problems, groups differ in the incidence of the problem, the severity of the problem, and the defenselessness of the population, its probable general responsiveness to any intervention, and its reachability. As outlined in this chapter, it is possible to make quantitative estimates of each of these factors and come up with an overall calculation on which to make relative allocations—which, in some cases, might turn out to be zero.

In the case of strategy formulation, the key determinants are the incremental costs and the incremental benefits of reaching each segment. These factors are, in turn, a function of segment size, differences in responsiveness to marketing mix elements, and the organization's ability to carry out the strategy. These factors, too, can be subject to prior research.

In order to choose among segments, marketers must first divide the population into possible groups. Segmentation bases used in commercial marketing differ depending on whether the measures used are objective or inferred from questionnaires and whether they are general or specific. Objective general measures such as age or place of residence are among the most popular bases because they are available in census data and other secondary sources. However, such measures tell the marketer little about the segment's needs, wants, and perceptions and how it might respond to a specific strategy. For this, inferred specific measures may be more helpful. One of the most valuable inferred measures is the stage of the decision process the target segment has reached. The stage specifies many of the intervention approaches discussed in later chapters in the book.

Chapter Six

Bringing the Customer to the Door: Creating Active Contemplation of New Behaviors

Once social marketers have decided what market segments to target, the next step in the strategic planning process is to figure out how to go about influencing the key behaviors. How does one begin? The answer, as usual, is found in the consumer behavior model outlined in Chapter Four. As we saw there, changing behavior means getting consumers to contemplate the action, then take it, and then (if relevant) to continue to act in specific new ways. Thus, the first cut at the strategic planning task is to ask, Where is the target audience in the behavior-change process: Precontemplation, Contemplation, Action or Maintenance? In the present chapter, I will address briefly the marketing problems involved at the Precontemplation Stage. In the next two chapters, we will get into the meat of social marketing, which comes most forcefully into play in the Contemplation Stage. Chapter Nine will then consider the Action and Maintenance stages.

Characteristics of the Precontemplation Stage

In the Precontemplation Stage, the fundamental problem is—quite simply—that the target audience is literally not contemplating the desired action. This may be a problem that afflicts an entire society or it may be a problem that affects specific subpopulations or segments. One can identify three basic reasons why individuals do not contemplate a new course of behavior. (I am not speaking here of people who do contemplate it but reject it—a problem for the Contemplation Stage.) The three reasons are the following:

- *Ignorance.* They are simply unaware of any need to give up a present course of action (as was the case for everyone in 1981 when no one had heard of something called AIDS or the human immunodeficiency virus).
- *Presumed irrelevance.* Although they have heard that there is a need for some people to change their behavior, they do not include themselves among those people (as is the case today where many heterosexual, non-drug-using groups see AIDS as someone else's problem).
- *Principles.* Although they are aware that there is a potential need for people like them to adopt a new behavior, their basic values prevent them from considering engaging in the behavior (as is the case when people refuse to consider using condoms because it is against their religious beliefs).

   Clearly, the challenges facing the social marketer are different in each case. In the first instance, the problem is creating awareness; in the second, creating interest; and in the third, changing inhibiting values. In all three cases, however, the principal tools are communications tools, either mass communications, "little" communications (posters, brochures, flyers), and face-to-face communications. These are tools that are also used at the Contemplation Stage, so that much of the discussion in this chapter has application there. The difference is that at the Precontemplation Stage the goal is primarily to communicate information to break through present complacency, while in the Contemplation Stage the objective is to obtain action. In the latter stage, strategy involves much more than communications. In Precontemplation, the tasks more often involve education and propaganda.

Creating Awareness and Interest

How, then, might a social marketer go about increasing awareness and changing values? There are two fundamental issues here. First, to decide on the objectives of the awareness campaign: what is it that the target should come to understand? Second, to figure out how to deliver this message. There is a great deal of literature on both these topics in the fields of health communication and public communication (for example, Backer, Rogers, and Sopory, 1992; Rice and Atkin, 1989; Atkin and Wallack, 1990; Salmon, 1990).

I will not repeat this material here but rather will suggest how a social marketer might approach the basic problem. The question is: how would a commercial sector marketer for Pepsi-Cola, Tide, or General Motors address the challenge? There are a number of clear steps that commercial sector communications programs follow. These are:

1. *Determine objectives for the communications component of the marketing strategy* that emerge from a careful analysis of the target audience (what Atkin and Freimuth (1989) call "preproduction formative research"), link the planned communications directly or indirectly to specific outcomes, and are measurable in concrete terms.
2. *Develop communications messages* that also emerge from the target audience, and that recognize the existence of message competition.
3. *Select channels of communication* that reflect known audience preferences and behavior, add the most communication power to the messages, and maximize impact while minimizing waste.
4. *Develop different communications for different markets* whenever possible.
5. *Pretest every message* to ensure that what is received is what was intended.
6. *Integrate every element* of the communications program internally.
7. *Integrate the communications program* with everything else in the marketing mix.
8. *Evaluate communications outcomes* in terms of the preset criteria.

Setting Objectives

Determining the communications objectives in the Precontemplation Stage is relatively simple at one level: the social marketer needs to communicate to the target audience whatever it will take to move them on to the next stage of the communications process, that is, lead them to begin to contemplate the proposed behavior. The question is: What will it take?

Obviously, the answer will vary by the situation. Marketers recognize that communications objectives with ultimate behavioral impacts must look at both the present behavior and the future behavior. That is, to get someone to contemplate a new behavior, the marketer must help the customer learn one or more of two things:

- That the old behavior (say, eating high-fat frozen dinners) is undesirable (leads to heart problems) and should be replaced by something else.
- That there is a new behavior that is superior to the old (if only that Healthy Choice frozen dinners have less fat than Swanson).

In the area of health behavior, a framework called the *Health Beliefs Model* has been proposed to help with this problem (Hochbaum, 1958; Becker, 1974; Rosenstock, 1974; Rosenstock, Strecher, and Becker, 1988). As recently indicated by Rosenstock (1990, pp. 42–43), the Health Beliefs Model is based on the assumption that individuals will change their present behavior if they are motivated by health concerns and if all of the following statements are true:

- They believe they are at risk of some undesirable outcome occurring if they continue their present behavior.
- They believe the severity of that outcome is substantial.
- They believe that there is a course of action available to them that would reduce either their risk or the severity of the expected outcome.
- They believe that the anticipated barriers to (or costs of) taking the action are outweighed by its benefits.

As one can see, this formulation sets three conditions that would have to be met for individuals to move on to contemplate the costs and benefits and to consider what others want them to do and whether they have the behavioral control to actually make the new behavior happen. Thus, the challenge for the social marketer at the Precontemplation Stage is to use preliminary research to answer three questions:

- What is the level of risk (if any) perceived by the target audience if they continue a present practice (overeating, not having a child vaccinated, having unprotected sex)?
- How serious are the negative outcomes (if any) perceived to be if the risk exists?
- Do they believe that there is a proposed action (if any) that will reduce the risk or decrease the severity?

The objectives of the communications strategy at this point, therefore, are to increase the perceived risks and severity of outcomes of the present behavior and make people aware of the existence of the new, potentially better alternative (Holtgrave, Tinsley, and Kay, 1995). Weinstein says that the perception of personal risk does not come about all at once. His Precaution Adoption Process model suggests that creating awareness of risk is a three-stage process (Weinstein, 1988; see also Kunreuther, Sanderson, and Vetschera, 1985).

- Stage 1: The audience members have heard of the risks of continuing with the present behavior, but regard them as unimportant or irrelevant.
- Stage 2: They believe that there is a significant risk for others, but not themselves.
- Stage 3: They acknowledge personal susceptibility.

One of Weinstein's major contributions is to point out the difficulty in getting audiences to admit that a new behavior is necessary for them. He cites a number of studies (including Perloff and Fetzer, 1986; Svenson, Fischoff, and MacGregor, 1985; Weinstein, 1980, 1984, 1987) that demonstrate that target audiences very often will recognize a serious problem but will deny that it applies to them. This "optimistic bias" can come from incorrect information ("one of my children has had polio, so the others will never get it") or from a need to protect self-esteem or avoid fear (Weinstein,

1988, p. 363). Optimistic biases occur for risks that are rare, that people believe are preventable, and that are believed to appear early in life. Weinstein argues that providing general facts about risks will seldom move people beyond Stage 2; individuals must receive information about personal risk. Experience with the risk is, of course, a critical source of such information—but personal or mass media communications can be effective. Being told that others are taking precautions can help people to see the true extent of their own risk (Weinstein, 1983).

Weinstein also argues that for target audiences to contemplate action, they must pass through similar stages with respect to the severity of the risk and the effectiveness of the precaution. He suggests that audiences may have *minimum cutoffs* for both likelihood and severity before they are willing to move on. This is consistent with the formulation that a minimum level of awareness and interest (that is, perceived personal relevance) is necessary for consumers to move from Precontemplation to the Contemplation Stage of the model. The challenge, as Lewin would suggest, is to "unfreeze" consumers from their present behavior (Lewin, 1935).

Developing Messages

Of course, the place to start in developing messages is to conduct research with the target audience to learn what they know and what possibly can be changed. In a recent review of the quantitative evidence surrounding the practice of protected sex, Gortmaker and Izazola (1992, p. 56) listed thirteen factors that influence unprotected sexual behavior. In each case, they indicated the extent to which the factors were (a) important and (b) changeable. These factors are reported in Table 6.1.

Three of these factors are determinative in the Precontemplation Stage:

- Lack of knowledge of paths of HIV infection
- Lack of knowledge of condom use as preventative
- Religious beliefs

The first two are important and highly changeable: the latter is very hard to change—although not impossible. But how does

Table 6.1. Factors Affecting Protected Sex Behavior.

Importance	Changeability	Factor
		Predisposing
Medium	High	Lack of knowledge of paths of HIV infection
High	High	Lack of knowledge of condom use as preventative
High	High	Belief that condoms fail
High	Medium	Unwillingness to use condoms
Medium	Low	Religious beliefs
Medium/High	Low	Demographic variables
		Enabling
High	High	Availability and accessibility of condoms
High	High	Skills in proper condom use
Medium	Medium	Cost of condoms
		Reinforcing
High	Medium	Partner reaction and fear of it
High	Medium	Bad previous experiences with condoms
Medium	Low	Media emission of "not-proven news"
Medium	Medium	Alcohol and drug use

Source: Gortmaker and Izazola, 1992, p. 56.

one develop messages to move target audience members on to the Contemplation and Action stages?

Much of the literature on message development is implicitly or explicitly based on the McGuire's (1989) hierarchical model of communications effects. McGuire states that, if a campaign is to achieve a permanent behavior-change goal, the target customers must pass through these twelve steps:

1. Be exposed to the communication
2. Attend to it
3. Like and become interested in it
4. Comprehend it (learn what it says)
5. Acquire necessary skills (learn how to do what it recommends)
6. Yield to it (attitude change)
7. Store the message content or agreement to it
8. Search and retrieve this information
9. Decide on the basis for action
10. Behave in accord with the decision
11. Reinforce the desired actions
12. Consolidate the new lifestyle after the behavior

The first four steps of the hierarchy are relevant at the Pre-contemplation Stage. However, one immediately recognizes a serious problem: How does one get target audiences to expose themselves to a message, pay attention to it, become interested, and comprehend it, unless the topic is already something they know about or have any interest in? It is a classic Catch-22: audiences have to first be (at least marginally) interested in the message topic in order to process a message that is intended to get them interested in the topic! The problem here is that consumers engage in *selective exposure* and *selective attention* all the time. In part, this is simply to allow them to navigate through an information-dense world (especially in highly developed media environments). But also, it is in part to help people avoid topics they do not wish to contemplate. This is often the social marketer's dilemma!

Selective exposure: Here target audiences actively avoid exposing themselves to the target message. Thus, villagers neglect to go to a town meeting to discuss sanitation or birth control. Or a family with traditional values refuses to listen to a radio soap opera with so-called modern values.

Selective attention: Even though target audiences may put themselves in front of a social marketing message, they may not actually see or hear it. Three factors can occasion this. First, the target audience member may not be interested in the topic. Teenagers seldom look at life insurance ads. Older white people ignore rap music. Second, competition or clutter in the media environment may overwhelm the message. Today, for example, consumers in the United States are deluged with a great many health messages from both public and nonprofit sector and commercial sector marketers promoting exercise equipment, diet foods, and rejuvenating lotions and potions. A new behavior-change message faces stiff competition. Third, the ad itself may not speak to the target audience.

There are many approaches to overcoming these problems. They fall into four categories:

1. *Careful selection of channels.* If social marketers are clever in their placement of messages, making sure they are found in channels the target audience says it normally uses, then the exposure problem will be minimized.

2. *Use of dramatic design elements.* To overcome selective attention, social marketers can create messages that are unusual. Dramatic colors, bizarre designs, clever headlines, loud music, and so forth can all prove arresting.

3. *Use of familiar spokespeople.* Audiences will often attend to messages delivered by prominent celebrities, important officials, or simply people very much like themselves. In Jordan, HealthCom found from focus groups that the best spokesperson for their breast-feeding program was "an experienced woman [who] would understand the emotions of breast-feeding not 'just the facts' as a doctor would." As a consequence, the program created Doctor Huda (which means "guide" in Arabic) as "an older female physician who has seen many patients and breast-fed her own children." Radio spots featured Doctor Huda counseling young mothers with specific questions about breast-feeding. (Roberts and Seidel, 1993, p. 63).

4. *Use of already-familiar themes and values.* The tendency to avoid a message about a new topic can be overcome by connecting it to an old topic. Thus, for example, a marketer could begin a message with a subject in which research has shown the audience

is already interested. In the commercial sector, for example, a marketer of a new brand of peanut butter or automobile may start a commercial by mentioning an existing popular brand, and only later—once the audience is hooked—mentioning the new brand that is the real subject of the ad. Similarly, a social marketing message about vaccinations might begin with an accepted, interesting topic such as the value of schooling to children. Then, once the audience is hooked, the message can go on to introduce the new behavior-change proposal.

Overall, the objective is to look for what Wells (1989) calls "apertures." As Lefebvre and his colleagues describe it, *apertures* are the "times, places, and circumstances when the target is most likely to be receptive to the message" (Lefebvre and others, 1995, p. 223). For instance, a young person might be most receptive to a message about AIDS in a bar setting; an overweight person might be receptive to weight loss messages in a supermarket, or a mother might be open to vaccination messages on a video player in a clinic waiting room. In each instance, the target's focus is on the general topic area of the message. Use of the aperture may then induce the target to begin to contemplate the recommended action.

A technique that has been found very effective in a number of developing countries has been the creation of radio and television ads in the form of mini-dramas, as a way of hooking audiences by mimicking a very popular form of local entertainment. Thus, a thirty-second TV spot for ORS in Honduras had the following format: "[The screen] shows a young husband and wife concerned about their daughter who has diarrhea. A passing neighbor explains the dangers of dehydration and briefly tells them how ORS can help. He tells them they can go to the health center any time for assistance" (Rasmuson, Seidel, Smith, and Booth, 1988, p. 108). Clearly, this is little different from many soap operas and can be engrossing to many otherwise busy mothers and fathers for whom the soap opera was an aperture!

Customer-Centered Creativity

In creating the messages, a customer-centered social marketer will involve the target audience as much as possible in the design process itself to make sure that the message truly speaks to them. Sometimes this is done in a multistep process where formative research is conducted and messages are developed and then pretested one or more times until they are ready for launch. The Secretariat for Integrated Rural Development (SEDRI) child health project in Ecuador carried out all three of these steps at the same time (Pareja and Salazar, 1993). The SEDRI project had two broad objectives. One was to improve child health in rural communities. The other was to strengthen the communities themselves, that is, to improve community participation, increase the degree of social organization, and initiate development projects chosen by the communities themselves. The design of social marketing communications provided an opportunity to achieve both goals.

In creating a program to control diarrheal diseases, SEDRI decided to use multiple communications channels, including radio, print, and face-to-face communications. The latter would be carried out both by the usual health worker involvement and by community representatives. The latter were important to the joint objectives of the program, improving health while strengthening the community. The community representatives would serve two roles: they would be distributors for oral rehydration salts and they would conduct information sessions for mothers in groups and one-on-one.

Because the community representatives were not at all expert in presenting information to others in a more-or-less formal way, it was decided to give them formal training and to provide visual aids, particularly in the form of a flip chart. To design the flip chart, SEDRI and its HealthCom consultants decided on a unique approach. They hired an artist with experience diagramming and illustrating educational texts and sent him out to interact with mothers and develop the flip chart in the field! Because Ecuador has two major cultures, mountain and coastal, two separate flip charts were needed. But the process was the same. For example, to develop the mountain flip chart, the artist and the facilitator went to Salcedo in Cotpaxi Province and met with thirty-four mothers. As recently reported, the sessions went as follows:

> As the first step in producing the panel, [the facilitator] explained that a child's personal hygiene and the cleanliness of its surroundings can affect the child's health. The facilitator then asked: "How

can our artists show a dirty community? What should appear in the drawing to show that there are sources of infection around that might cause a child to get diarrhea?" The mothers suggested drawing the image of a child about three or four years old playing on the ground. Another mother suggested that the child should be shown eating from a plate on the ground. Another suggested showing a dog licking the child. The artist then sketched these different elements. One mother pointed out that the child should be pantless and that the child drawn was too fat. The artist corrected these elements in another draft. Another mother suggested that the scene should be set on the patio of a hut or house. Others suggested showing a chicken walking about and some flies on the food. [Pareja and Salazar, 1993, p. 122]

As a result of this process, nineteen panels were produced and tested with two other groups of mothers for:

- Comprehensibility
- Acceptability
- Attractiveness
- Relevance

The researchers considered relevance to be very important. "It is not enough that a mother comprehend the message. She must somehow make a connection between the picture and her own life. This is especially true when a program encourages behaviors that are quite different from those that have been traditionally or habitually accepted" (Pareja and Salazar, 1993, p. 124).

The Role of Emotions

There are a number of circumstances under which an emotional appeal may serve to move a target audience member to the Contemplation Stage (Monahan, 1995). Fear appeals have long been suggested as a way to get consumers' attention and interest (Janis, 1967; Averill, 1987; Peter and Olson, 1993). The difficulty here is that fear can have two competing effects (Hale and Dillard, 1995). On the one hand, when attended to, fear appeals can be motivating in encouraging people to think about taking precautionary actions (Rogers, 1975, 1983; Kunreuther, Sanderson, and Vetschera, 1985). On the other hand, fear can serve as a powerful force preventing attention from taking place. For example, women may avoid considering breast self-examination—and messages about it—simply because of the fear of what such an examination will find.

The literature seems to make clear that if fear is to be used, only a moderate level of fear would be effective in inducing further contemplation. It is necessary to balance the potential attention-getting and inhibiting effects of the fear-based message. What exactly constitutes the optimum level of fear to use in a given case is, of course, an empirical question to be addressed in the pretesting phase. Further, the literature suggests that, if fear is used, it should be directly coupled with some mechanism for its reduction.

However, there are many researchers and practitioners who feel that fear appeals will not be effective at all. In a recent review of health communications campaigns, Backer, Rogers, and Sopory conclude that "Campaigns for preventive behavior are more effective if they emphasize positive behavior change rather than the negative consequences of current behavior. Arousing fear is rarely successful as a campaign strategy" (1992, p. 30). Weinstein (1988) suggests that fear may be particularly counterproductive when dealing with existing problems rather than getting audiences to take precautionary actions against future problems.

Selecting Channels

Given that the broad objectives of the communications program have been identified—including a specification of the target audience to be reached—the next critical decision is the selection of channels through which the communications will be delivered. The decision is a very difficult one because channels vary enormously in their ability to be effective and efficient in achieving the program objectives. Basically, there are two broad formats that marketers can use: *impersonal* and *personal*. Each of these can be further divided into *advocate* and *independent*. Table 6.2 suggests the resulting options.

Of course, there are great variations within the individual options in each of these cells. For example, paid media include radio, TV, newspapers, magazines, billboards, posters, transit cards, and so forth. Finally, channels can vary depending on whether they

Table 6.2. Alternative Communications Vehicles.

	Advocate	Independent
Impersonal	Paid media advertisements	Newspaper columns
	PSAs	*Consumers Report* reviews
	Direct mail pieces	Magazine articles
	Videotapes, audiotapes	Soap operas
Personal	Professional consultations	Peers
	Work site lectures	Newscasters
	Fairs, events	Family members
	In-home "sales" visits	Religious figures
		Traveling entertainments

are highly *individualized* (direct mail, professional consultations, or peer discussions) or address consumers *in groups* (work site lectures and mass media advertisements).

Channels vary significantly in their ability to meet strategy objectives. In choosing among them, social marketers typically ask the following questions:

Is the channel best for the type of messages the program will use? Table 6.3 outlines some of the pros and cons of various types of mass media.

Will the channel enhance the message or detract from it? For example, a message describing the negative consequences of some existing behavior may have enhanced credibility if emanating from a newspaper article and, in some countries, have diminished credibility if it comes from a paid advertisement or a public health worker.

Will the channel efficiently reach the target audience? Will it reach a lot of people who are not part of the strategy? This criterion requires that, in choosing among alternative channel vehicles, commercial sector marketers carefully consider four factors:

Table 6.3. Strengths and Weaknesses of
Alternative Media for Nonprofits.

Strengths	Weaknesses
Television	
High Impact	High production costs
Audience selectivity	Uneven delivery by market
Schedule when needed	Upfront commitments required
Fast awareness	
Sponsorship availabilities	
Merchandising possible	
Radio	
Low cost per contact	Nonintrusive medium
Audience selectivity	Audience per spot small
Schedule when needed	No visual impact
Length can vary	High total cost for good reach
Personalities available	Clutter within spot markets
Tailor weight to market	
Magazines	
Audience selectivity	Long lead time needed
Editorial association	Readership accumulates slowly
Long life	Uneven delivery by market
Large audience per insert	Cost premiums for regional or
Excellent color	demographic editions
Minimal waste	
Merchandising possible	
Newspapers	
Large audience	Difficult to target narrowly
Immediate reach	Highest waste
Short lead time	High cost for national use
Market flexibility	Minimum positioning control
Good upscale coverage	Cluttered
Posters, Billboards	
High reach	No depth of message
High frequency of exposure	High cost for national use
Minimal waste	Best positions already taken
Can localize	No audience selectivity
Immediate registration	Poor coverage in some areas
Flexible scheduling	Minimum one-month purchase

Source: A Program Manager's Guide to Media Planning. Washington, D.C.:
SOMARC/The Futures Group, n.d. Used by permission of the publisher.

Reach: The number of different target audiences members who will encounter the message at least once.

Frequency: The number of different times a given reached person encounters the message.

Impact: The relative effectiveness of the given messages delivered through that medium.

Cost: The amount expended for each unit of communication—each ad, each lecture, or whatever.

If the various alternative channels have the same role to play, one can use a computer program (or some back-of-the-envelope calculations) to translate data (estimates or hard numbers) for each of these four variables into recommended courses of action based on some criterion. One frequently used criterion would be "cost per thousand target audience members reached at least four times" with the reach figure weighted by the estimated impact through the given medium. The result inevitably will be a mix of channels that collectively will either *maximize* the effectiveness of the communications outcomes for a given budget level, or *minimize* the level of expenditure for a given effectiveness level.

The more difficult case—and the more typical case—is where the different channels are assigned different communications roles. Thus, health workers might train householders in necessary skills, while radio advertisements teach people where to obtain required products or services and posters identify sales and service locations.

New Channels

Often imagination can suggest new channels that can be effective as program communicators. An example of such a program is that devised by the National Cancer Institute in the 1980s to work through dentists to reduce the incidence of smoking in America. The material in the next few paragraphs is drawn from Mecklenburg and others (1990).

As then-Surgeon General Louis Sullivan noted: "Tobacco use adversely affects both a patient's oral health and his or her overall health and well-being. . . . Dentists are trained to detect adverse oral conditions associated with tobacco use. Routine interactions with patients [provide opportunities] for dentists to describe to patients how tobacco use affects their health and advise them to stop. Simple, brief tobacco use interventions can be merged smoothly and appropriately into clinic schedules."

To make this channel effective, the National Cancer Institute had to first market the idea to the dentists. They did this using principles central to this book. They pointed out the benefits of this behavior to their dental practice and profits, their reputation in the community and among other health professionals, their skills in dealing with addictive behaviors, and their sense of personal contribution to a solution of a major social problem. They sought to minimize the perception of costs by noting that "dental practice abounds with 1- and 2-minute opportunities that can be used to provide practical bits of tobacco-related preventive and cessation information." And they sought to increase dentists' sense of self-efficacy by providing them a vast array of tools to work with, emphasizing that they can be effective because "oral health personnel usually have established a longstanding rapport with their patients" (a phrase dentists could appreciate) and noting that "There is evidence that many individuals will stop using tobacco simply because they are asked to do so in a positive, caring, and nonthreatening manner by a respected health professional." The program also kept the dentists' expectations for success low so that their sense of self-efficacy would not decline once they saw that perhaps three-quarters of those whom they induced to quit returned to smoking.

As recommended in the present volume, the program sought to get dentists to intervene in different ways depending on where the patient was in the behavior-change process. Thus, dentists were given different instructions for preventing a young person from initiating tobacco use, causing a tobacco user to contemplate stopping, motivating a tobacco user to stop, and sustaining tobacco-free behavior by a former smoker.

To assist these new channel members in this intervention, the National Cancer Institute also provided Tobacco Use Assessment forms for the dentist or the office coordinator for the program. They provided cessation information pamphlets, booklets, and self-help manuals to be given to patients. These materials were specifically designed for segments of the market such as smokers and smokeless tobacco users, youth, pregnant women, and minorities. They also provided doctors with names and addresses of other organizations that could provide other materials or support such as STAT (Stop Teenage Addiction to Tobacco) or DOC (Doctors Ought to Care). They also provided lists of community sources of withdrawal help for smokers unable to break the habit on their own, and templates for "Smoke-Free Office" notices.

One major virtue of this approach is that it uses personal channels of communication, which are particularly effective because they permit rapid feedback. A well-trained presenter can usually tell if the audience is understanding and retaining what is being communicated. He or she can probe the target audience and adapt the style and content to fit interests and processing capabilities. The downside of such channels is that marketers lose a fair bit of control. A message can be badly distorted, often in very subtle ways. For example, a lecturer using flip charts can very easily affect the apparent importance of various topics simply by the speed at which charts are flipped!

Popular Media

One approach that has been very effective in overcoming the problems of selective exposure and selective attention on the part of indifferent target audiences has been the use of popular forms of entertainment. This has come to be called the *Entertainment-Education Approach* (Rogers and others, 1989). It began in the 1960s with a soap opera in Peru called *Simplemente Maria,* which discussed family planning, among other topics. Miguel Sabido— a Mexican television writer-director who created six soap operas on social issues used throughout Latin America from 1976 to 1983—was an early exponent of the medium (Backer, Rogers, and Sopory, 1992, p. 168). More recently, the Johns Hopkins Population Communications Services group developed very effective episodes that brought family planning themes into a television variety show in Nigeria (Winnard, Rimon, and Convisser, 1987). In another instance, a radio soap opera in Jamaica, *Naseberry Street,* reached 40 percent of the country's audience promoting family planning (Rogers and Singhal, 1990).

Popular songs and popular singers have also been used to attract interest and attention. For example, HealthCom developed songs about breast-feeding for their program in Honduras (Rasmuson, Seidel, Smith, and Booth, 1988) and Swaziland (Roberts and Seidel, 1993, p. 59) and a song for schoolchildren in Swaziland on "the six killer diseases" (de Fossard, 1993). The latter was designed to get the children to bring the need for immunization to the attention of their parents. Perhaps the best known social marketing songs were developed by Johns Hopkins University's School of Public Health, first "Cuando Estamos Juntos" sung by Tatiana and Johnny in Mexico and Latin America and "I Still Believe" sung by Lea Salonga in the Philippines (Kincaid, Jara, Coleman, and Segura, 1988).

Traveling entertainers (puppeteers, actors, singers) have been used in developing countries to bring social messages out to remote villages. Comic books and foto-novellas have also been extensively used. An example of the latter was a foto-novella developed by the Ministerio de Salud Publica de Honduras called *You Saved Your Little Sister!* "This 21-page black-and-white photo novel tells the story of a baby girl, Estela, who has diarrhea and becomes dehydrated. The story is told from the point of view of her older brother, Mario, who first notices she is ill. As the drama unravels, Mario and his family learn how to identify dehydration and what to do about it. Discussion questions are included with the book" (Rasmuson, Seidel, Smith, and Booth, 1988, p. 117).

In the United States, various projects have attempted to get movie and television scriptwriters and directors to include social marketing messages in their productions. For example, the Harvard Alcohol Project convinced thirty-five prime-time television series to include "designated driver" themes in their programs during the 1989–1990 season (Winston, 1990). So-called Hollywood lobbyists are now seeking to have drug, AIDS, mental health, and environmental issues incorporated routinely in movies and television (Montgomery, 1988).

Repetition in Multiple Channels

In their recent review of effective health communications campaigns, Backer, Rogers, and Sopory (1992) offer twenty-seven generalizations about health communications campaigns. Five of these relate directly to the use of multiple simultaneous approaches to achieving campaign goals:

- *More effective campaigns use multiple media* (television, radio, print, and so on).
- *More effective campaigns combine mass media with community, small group, and individual activities,* supported by an existing communication structure (this involves using a "systems approach" to campaigns).
- *Repetition of a single message makes for a more effective campaign.* It may be in the form of retransmission of a specific message or transmission of slight variations on a basic theme.
- *Public service announcements alone generally do not effectively bring about behavior change.* PSAs should be combined with other campaign activities.
- *More effective campaigns use the news media* as a means of increasing their visibility.

All of these findings are consistent with the more general conclusion that the most effective communications are those that use multiple repeated messages in multiple channels, both paid and unpaid. This is true of communications at all stages of the behavior-change process, but particularly in the Precontemplation Stage, where one must break through barriers of ignorance and indifference.

Different Communications for Different Markets

As indicated in the previous chapter, markets must be segmented at the Precontemplation Stage as well as at any other time. There may, for example, be markets that are unaware of different things. For example, research on condom use among college students has indicated that the two sexes had different gaps in their awareness. Young men were unaware that many men were using condoms. They believed that if they did, they would seem to their dates to be "weird." Women, on the other hand, were unaware of ways in which condom use could be proposed as a means of enhancing the sexual encounter. Clearly, different information was needed for each gender group before they would seriously contemplate trying to use condoms in a given encounter.

Pretest Every Message

Several methods for pretesting ads were presented in Chapter Three. At the Precontemplation Stage, the most important trait to pretest in ads is *comprehension*. Social marketers need to communicate information—often substantial amounts of it, as in the early days of the AIDS epidemic. There are a number of computer-based programs that will assess the readability of text (for example, the "Fog Index"). But the final arbiter—as always—is the target consumer. Messages that treat delicate, complex subjects in sometimes complex language—for example, talking to your children about drug use—must be exposed to target audiences, and their recall and understanding carefully assessed. Tests should be performed on all segments of the market: a message on drugs that is clear to African-American parents may not be so clear to Asians, who come to the communication with different values and experiences.

Integrate Messages Internally

Campaigns have multiple communication elements—brochures, posters, public service ads, public relations releases, and so on. Each and every one of these elements must have the same basic message. Messages should not say something is easy in one medium and hard in another, even if the two messages are talking about different aspects of the topic. This is an easy error to fall into, because the marketer's knowledge of the field makes both messages make perfect sense. For example, one message in a program about family discussion of drug use may say that it is easy to discuss the different kinds of drugs that are out there and which ones are particularly bad—most kids today know this, even in elementary school. But another message may say that it is not easy to discuss why and how kids should resist temptations to get involved with drugs. Audiences exposed to both messages may simply be confused and unwilling to contemplate action because they think "Hey, those people don't know how to deal with this drug problem. What makes me think I can!"

Integrate Messages with the Rest of the Marketing Mix

Of course, communications are only one element of the overall marketing mix, albeit especially important at the Precontemplation Stage. Good marketers constantly seek out ways to make other elements of the mix reinforce the communications message. A good example is family planning campaigns that emphasize condom use. As noted earlier, one problem in getting teens and college students to use condoms is that they think this is a rare act that, if adopted, will make them stand out as odd. Constant repetition of condom promotions in many, many forums will help break down the sense that condom use is atypical. Unique packaging and point-of-sale displays can do a lot to reemphasize a message proclaiming the ubiquity of condom use. A campaign that uses brilliant package colors and includes package photos in all print and TV material is setting the stage for each exposure to a package or a display in a grocery store or pharmacy (or anywhere else they can be displayed) to significantly reinforce the primary thesis that "everyone is doing it!"

Evaluate Outcomes

It is important that social marketers continually monitor how they are doing so that they can adjust message campaigns as they go. Often such evaluations can reveal important omissions or misdirections in campaigns. For example, the PREMI vaccination campaign in Ecuador in the 1980s repeatedly used a logo that portrayed two adults and two children in stylized form. The children were known as the Premi kids. One of the objectives of the campaign was to make mothers aware that they had to get their children immunized when they were under one year of age. However, early evaluations of campaign messages revealed an important problem: mothers saw the Premi kids as relatively older—say, aged three or four. Thus, they concluded that vaccinations were not really necessary until the child was three!

As a result of that evaluation insight, the Premi kids were soon joined by a baby brother, named Carlito, who got across the message that vaccinations were indeed for the very young.

Changing Values

As Gortmaker and Izazola (1992) have indicated, changing basic values such as religious beliefs that militate against undertaking a new behavior can be highly important in social marketing campaigns, especially those involving family planning, child care, and the role of women. However, such values are difficult to change. There are typically only two possibilities for change. First, it may be the case that the target audience believes that they are adhering to some sort of prevailing religious or social norms but misunderstand those norms. Here, a simple correction, preferably by a religious or community leader, is all that is required.

The alternative scenario is that the norms are correctly perceived by the target audience but can be shown to conflict with other superior norms that support the proposed action. An example would be the mother who refuses to contemplate family planning because her husband does not want her to do so and she holds obedience to her husband as a very important value. There are several possibilities here—all of them difficult. First, the mother could be encouraged to value her role as household manager more highly than obedience to her husband. She could be shown that having too many children too rapidly makes her ill too often, and this in turn makes it impossible for her to take care of the house, feed her family and her in-laws, shop, tend the garden, and so on.

Other values that could be elevated are the mother's devotion to her children or her sense of her own self-worth. In the former case, if she can be shown that her existing children will suffer if she continues to have children (for example, because there will be less food to go around), her reaction may overcome her obedience to her husband. The latter case is more difficult but more profound. An increasing priority of a number of world health programs is empowering women in developing countries. It is argued that many present health problems stem from mothers not standing up for their own rights. Because they give in too often to husbands, mothers-in-law, traditional healers, village leaders, and so on, they do not take actions that are in their own—or their children's— best interests. The Academy for Educational Development is currently embarked on a project using social marketing techniques to increase the number of women in Bangladesh who are sent on to secondary school, a relatively rare event in a male-dominated society where the education of women has historically been seen as a waste of society's resources.

Summary

Social marketing strategies must adapt to the stage at which their formative research finds their target audience. In a great many situations—especially with new social issues—most target audience members are simply not thinking about the proposed behavior, that is, they are in the Precontemplation Stage. Three reasons target audience members do not move beyond this stage are that they are: (a) unaware of the new possibility, (b) believe that it is not appropriate for them, or (c) believe that it is against their basic values. The social marketer's challenge is therefore to create awareness, create interest, and (where necessary) change values. The tasks are primarily matters of education and propaganda.

Social marketers recognize that a major problem at the Precontemplation Stage is that they are competing with existing, often comfortable behavior patterns where change, *per se,* is undesirable. For health problems, it is possible to overcome such inertia by convincing consumers that they are at risk of some undesirable outcome if they continue their present behavior, the outcome is severe, and there is a course of action that can reduce the risk or the severity of the outcome. Once customers are convinced, they can then move on to the Contemplation Stage where they can factor in other considerations, such as the cost of the change, what others want them to do, and whether they believe they have the behavioral control to make it happen.

In order to reach Precontemplation consumers with messages advocating the consideration of a new course of action, social marketers must overcome two communications barriers, selective exposure and selective attention. People unaware of or uninterested in a topic may consciously avoid exposure to messages about it—or simply screen out messages when they are exposed. Careful choice of message channels, message designs, spokespeople, and message themes can often overcome these selectivity problems. Fear appeals can often be effective, but some social marketers regard them as likely to backfire.

Research has suggested that the most successful campaigns use multiple channels, combine mass media with small group and community activities, repeat the message frequently, and make use of the news media. Among the channels that can be particularly effective are the popular entertainment media. Messages about new behaviors can be inserted in traditional vehicles such as soap operas, plays, popular songs, comic books, and foto-novellas to great effect.

Changing values is probably the most difficult challenge at the Precontemplation Stage. These values are usually drawn from the individuals' upbringing or from the community surrounding them. The greatest effects can be achieved if target audience members can be shown that they misunderstand community values or if they can be shown that the new behavior is compatible with higher social values, such as being a good mother or supporting the community.

Chapter Seven

Making the New Behavior Attractive and Low Cost: Benefit and Cost Strategies

Our concern in this and the chapters to follow will be the Contemplation Stage of the behavior-change process. Thus, we will focus on individuals who are already aware of the possibility of action and who are not opposed to it on the basis of important religious or social values. At the beginning of the Contemplation Stage, they may have limited information and will have formed only vague intentions. However, as they progress, they will become more and more involved in the issue, gather more and more information, and take a reasonable length of time before deciding to go ahead. During the Contemplation Stage, there are four major things they think about:

- What will I gain if I undertake this proposed behavior?
- What will it cost me to do it?
- What do those who are important to me want me to do?
- Can I actually carry it out?

Of course, they think about these things not only for the proposed behavior but also for its competition (most typically, the status quo). From the marketer's standpoint, other things equal (which I will discuss below), behavior is likely to occur if and when the outcome of this thought process leads consumers to conclude that, on balance, it is better to go ahead with the recommended behavior than with its competition. Consumers believe they can undertake the behavior and conclude that they should pay the costs in order to get the expected gains or to accede to social pressure.

The marketer's task is "simply" to make this outcome occur! The overall approach can be summarized in the acronym *SESDED*. What the marketer must do is:

CREATE A *S*UPERIOR *E*XCHANGE (COMPARED TO COMPETITION) THAT IS *S*OCIALLY *D*ESIRABLE AND *E*ASILY *D*ONE.

There are five principal strategies that the marketer can take to induce a given target population to undertake the desired exchange:

- Increase the expected gains.
- Decrease the expected costs.
- Increase the present social pressure.
- Improve the consumers' ability to act.
- Decrease the desirability of competitive alternatives.

In the commercial sector, the fifth strategy is very often chosen because the marketplace is essentially a zero-sum game. One firm's gain in market share is another firm's loss. So one can often increase market share, not by pointing out the good features of one's own product or service or reducing its negative features, but by pointing out the weaknesses of competitors' offerings. Classic examples of this strategy are found in the marketing wars between AT&T and MCI, where each side accuses the other of wasting customers' money! However, fighting the competition in the social marketing world is a tricky proposition. At some levels (such as competing with unhealthy current practices) it is a good thing—but at others (such as competing with other brands or types of oral rehydration solutions) competition makes little sense. In the former case, it is a zero-sum game; in the latter, it is clearly a positive-sum game. My subsequent discussion assumes that the only competition is an undesirable present behavior.

For social marketers, the choice among the five strategies depends on two factors: (a) where the target audience stands now and (b) what leverage exists for each alternative. This is why research is so important at the formative stage of any strategic process.

But one might first ask: Why not just do everything? That is, a marketer could attempt to change gains, losses, social pressures, and behavioral control all at the same time while simultaneously bad-mouthing the competition. Surely this would work! But there are three problems here. First, most social marketers will not have the funds or the energy or the consensus to do everything at once. Second, a core strategy that does everything will have no focus and consumers will be confused about what the marketer is really try-ing to get at. Finally, there is the serious danger that the strategies will be incompatible. For example, suppose a marketer decides to increase both group pressure and perceived gains. If the group does not perceive the gains in the same way as the marketer is proposing to the individual, the result will most likely be, at best, confusion on the part of the consumer or, at worst, distrust of the marketer for saying things with which others (who are probably more trusted) disagree!

Given, then, that most social marketers will not want to try everything at once, what should come first? The ultimate answer in each strategic situation will depend on the behavior in question and on the target audience. However, some generalizations can be offered based upon past experience and what is known about con-sumer decision making:

The relative importance that consumers place on benefits and costs shifts over the stages (Prochaska and DiClemente, 1984a). In early stages, they emphasize benefits; in late stages they emphasize costs. Thus, we may expect that consumers who are early in the Con-templation Stage will probably be most responsive to *benefit-centered* strategies. They will:

- Place more emphasis on benefits than costs
- Be aware of relatively fewer benefits
- Not yet have thought seriously about efficacy or behavioral control issues

Consumers who are late in the Contemplation Stage will prob-ably be most responsive to *cost-centered* or *behavioral-control-centered* strategies. They will:

- Be aware of most of the major costs and benefits
- Place more emphasis on costs than benefits
- Be concerned about their abilities to carry out the behavior (see Prochaska and DiClemente, 1985)

Consumers who are members of tightly knit social settings who have limited personal autonomy will probably be more responsive to *social pressure* strategies.

Consumers with greater information-processing skills (that is, the more literate or more educated consumers) will be more responsive to *benefit/cost* strategies.

In the remainder of this chapter, I will consider how to go about creating benefit-based or cost-based strategies. I will show how marketers can analyze the type and importance of various costs and benefits and how to use that information to develop different strategies. In the next chapter, I will consider strategies that focus on social norms and behavioral control.

It should be noted that the alternatives discussed in these chapters are of three broad types. First, information has an important role to play in telling consumers about the reduced costs and improved benefits of options and their alternatives, and about the behavior of others whom they consider important. Second, market conditions have a role to play in making it possible for the behavior to take place. Consumers cannot have behavioral control over AIDS-preventing behavior if they cannot easily and cheaply acquire condoms. Third, skills play an important role, again in giving the consumer a sense that he or she can actually accomplish the desired behavior.

Benefit-Based Strategies

Benefits are the positive consequences that target consumers believe will occur if they undertake a proposed behavior. As shown by the discussion of consumer behavior in Chapter Four, one can think of each of these benefits as having two characteristics: the likelihood that it will occur, and the value or importance that the consumer places on the outcome.

This means that there are basically three alternatives that social marketers have available to them to increase the total perceived positive outcomes of an exchange.

1.   *Take a positive outcome that the consumer thinks might happen if the action is undertaken and increase the perceived likelihood that it will occur.* For example, the marketer could learn that a target mother believed that a better diet might make her child grow up stronger and be a better worker in the family fields as a teenager. The marketer could provide growth chart information showing the difference that a better diet makes.

2.   *Take a positive outcome that a consumer thinks is very likely to happen but is not very important and increase the importance or desirability of that outcome.* For example, the mother may think that a better diet will almost certainly cause the child to be healthier and happier, but, given all of her other concerns in life, this is not her most important objective. Here, the marketer could point out that a healthier and happier child is likely to take up less of the mother's time because the child is less often lazy, irritable, and confrontational, and more often will volunteer to take on extra chores.

3.   *Add a new positive outcome.* Here, a marketer might reward visits to a health clinic with periodic food supplements that would increase a child's health and that would also reduce the household's food expenditures.

Determining What to Do

The starting point for crafting a *benefits approach* is to ask customers at the formative research stage two very simple questions: What positive things do they think will happen if they undertake the desired behavior? and How important are these things to them?

This should first be done in an informal setting as part of pilot research. If done thoroughly by a trained researcher with a very wide cross-section of possible target customers, it will yield marketers a list of the possible benefits that consumers think about. When soliciting this information, there are two important considerations to keep in mind:

• *Ask about benefits, not attributes.* Naive researchers in both the commercial and nonprofit sectors often ask consumers to describe their ideal product or service. Thus, one might ask, What would an ideal health clinic in your village be like? or What would an ideal weight-loss program be like? Such questions typically yield a list of attributes, not benefits. For example, in response to the question about a weight-loss program, a respondent might mention wanting:

A small group

Low costs

A group comprised of people of similar sex and age

Fast results

A female leader/instructor

No criticism of participants' past behavior

The problem with this list is that it does not tell the marketer why the individual wants the particular attribute. Each attribute must be linked to an underlying benefit (or set of benefits) so that the marketer will know how to make the experience more closely meet the consumer's needs and wants. *Attributes data* can be very ambiguous. Take, for example, an individual's desire for a small group in a weight-loss program. The mention of this attribute could mean that he or she is seeking any one—or several—of the following benefits:

The chance to make new friends

Having more time spent on my problems

Being able to speak up more easily about my problems

Having the leader get to know me and my problems better and so provide better help

The chance to stand out if I'm successful in losing weight

Clearly, a marketing program designed to induce this person to join a weight-loss program that emphasized the fact that groups were small and that this would mean "more attention to your problems" would be well off the mark for the target customers who wanted small groups so they could make new friends. These customers might feel that having too much attention paid to their problems might interfere with their ability to make friends because it could single them out as having serious problems.

Changing the benefits of a behavior often means changing its attributes. Marketers can manipulate attributes relatively easily. Packages can be made easier to open, health clinics can be decorated in warmer colors, staff can dress more professionally. What is critical, however, is not that attributes are changed but that these changes deliver real benefits to consumers. It needs to be stressed again: *consumers do not seek attributes,* they seek benefits.

In formative research, the key to learning about benefits is always to ask consumers who mention attributes why they want these particular attributes.

- *Link benefits to deeper values wherever possible.* The question *why* is very helpful not only in revealing the benefits that underlie attributes but also in revealing the values that underlie particular benefits. Values are "the mental representations of our underlying needs, after they have been transformed to take into account the realities of the world in which we live" (Wilkie, 1990, pp. 213–214). Behaviors ultimately are means we take to achieve particular ends. Value researchers believe that we can construct better behavior-change programs if we can link the desired behaviors to fundamental life-objectives. Such a linkage will help marketers understand why particular benefits are important or unimportant to consumers.

Value researchers distinguish between two kinds of values (Rokeach, 1973): *terminal* or end-state values and *instrumental* or means values. Examples of the former would be personal happiness or wisdom. Examples of the latter would be behaving honestly or caring for others' needs. The set of values that most individuals strive for is determined in large part by culture or subculture and is relatively enduring. Thus, respect for elders is an important instrumental value in Japan but much less so in the United States. By contrast, excitement would rank high as a terminal value in the United States but less so in Japan. The importance of various values is not permanent over one's lifetime. Young people may place emphasis on excitement and fun and enjoyment in life while those over sixty might stress security and self-fulfillment. There are many lists of values. One that has been used in marketing is Lynn Kahle's List of Values (Kahle, 1984). Kahle lists nine basic terminal values:

- Self-respect
- Sense of accomplishment
- Self-fulfillment
- Fun and enjoyment in life
- Security

- Being well respected
- Sense of belonging
- Warm relationships with others
- Excitement

One of the research techniques that help commercial sector marketers to follow the linkage from attributes through benefits to values is called *laddering* (Reynolds and Gutman, 1988). Researchers begin by asking consumers what attributes they would like to see, say, in a new health clinic. Then they ask them why they would like to see that attribute. This typically leads to a listing of one or more benefits. For each benefit, the researcher then asks why the consumer would like to have that benefit. This may yield more benefits, which should prompt more *why* questions. One continues asking *why* questions until values are expressed and until there appears to be no deeper level of explanation possible. Such values research would allow social marketers to position new offerings or new attributes as meeting basic values that are extremely important to their target audiences.

An example of laddering research used to generate message themes for promoting breast-feeding (Gengler, Oglethorpe, and Mulvey, 1995) is reproduced in Figure 7.1. In this study, interviews of a sample of breast-feeding mothers revealed a number of attributes of breast-feeding they considered important: no bottles; inexpensive; provides natural nutrition, including immunities; and offers phsycial contact with the child.

Further, as the figure shows, the attribute "no bottles" leads to the benefit of "convenience," which in turn is linked to another benefit, "saves time," which along with the benefit of "reduces stress" yields an important basic value, "a better family life." As can be seen, seven basic values were identified in the study. The two mentioned most often (as indicated in the size of the circles) were that the mother would see herself as a good parent and that she would have a close, bonded relationship with her newborn. These basic values can then be the basis of a message strategy that links the behavior of breast-feeding to being a good mother and developing a great relationship with the baby. The reader can easily imagine the warm, fuzzy images that could accompany such themes.

- *Pay more attention to benefits of the behavior itself than to the long-*

Figure 7.1. Reasons Why Mothers Choose
Breast-Feeding over Bottle-Feeding.

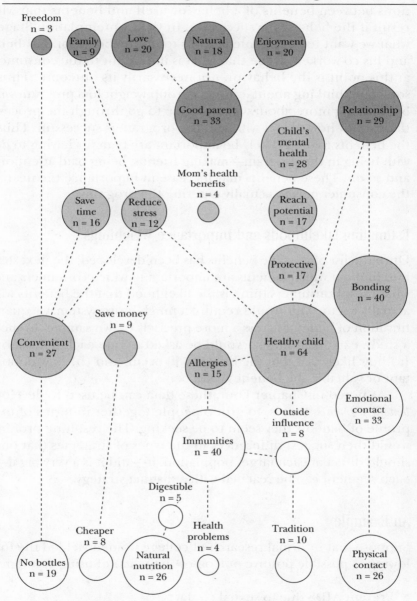

Source: Gengler, Oglethorpe, and Mulvey, 1995. Used with permission.

term outcomes of that behavior. Just as it is useful to make distinctions between instrumental and terminal values, one can make distinctions between benefits of a behavior itself and benefits that will result if the behavior is successful. In the Contemplation Stage, what we want to get people to do is to try the behavior. Fishbein and his co-workers argue that what is important to the consumer at this point is the behavior, not necessarily its outcome. Thus, someone thinking about joining a group weight-loss program will be thinking more about what it is like to go through the process than about how nice it will be if the program is successful. Thus, the benefits that will likely be important are benefits having to do with being in the program—making friends, being paid attention, and so on. These benefits may increase in importance the nearer the consumer gets to actually entering the program.

Estimating Likelihoods and Importance Weightings

Once the list of possible benefits has been developed, the next step is to find out which benefits are important to which consumers and what these consumers think is the likelihood that the benefits will actually occur. This would require a much more systematic quantification of benefits across a more precisely drawn sample. In such a study, each respondent would be asked to rate each benefit on (a) how likely is it that the benefit will occur, and (b) how important or valuable the benefit would be.

As noted in Chapter Four, these data can be used to develop *benefit segments,* that is, to group people together in terms of the profile of benefits they seem to be seeking. The resulting profiles would then suggest differences in the types of strategies that one should direct at each target population, if—and it is a very big if—each segment can be reached with a distinct strategy.

An Example

Suppose that informal research of college women yielded the following as possible positive outcomes (benefits) of using condoms:

- Prevent AIDS due to sexual contact
- Prevent other STDs due to sexual contact

- Assert control over the woman's own body and health
- Assert power in the woman's relationship with her partner
- Increase the depth of the woman's relationship with her partner
- Increase possibilities for foreplay
- Demonstrate up-to-date knowledge and behavior ("be cool")
- Demonstrate a sense of responsibility

Further, suppose a follow-up study of a random sample of women enrolled at Whitman College (fictional name) rated the likelihood of each outcome and its importance to them as shown in Table 7.1 (each measure is on a seven-point scale).

What then does one learn from this information about possible benefit strategies? One way to view the data is in a two-by-two table, plotting likelihood on one axis and importance on the other. Table 7.2 helps us consider the implications of Table 7.1.

Cell 1: Likelihood High, Importance High. Three benefits fit this category: preventing AIDS, preventing STDs, and being responsible. This set would comprise benefits that the program would want to maintain. That is, the marketers would particularly want to make sure to find out quickly and take corrective action if consumers at some point begin to doubt that condoms would be effective against AIDS and STDs. For example, program managers should be alert

Table 7.1. Benefits of Using Condoms.

Consequence	Likelihood	Importance
Prevent AIDS	6.35	6.62
Prevent STDs	6.11	6.65
Assert control	5.39	3.41
Assert power	2.89	3.66
Better relationship	3.28	6.94
Better foreplay	2.05	5.88
Be cool	3.93	5.95
Be responsible	5.11	5.62

Table 7.2. Likelihood and Importance of Benefits.

	High Likelihood	Low Likelihood
High Importance	1. Maintain	4. Increase likelihood
Low Importance	3. Increase importance	2. Ignore

for rumors in the community or new research studies showing failure rates (which there are) that might affect perceived likelihoods.

Cell 2: Likelihood Low, Importance Low. One benefit falls into this sector: Asserting power in the relationship. Presumably, among these students, power is not an important objective in male-female sexual relationships (although it may be very important in other parts of the relationship). As a consequence, this may well be a benefit that the social marketer may wish to ignore.

Cell 3: Likelihood High, Importance Low. One benefit fits here: asserting control over one's own body in the relationship. Condoms are seen as likely to give the young woman more control. Unfortunately (from the marketer's standpoint), college women do not rate this benefit as particularly important. The issue facing the marketer at this point is whether to attempt to increase the importance of this benefit. In general, it is difficult to change importance "weights" for a benefit, in part because these weights are tied to more fundamental values of the individuals. These deeper values are likely to be linked to a wide range of behaviors. For example, asserting control over one's body may be linked for many women to fundamental values about male-female relationships and about fairness. (Of course, this would need to be researched.) For example, female body control may be related to female equality (to men); those who value female equality high will also value asserting control over one's body highly and vice versa. Thus, a low importance score in the example here may reflect low interest in female equality on this particular campus. Presumably, this low interest in female equality on the campus will be linked to other campus behaviors such as attendance at Women's Study courses, membership in radical women's groups, attendance in date-rape seminars, and so on. For the marketer to change the importance score for a specific benefit buried within this complex set of values and behaviors would seem to be a particularly difficult task. However, it should be noted that this is not always the case.

Cell 4: Likelihood Low, Importance High. There are three benefits falling into this category: improving the relationship with one's partner, improving foreplay, and "being cool." In each of these cases, the benefits are important to the young women, but they do not think that using condoms can yield the desired outcomes. The marketer needs to take one additional step at this point, and assess whether the perception of low likelihood is a *reality problem* or a *perceptual problem.* That is, is it that there really are few possibilities to improve foreplay with condoms, or is it a matter of knowledge and belief? Depending on the answer to this question, the marketer's options differ:

- *A Reality Problem.* If the behavior does not really meet the target audience's needs, the marketer can consider improving the product or service just as they would in the commercial sector. In the case of condoms and foreplay, the marketer will have to find ways to really increase the possible benefits. Thus, the marketer might consider researching the use of condoms in foreplay to see whether innovative options could be created to increase college women's beliefs that condoms do, in fact, meet their needs for better foreplay.

- *A Perception Problem.* If exciting foreplay options already exist and the college women simply do not know about them, the marketer's problem is much simpler. A perception problem is more a problem of effective communication.

There are a great many ways to increase the real benefits that a behavior will generate. Some are inherent in the behavior itself, as in the case of increasing the foreplay pleasure from using condoms. Others involve associations with the behavior. There is a long history in commercial sector marketing as well as in the broader world of social behavior and politics where behaviors have changed because their associations change. Many young people took up smoking in the mid-twentieth century because the behavior was associated in the movies with specific sophisticated actors, with sexual prowess, and with tough-guy machismo. Today, the clothing styles and speech patterns of young people are strongly influenced by what rock musicians do.

Commercial sector marketers make use of this phenomenon all the time, most dramatically with the use of prominent spokespeople. Nike running shoes and Gatorade use basketball superstar Michael Jordan in their commercials because research has undoubtedly shown them that customers buy and use the products so they can "be like Mike!"

Choosing the Best Benefit Strategy

Asking target consumers about the good things that might occur if they undertake a desired behavior can be a very useful basis for a behavior change strategy early in the Contemplation Stage. And the framework in Table 7.2 offers the social marketing manager a way of thinking about the strategic possibilities. However, it does not offer enough information to make a final choice. There are four additional factors the manager must consider:

1. *Can I believe the data?* I have assumed that the research findings outlined above were perfectly valid. However, this may be a risky assumption, especially with respect to (a) high-involvement, potentially embarrassing behaviors and (b) many behaviors in cultures discouraging candor with relative strangers—such as interviewers.

2. *Are benefits that respondents say are important predictors of present intentions to act the same benefits that will get the target audience to change behavior (or increase their intentions)?* One possibility that would confound that conclusion is if the two dimensions, likelihood and importance, were correlated. Indeed, some researchers have argued that measuring consumer importances is unnecessary because consumers implicitly fold importances into estimates of likelihood. That is, they say to themselves: if it is not going to happen, it is not important—and vice versa.

In the example, I noted that the likelihood that using condoms would allow a woman to exert power in a relationship was low and, in sexual settings, the importance of exerting power was also low. But suppose the social marketer could develop a campaign to induce college women to believe that they could exert more power by insisting on the use of a condom in sexual encounters. Is it conceivable that now, because the women believe that it is possible to exert more power in a sexual encounter, they are willing to entertain the possibility that exerting power in this aspect of their relationship might be a very important thing to have happen, as in other aspects of their relationship (chore sharing, bill paying, leisure decision making, and so forth). In this case, we would have to conclude that the "power" benefit may not be (presently) important, but it may be *determinative,* that is, be the one that determines what course of action will be taken.

3. *Can I change the beliefs about likelihood or the importance weights?* As suggested earlier, a benefit may be important, but if the marketer cannot conceive of a way of changing the attributes that generate it (for example, the unsexiness of condoms), this benefit is not going to be determinative either. In the same sense, an unimportant benefit may be perceived to be very likely if the behavior could be undertaken but it may be impossible to change its weighting. For example, condoms may allow a woman to exert power, but today in many third-world cultures, a woman would not even think about exerting power. In fact, in such cultures, the "power" benefit may never appear in the set of relevant benefits!

4. *What will it cost to change beliefs or importances?* This is an issue of both dollars and time. Changing some beliefs may be relatively easy, especially if it is merely a matter of correcting misinformation or misperception. However, changing other beliefs and changing most importances may take a very long campaign and a very large budget. In part, the ability to change benefits is a function of three things:

The target audience's willingness and readiness to change

The immutability of the belief or importance

The social marketing organization's own capabilities to create the change

A final consideration, of course, is whether a benefit-based strategy should be carried out alone or in conjunction with components from one of the other three strategy domains: cost, social pressure, and behavioral control.

It is at this point that managers who face decisions about benefit strategies earn their salaries! In the commercial sector, marketing managers are often paid very high salaries to make bet-the-firm decisions about basic strategy on the basis of incomplete, conflicting, and potentially inaccurate data. Good managers know that the odds of making good decisions are significantly increased if one becomes totally immersed in the available data, particularly data on the target customer. While managers like to think that good decisions are made on the basis of good instincts (the "golden gut"), these instincts may simply be the result of the subconscious calculations of a mind thoroughly steeped in market data.

Cost-Based Strategies

The other side of the customer exchange is, of course, costs. For everyone on every occasion, taking an action involves some kind of cost—at minimum, the effort of overcoming routine practices and avoidance of the issue. Evidence from Prochaska and DiClemente's long series of studies makes clear that the closer consumers come to undertaking action—that is, the further along they are in the Contemplation Stage—the more important costs become in their decisions. And as Weinstein (1988) points out, costs—particularly short-term costs—are certain, whereas many of the benefits of social behaviors are hypothetical. Taking time to go to a clinic for a vaccination is a very real near-term cost, whereas protecting a child from a relatively rare disease may seem to many mothers as only hypothetical—they see no clear evidence that vaccinations work. Vaccinated children do not get disease, but who knows what causes this? For consumers in the late Contemplation Stage, the social marketer's principal focus must be on cost-reduction strategies—often along with efficacy-enhancing strategies, as I will discuss in the next chapter. It may be, as Wright and Weitz (1977) have pointed out, that marketers should focus on short-term costs. Consumers do appear to weight these costs more heavily in decisions, as economic theories of discounting and approach-avoidance theory (Ajzen, 1985) would suggest. However, as Weinstein concludes, "Prevention campaigns try hard to make long-term benefits salient and often ignore short-term costs" (1988, p. 374).

The approach to evaluating the cost-based options and determining a precise strategy is virtually identical to that suggested for benefits in the previous section. We shall proceed through the steps one would take to develop cost data for the hypothetical Whitman College women.

1.   *Develop a list of the kinds of costs that consumers may think about when considering a particular course of action.* This can be achieved through informal research such as depth interviews or focus groups, preferably with consumers relatively far along in the Contemplation Stage. The marketer must be sure to ask target consumers (a) to indicate costs related both to the behavior itself (*instrumental costs*) and costs related to the outcome, should the behavior turn out to be permanent (*terminal costs*), and (b) to indicate why each cost is important to them, to shed light on the way specific costs are linked to more fundamental values.

2.   *Carry out more formal research with a representative sample of target consumers,* asking them to indicate for each cost (a) how likely they think it is that the cost will occur, and (b) how important the cost would be to them should it occur. Let us assume that the set of costs that the hypothetical Whitman College woman says she is considering are the following:

- Cost money that could have been spent on other things
- Interrupt personal pleasure during sex
- Reduce partner's pleasure during sex
- Offend partner by implying he might have AIDS or an STD
- Force unwanted discussion about sexual history and sexual attitudes
- Create impression of being too easily frightened, a worrier
- Create impression of being undesirably experienced in sex
- Cause worry about parents discovering condoms

3.   *Determine whether the target audience should be segmented into subgroups on the basis of cost profile.*

4.   *Develop final strategies by calculating mean values for each cost on likelihood and importance dimensions.*

5.   *Plot each cost in a four-cell diagram* like Table 7.4. Hypothethical means for the Whitman sample are given in Table 7.3.

6.   *Consider possible strategies for each of the four cells plotted in Step 5.* In this case, it is useful to consider the cells in a different order (though the cell numbers are the same as before, for consistency).

Cell 2: Likelihood Low, Importance Low. This is the ideal situation, but it still needs monitoring. In the example, it applies to concerns about seeming like a worrier or seeming too experienced.

Apparently, the Whitman women think these costs are unlikely to occur and are not very important. However, social marketers should be alert to changes in the environment or competitors' actions that may increase the salience or perceived likelihood of these costs. For example, suppose *USA Today* headlined a study that says "Girls Who Have Lots Of Sex Most Likely To Insist on Condoms!" Assuming that for the sample, the cost of "seeming too experienced" is linked to an important underlying value like "wanting enduring male relationships," the *USA Today* headline might significantly increase the importance the target audience places on the cost of appearing too experienced. This change in weighting might be enough to keep many women from beginning to use condoms—and might, in fact, cause some of those who have already been insisting on their use to discontinue doing so.

Cell 4: Likelihood Low, Importance High. Vigilance is even more critical here. Costs are not perceived as very likely but are high in importance. At the moment, the one cost in this cell should not be a major deterrent to behavior, because it seems unlikely to occur. However, because it is a cost dimension that is quite important to the consumer, it is probably one that she is consciously or unconsciously monitoring very closely. In this category is the perceived cost of having the use of a condom spoil the woman's pleasure. Presumably, the sample of women have learned, either

Table 7.3. Costs of Using Condoms.

Consequence	Likelihood	Importance
Cost money	6.35	1.62
Spoil own pleasure	2.11	6.65
Reduce partner's pleasure	5.39	6.23
Offend partner	5.89	6.61
Force unwanted discussion	5.28	3.94
Make me seem a worrier	2.05	2.88
Make me seem too experienced	2.93	2.95
Must deceive parents	5.11	3.12

through their own experience or through word-of-mouth from their peers, that using a condom will not interrupt their pleasure significantly. Suppose that the major reason for this is that men on the Whitman campus have generally been thoughtful about discretely putting on a condom before sex begins. Suppose, however, that men change their behavior for some reason. The women may then begin to find (or expect) that future sexual encounters are going to be ruined because their partners will have to stop to put the condom on. Again, this changed cost circumstance may significantly decrease condom use.

Cell 3: Likelihood High, Importance Low. This too is a situation to watch closely because it could explode into a serious impediment to program success. In the example, the scenario applies to the economic cost of condoms, the question of deceiving parents, and the perceived cost of having to have a discussion of each partner's sexual history and attitudes toward sex. In the latter case, the women in the sample apparently feel that, yes, it is going to happen, but, no, it is not a big deal. Vigilance on the part of marketers is still important. For example, suppose sexual politics heats up as a campus issue and sexual partners now feel compelled to "work it all out" before using condoms. Many women may now think that this is going to be a major cost and avoid bringing up condom use because they do not want to "get into all that sexual politics stuff."

Cell 1: Likelihood High, Importance High. This, of course, is the major category that the social marketer needs to worry about and the one that is most likely to be preventing women from asking men to wear condoms. There are two cases like this in the sample, reducing the partner's pleasure and offending the partner. As with benefits, the social marketer has two options here:

Table 7.4. **Likelihood and Importance of Costs.**

	High Likelihood	**Low Likelihood**
High Importance	1. Reduce cost	4. Be vigilant
Low Importance	3. Be vigilant	2. Ignore

- *Reduce the importance of the costs.* This may be difficult to do, particularly if the costs are tied to important underlying values. In the example, both costs in the cell may be related to the value of "being considerate of others." To reduce the importance of the costs, the social marketer would, in effect, have to get the women to be more self-centered. This would seem like a particularly difficult challenge but one that some marketers may believe ought to be undertaken. That is, the marketer may feel that the women are putting themselves at risk by putting too much weight on pleasing men. The social marketer may feel that the socially responsible strategy is one that evens the playing field.

- *Reduce the perceived likelihood.* This, in many cases, may be the best strategy. However, there are two possible realities that the social marketer could face. One is that the perceived likelihood is accurate: Men at Whitman may feel that their pleasure is really reduced with a condom. They may really be offended if a woman asks them to wear one. Here, the social marketer's challenge is to change the men. In the case of sexual pleasure, it may be a matter of teaching women to give pleasure from using a condom. In the case of personal offense at being asked to wear the condom, perhaps a campaign aimed at men to make them more thoughtful of women's concerns would reduce the frequency with which they would indicate that they were offended by being asked to wear a condom.

The second possibility is that the women simply misperceive men's responses to wearing, or being asked to wear, a condom. The appropriate marketing campaign could involve getting men to talk more with their partners and tell them the truth about these two issues. Alternatively, it could involve some sort of media campaign to inform women about the men's true feelings. In the latter case, the use of spokespeople—especially if they are real, preferably well-known, campus figures—can be very effective.

Combined Strategy

Of course, in most situations, the target customer will be looking at both costs and benefits, and trading off one for the other. Indeed, one of the problems with the approach cited above is that it involves focusing on individual costs or benefits, on the assumption that a change in a single belief or importance will yield the desired outcome. This is probably rare. As discussed in Chapter Four, individuals are more typically making choices between bundles of benefits and bundles of costs. They may often be willing to give up some amount of a desired benefit if this also means that they can avoid or minimize an important cost. Alternatively, they may be willing to put up with an additional cost if it means that they get an additional important benefit. It is the combination that is important.

Economists have a useful framework for thinking about this problem. It involves utility theory and indifference curves. While the complexities of this framework are beyond the scope of this book, the model implies that, in designing their final strategies, social marketers should seek out the ideal combination of costs and benefits that will yield the maximum total expected satisfaction by the target audience.

Take the example of immunization services. Let us assume that research in an underdeveloped country has shown that consumers in a district typically consider two benefits and two costs when thinking about having their children immunized. These are:

- *Benefits:* Each child will require less illness-care in future (terminal benefit), and I will be treated well (respected, listened to) during the immunization visit (instrumental benefit).
- *Costs:* It will take a large amount of time to go to the clinic (instrumental cost), and it will take a large amount of time to be served when I get there (also an instrumental cost).

Assume further that the social marketer with a limited marketing budget is considering setting up an immunization program in the district. The district has, say, twenty-five villages and ten thousand target mothers spread over a fifty square mile area. The marketer has a number of alternative ways to spend the marketing budget. (Note that everything on the following list is a marketing activity, and that, in the last two cases, the marketer would be changing an attribute that is assumed to be linked to a specific cost.)

- Mount a media and village lecture campaign promoting the joys and the time and effort saved due to having a healthy child, thus increasing the first benefit.

- Conduct extensive training and follow-up of health care workers to induce them to be more customer-centered and respectful of their clients, increasing the second benefit.
- Place more clinics in more villages, decreasing the first cost.
- Increase the amount of volunteer staff at each clinic and improve the efficiency of the immunization process, decreasing the second cost.

Given that the marketer can't work on all four possible areas to the same degree, the question becomes one of deciding which area—or, more probably, which combination of areas—to develop. Let us assume that there are three realistic levels of action for each of the variables at the marketer's control:

- *Health Promotion:* Add minimal, modest, or significant amounts to the promotion budget.
- *Training:* Do nothing, or add modest or significant amounts.
- *Additional Clinics:* Place clinics in 5, 8, or 10 villages.
- *Volunteer Staff:* Leave unchanged, or increase by 10 percent or 20 percent.

This gives the marketer eighty-one possible marketing campaigns. Here are three of the possibilities:

Combination 1

A modest campaign directed at increasing perceived favorable illness outcomes a modest amount

An extensive training program for staff to make them very respectful of patients

Clinics in five villages

Increasing volunteer staff by 10 percent

Combination 2

A major campaign directed at increasing perceived favorable illness outcomes a significant amount

A minor training program for staff to make them somewhat more respectful of patients

Clinics in eight villages

Increasing volunteer staff by 20 percent

Combination 3

A modest campaign directed at increasing perceived favorable illness outcomes a modest amount

No training program for staff, as they are already respectful of
patients

Clinics in ten villages

Increasing volunteer staff by 20 percent

Faced with all of this—and seventy-eight other possibilities—
how is the marketer to make a choice? One obvious solution is to
return again to consumer research (the reader must be accustomed to this answer by this point in the book) and ask consumers
for their preferences among combinations of benefits and costs.
Fortunately, one need not present consumers with all eighty-one
combinations. In cases like this, commercial sector marketers and
researchers take advantage of a technique called *conjoint analysis*
(Green and Srinivasan, 1978; Green and Krieger, 1991), which
requires consumers to rank only a specific subset of the combinations. One reason the number of combinations can be reduced is
that one can assume that consumers would always like more of
each benefit and less of each cost.

The conjoint technique produces three kinds of information
that will be particularly valuable to the marketer. It will indicate
which of the given combinations is preferred (overall and by individual segments), and it will estimate the importance weighting
of each of the four variables (two costs, two benefits) that the
entire group of respondents (but not each individual) is implicitly using when they rank the combinations offered to them. Most
important, by assuming a linear progression of values between levels that were offered to consumers, it can indicate optimal levels
of the variables for each segment or the population overall—even
when those levels were not among the specific options offered for
consideration.

For example, a computer programmed for conjoint analysis

might extrapolate from the combinations offered the villagers in the hypothetical study and say that the combination that, if offered, would have been ranked the highest is:

Between modest and significant health promotion

Close to significant health worker training

Clinics in seven villages

An increase in volunteer staff of 12 percent

This combination is optimal only from the standpoint of the target consumers. It assumes that unit increases along each dimension cost the same to produce—which is not likely to be the case. To increase the number of clinics by 20 percent may cost four times as much as a 20 percent increase in health promotion. However, if the social marketer can specify the cost function for each marketing variable (that is, the dollar change in cost for each unit increase in the marketing variable), then another technique called *linear programming* can be used to estimate one of two things:

- The combination of levels of variables that will yield the maximum impact on the target consumer group for a given budget (an *effectiveness* criterion)
- The combination of levels of variables that will achieve a given impact for the least cost (an *efficiency* criterion)

Finally, the marketer may wish to explore the impacts of reducing total costs by working only on one or two variables at a time, given the management time involved in more complex solutions. Strategies that strongly emphasize one or two variables would be consistent with earlier recommendations for social marketers to intensely focus their limited resources.

Adding Benefits

It very often turns out that a large proportion of a target market is unlikely to undertake the desired behavior given their current perceptions of the costs and benefits. It can be excessively difficult or costly for the social marketer to improve existing costs or benefits enough to produce action. It is at this point that a marketer will think of adding benefits as a tactic for bringing about the desired behavior change.

There are a great many possibilities here and, inevitably, both the alternatives available and the best choices among them will depend on the situation. Further, as I will note in a moment, there are important ethical considerations. However, the classes of added benefits that a marketer might consider are the following:

- *Unrelated Material Bonuses.* A great many social marketing programs have offered material bonuses to consumers to get them to undertake desired behaviors or to get them to expose themselves to information or skill training that will move them closer to action. These can be material bonuses for all participants such as the plastic water container a mother gets for attending a workshop on how to mix oral rehydration solution or the radios the People's Republic of China gave out to women who had tubal ligations and that India gave out to men who had vasectomies. Sometimes they can be merely chances to get material bonuses, as when the HealthCom Project in The Gambia offered women who attended an ORS mixing clinic a chance to win a radio.

- *Related Material Bonuses.* Bonuses need not be unrelated to the behavior being promoted. Thus, a woman attending a child health clinic could receive free ORS packets, food supplements, or Vitamin A capsules. Women or men attending a condom skills training program could receive free condoms. Drug addicts attending an AIDS information presentation could get free clean needles. And so on.

- *Unrelated Services.* It is very common in the United States to make magazines and television available in the waiting rooms of hospitals. In the United States, this is generally regarded as a technique for reducing perceived waiting time. (And it is the perception that counts! Many hotels have installed television monitors near elevators, having found that this reduces complaints about slow service.) In developing countries, such entertainment services may be very much appreciated by men and women who otherwise have little access to such treats. They also welcome other forms of entertainment, including movies and comic books.

- *Related Services.* In many situations, marketers can achieve a behavioral goal by combining it with some other service the target customer would appreciate. An example would be the opportunity for a mother taking her child to be immunized to:

Have the child weighed and have the weight compared to a growth chart

Receive information on other child health issues

Receive instruction on child care skills such as deworming, lice control, mixing of baby formula, and so on

Ethical Issues

As many readers are aware, there is an important practical and ethical issue here. The problem is that an extrinsic reward or benefit is likely to cause behavior that is carried out primarily in pursuit of the reward. The result is behavior that is not likely to be permanent (because it is not internalized) and that is very often not in society's interest. There are many examples of the socially deleterious effects of providing extrinsic rewards for behavior. For many years, commercial blood donation clinics paid individuals for donations. Over time, these clinics became major sources of Hepatitis B infections and major sources of worry in the early days of AIDS. The problem was that many donors who needed the money would lie about whether they had conditions that would make their blood potentially dangerous.

Another well-publicized case is the use of radios to promote vasectomies in India. It was the feeling of many observers that many of the men having the procedure did not really understand—or did not want to understand—that the procedure was not reversible. They were so pleased to have the chance to obtain a cherished good, they acted against what they saw as their family's long-term interests.

Thus, program managers need to be extremely careful in their use of extrinsic rewards to promote desirable social behavior. This is especially so when the rewards are unrelated to the behavior in question—although it does apply to all extrinsic rewards. It is no more unethical to persuade an unsuspecting man to get a vasectomy because he will receive a five-year supply of condoms to fight AIDS than it is to offer him a radio.

In my view, this caution is particularly important for social marketers. As noted in the Introduction, many critics associate marketing with manipulative commercial sector techniques that get people to buy wasteful, unneeded products and services. It would do great damage to the cause of social marketing if we in the field are tainted in the future with scandals like those of the blood clinic and the Indian vasectomy program.

Summary

Once target consumers have moved to the Contemplation Stage, they begin to think about four sets of factors, the benefits and costs of the proposed behavior, the wishes of friends, relatives, and colleagues, and whether they have the behavioral control to actually make the behavior happen. With respect to benefits and costs, the social marketer simply (or not so simply) has to convince the target audience that the cost-benefit trade-off or exchange is superior for the behavior than for its competitors (including inertia). Because the relative importance of benefits and costs varies over the Contemplation Stage, consumers who are in the Early Contemplation Stage will likely be most responsive to benefit-centered strategies while those in the Late Contemplation Stage will likely respond most to cost-centered strategies. A benefit-cost focus is probably best for consumers with good information-processing skills. Social pressure strategies are better for consumers in tightly knit social settings or with limited personal autonomy.

Benefits-based strategies can have one or more of three possible objectives: increasing the consumer's perception that particular positive outcomes will occur, increasing the importance or desirability of those outcomes, and adding new positive outcomes. Formative research is the best source of information on which of these approaches is likely to be most effective. When conducting such research, it is important to look for benefits and not for attributes, to try to link benefits to deeper values, and to focus on the benefits of the behaviors themselves rather than the longer-term outcomes to which they will eventually lead.

Strategies will vary depending on whether particular benefits are rated by target consumers to be high or low on likelihood of occurrence or high or low on importance. In some cases, the problem is to change customer perceptions of the benefit; in others it is a matter of changing its reality. Cost-based strategies can be approached in the same way. Marketers need to assess whether consumers think particular costs are likely or unlikely, important or unimportant. Again, the strategic options can involve changing realties or changing perceptions. Very often, marketers will want to combine benefit and cost strategies because, for consumers, life involves constant trade-offs between choices that always have some costs. Conjoint analysis is a technique that can be helpful in understanding how consumers make these assessments.

A final approach in a benefit-cost strategy is to add benefits. Among the options the marketer can consider are related or unrelated material bonuses and related or unrelated services. Where the added benefit is unrelated to the behavior in question, social marketers must consider the ethical implications of what they are doing. They must ask: Is it right to use extrinsic rewards to induce a behavior that a society thinks is desirable but that the target audience member at the moment may personally prefer to avoid?

Chapter Eight

Bringing Social Influence to Bear and Enhancing Self-Control

Persuasive marketing strategies that focus only on costs and benefits can be very effective in bringing about desired behavior change. However, if social marketers stop there, they make a number of very critical assumptions, which they may not even notice. Pure cost-benefit marketing assumes that research can reveal all the needed information on perceived costs, benefits, importance weightings, and competition. More importantly, it assumes that the behavior in question is totally under the control of the target consumer, that is, that he or she is free to carry out the behavior at will, without regard to the opinions of others. It further assumes that the target customer believes that he or she has the capacity to carry out the recommended behavior.

In many cases, these conditions may prevail. A good example would be a social marketing program designed to induce sedentary consumers in a developed country to undertake an exercise program. Such behavior is primarily under the individual's personal control and requires little or no equipment. The target audience will be reasonably articulate about its perceived costs and benefits and how this information is processed. And many target audience members may undertake this behavior for reasons independent of what others think, that is, they do it for themselves. (This does not mean they do not appreciate or respond to positive feedback from others.) The only possible problem is that some may believe that they do not have the willpower to make it happen!

Under this very specialized scenario, the behavior may be said to be *under personal cognitive control.*

Alternative Scenarios

This specific set of conditions is, however, likely to be relatively rare. Three alternative scenarios may be much more common.

1. *Perceived lack of capacity.* For a great many behaviors of special interest to social marketers, action will not be undertaken even though the target audience personally prefers to do so because they do not believe they can carry it out and stick with it. This is typically the case for smoking cessation or weight-loss behaviors. Here, consumers would like to quit smoking or overeating, but feel that they just aren't capable of doing so. It is a scenario in which personal preferences are not enough to make the customer go forward.

2. *Perceived opposition.* For other behaviors, action will not come about even though the target audience personally prefers to do so because other individuals or groups that are important to them do not support the behavior. Examples here would be family planning behavior, alcohol or drug recovery, and safe sex. Here, the target consumer would like to, say, practice family planning—but spouses, relatives, even village leaders do not at all approve.

3. *Perceived social mandate.* For a final class of behaviors, action will come about despite target audience members' personal preferences—in the face of their outright opposition, reluctance, or indifference—because they believe they must conform to what others expect of them. In many cases, personal preferences may adjust to support the conforming behavior after it is taken on. For example, one may argue that current reduction in smoking by those employed adults in the United States who still smoke is being driven mostly by social pressure and does not necessarily result from smokers' personal decisions.

These distinctions have several implications for the social marketer. First, in a great many social marketing situations, the initiation of desired behavior will not take place unless the social marketer ensures that target consumers have the necessary skills and self-confidence in their own abilities to take action. But this may still not be enough. Social marketers may also have to ensure that other individuals who are important to target audiences support the proposed behavior change. In addition, there may be some situations in which the marketer can largely ignore individual consumer preferences by making social pressure irresistible.

Increasing Social Influence

Behavior change does not take place in a social vacuum. The broader society and its cultural norms and values have important roles to play, as do individual co-workers, friends, and family. The impact of cultural norms is largely accounted for in Chapter Six through their influence on individual cost and benefit criteria and on the weightings given them. But cultural norms and values also have an impact on the extent to which target audiences pay attention to and succumb to the wishes of others. Others are almost always involved, playing several roles—providing information about the potential benefits and costs of taking the action, serving as role models, and bringing direct pressure to act in the desired way.

Others as Sources of Information

In a seminal study of political behavior fifty years ago, Lazardsfeld, Berelson, and Gaudet (1944) asked voters how they acquired information that influenced their political preferences. Because there was an explosive growth of mass media during this period, researchers expected people to report that they got their information from newspapers, magazines, and the radio. But they were surprised to learn that most people reported that they learned about candidates and positions from somebody else. The researchers hypothesized that the role of the mass media was to transmit important information to key people who, in turn, would pass it on in a subsequent step to the masses. They termed this process the *two-step flow of communication*.

This finding was replicated in a wide range of studies on the diffusion of innovations (Rogers, 1962, 1983). This research found that most target populations had a set of *opinion leaders* who were among the earliest adopters of new ideas and behaviors, and who subsequently influenced followers among the *early majority* who rapidly accelerated the new behavior's adoption and acceptance.

This body of research makes it clear that, in each strategic situation, social marketers need to determine whether interpersonal communications are important channels through which individuals receive information about social behaviors (see Kunreuther, Sanderson, and Vetschera, 1985). If so, the marketers need to find out who in these social networks are likely to be the major *forwarding stations* for the messages. In situations where these interpersonal networks are important, even crucial, decisions about communications campaigns based on the media preferences and exposure of the final target audience may be irrelevant. The only thing that may be relevant is the media preferences and exposure of the network's opinion leaders!

Fortunately, there is a methodology available for detecting these opinion leaders. Actually, there are three approaches. The first and most expensive is to develop a sociometric diagram of the connections among the people in the social system. Sociometric studies may be feasible in small social systems like villages in developing countries and tightly knit neighborhoods in larger cities. The ethnographic technique involves asking people such questions as:

- To whom do you turn for advice with respect to the behavior domain in question?
- To whom do you give advice?
- With whom do you talk about other subjects of importance to you?
- To whom do you turn when you need help in the behavioral area?
- With whom do you socialize?

Where sociometry is not feasible, a second approach is simply to ask people to name those who have the reputation for being influential in the behavioral subject area. Finally, one can ask for self-reports wherein individuals indicate whether others turn to them for information or advice.

At first glance, all three techniques may seem entirely too costly for low-budget social marketing programs. However, it may be the case that formative studies in a target market will reveal consistent patterns that identify opinion leaders not by idiosyncratic characteristics but by their role or status in each society. Thus, in the area of health care in developing cultures, it may be found that the opinion leaders are:

- Village elders
- Traditional healers
- A few older women with large families
- Elected leaders
- Senior doctors (if any)
- Heads of local clinics (if any)
- Pharmacists
- Employers

In this case, social marketers need only to discover who these people are in all of the villages in their target market and, more importantly, discover how to reach them with what message.

Information about opinion leaders may also be useful to social marketers planning a regionwide mass media campaign. If the social marketer knows what kinds of people are looked up to as opinion leaders, these kinds of individuals can become characters in social marketing soap operas or can be characters in posters or advertisements. They are the kinds of people social marketers should use to endorse a product, service, or new behavior. Experience has shown that the ideal traits for endorsers are:

- *Expertise.* Good endorsers know what they are talking about. The former basketball superstar Michael Jordan is the ideal endorser for Nike sneakers and Gatorade high-energy drink. He would be less effective as an endorser for computers or TV dinners!
- *Trustworthiness.* Some individuals are good endorsers not for what they know but because the target audience believes that anything they vouch for is likely to be good. This undoubtedly explains the effectiveness of Bill Cosby, who over the years has been an endorser for computers, Ford automobiles and Jello pudding! Presumably endorsements from trusted newscasters like Tom Brokaw or Peter Jennings for just about anything would be highly effective.
- *Empathy.* A final trait that affects effectiveness is the endorser's similarity in values to the target audience. Thus, movie

director Spike Lee is an effective endorser for Nike not because he is a shoe expert or because he has some inherent trustworthiness but because he shares many of the values of young black males who are prime customers for Nike gear.

When attempting informational campaigns across entire markets, social marketers would do well to test alternative spokespeople with representatives of the target market across these three critical traits. Neglecting such research can lead to much wasted— even counterproductive—effort. A U.S. campaign by a headache remedy many years ago used John Wayne as its endorser. After many months on the air, the sponsor pulled the ad because it was having absolutely no effect on sales to the target audience. The advertising agency presumably was surprised at this turn of events because Wayne was extremely popular and had a reputation as being a straight shooter both in his movie roles and in his private comments. Subsequent evaluation of the campaign illuminated the problem. Wayne clearly possessed the second and third traits of an ideal endorser. The problem was: no one believed that John Wayne ever got headaches, or that if he did, he would do something so craven as take a painkiller. People figured he would just tough it out as he did in all his movie roles.

Others as Role Models

Earlier sections of this chapter illustrated how other individuals can serve an important function in social marketing campaigns by acting as role models. Role models are individuals who communicate to target consumers not only what can and should be done but also how to do it. The latter is particularly important in helping consumers build self-efficacy. The best people to serve as role models may or may not be the same people the social marketer uses to provide information. Probably, an elderly male village leader who could be very important in telling families about the importance of giving oral rehydration solution to children with diarrhea cannot serve as a role model for mothers as to when and how to carry out the behavior. A separate piece of research may be necessary to establish who is best for this purpose.

However, if the social marketing campaign lacks the budget for such research, a number of principles can be applied to the selection of the best role models. Private sector marketers have known for a very long time the importance of choosing the proper role model. Many of the same principles apply to social marketing. Basically, private sector marketers look for three characteristics in an ideal role model:

- *The role model must be someone the target audience can identify with or look up to.* That is, they must belong to either a *normative* or *aspirant* reference group. This means that the role model should share similar values with the target audience or hold values that the target audience would like to share some day.
- *The role model should be someone who is respected* by the target audience as someone who has time and again provided good guidance on new behaviors.
- *The role model should be in similar circumstances to the target audience* with respect to the target behavior.

The last characteristic would appear to be a necessary condition. That is, the best role model for a child health campaign would be someone who has children of the appropriate age. A good role model for a condom-use AIDS campaign directed at sexually active gay males would be a gay male. And a well-known juvenile Hollywood actor or actress would be the best role model for a campaign designed to cut down on teenage drinking. Such people could not only help explain the appropriate behavior to target audiences and show how it is actually done, but implicitly give their approval or endorsement to its being undertaken.

Others as Sources of Social Pressure

In a classic research experiment in the 1950s, Solomon Asch asked groups of college students to compare two drawn lines and to indicate which one was longer (Asch, 1952). All members of each group except one were confederates of the researcher and were trained to (incorrectly) vote for the shorter line. The target group member then faced the choice of voting on the basis of his or her own perceptions or going along with the group. While not the majority, a very significant number of these students submitted to group pressure and chose the shorter line contrary to the evidence their own eyes presented them.

The willingness of individuals to subvert their own judgments to the collective will has a very long history. In its scariest incarnations, it explains the success of demagogues like Hitler, Mussolini, and Saddam Hussein in recruiting citizens to take actions that are against their own moral codes and their own expectations and preferences. In more mundane settings, it explains the willingness of individuals to go along to a movie starring their least-favorite actor because it is the preference of the other members of the group. It partially explains the behavior of the individual in a restaurant who waits until everyone else orders and then makes a choice that, in some sense, conforms—if not mimics—the choices of the other diners. It also explains a number of behaviors that individuals avoid. In the United States, men do not wear shorts to work in banks or dresses while selling shoes in the mall! And it explains the behavior of the smoker who finally tires of having to go outside on the front porch during a party in order to have that important cigarette and gives up the habit.

These situations vary in a number of important respects. They differ in terms of whether the behavior:

- *Requires group consensus* in order to be carried out. This is the case of the movie decision.
- *Requires group permission* to be undertaken. This is the example of the shorts in the banking environment. If an individual undertakes the forbidden behavior, he risks being fired. Of course, management can decide to change its corporate culture and permit this new behavior. Many firms, indeed, have "casual clothes days," especially in hot summer months. Firms such as Apple Computer pride themselves in their lack of sartorial conformity. Again, for the individual to change, the larger collectivity must change.
- *Is designed to provoke group approval.* This is the situation in the restaurant, where the individual has an opportunity to make an oddball choice but may prefer—or be driven—to make a choice others will applaud.
- *Is subject to group pressure.* This is the case of the smoker suc-

cumbing to the wishes of friends and strangers who frown upon the undesirable behavior and, on the other hand, are likely to praise the turnaround in the person's actions.

A wide range of cognitive theories about consumer choice and behavior incorporate a role for social influence. For example, in the Theory of Reasoned Action (Fishbein and Ajzen, 1975), behavioral intentions are seen as driven by two sets of factors. The first is the individual's perception of personal consequences of taking the behavior. This component is often called "the attitude toward the act." The second component is the influence of others, or what they call *subjective norms*. In their model, Fishbein and Ajzen suggest that the subjective norms factor has two components. First, there is what they call *normative behavior*. This is what the consumer believes to be expected by groups whose opinions matter to him or her. There may be many such groups, including immediate family, parents, peers, co-workers, religious figures, and so on. What is important is not what these groups really want the person to do but what the person thinks that they want.

In the Theory of Reasoned Action, normative behavior (what others want) is treated as a dichotomous variable. Either the group wants the individual to do the target behavior or not. However, in reality, all of us are familiar with situations in which someone important to us wants us to do something and makes it very clear that this is something wanted a great deal. The wife who threatens to move out if the husband does not "quit trying to kill himself by smoking (eating high cholesterol foods)" is certainly sending a much stronger message than if she said "Gee, dear, it would awfully nice if you quit that (those) bad habit(s)." It is clear that there is a quantitative difference between influence and pressure.

The second component of subjective norms in the Theory of Reasoned Action is called *motivation to comply*, defining the extent to which the individual is likely to go along with the wishes of each particular group. The overall Subjective Norm is then a sum of Normative Behavior times Motivation to Comply for all of the significant groups, which in effect makes this a component in which the elements are compensatory. That is, a negative norm from one important group can be counterbalanced by a positive norm from another.

Thus, in the Theory of Reasoned Action, there are two major determinants of behavioral intention, the individual's personal attitude toward the act (that is, beliefs about the likelihood of various outcomes times the value of those outcomes) and the subjective norms affecting the individual. However, the relative importance of these two components may differ depending on two factors: the individual and the type of behavior.

With respect to individual differences, sociologist David Reisman pointed many years ago that people differ significantly in terms of the source of values by which they guide their lives. Some people, those Reisman called *Inner-Directed,* have internal gyroscopes that tell them what to do. They pay little attention to other individuals and groups. A second group, called *Other-Directed,* are individuals who have large and sensitive antennae paying close attention to what others expect of them. They do not make a move without checking it out with those who count in their environment. (Reisman proposes a third class of individuals whom he labeled *Tradition-Directed.* These are people who proceed through life guided by the lessons of the past. In the model proposed in this volume, this set of influences would have already been incorporated in the set of importances that individuals attach to various consequences.)

In the context of the Theory of Reasoned Action, an Inner-Directed individual would be driven largely by the Attitude Toward the Act component whereas Other-Directed individuals would be driven by the Subjective Norm component. Thus, the relative contribution of social influence will vary across individuals based upon more enduring personality traits. It will also vary across behavior types, particularly whether the behavior is public or private and whether it involves others directly or indirectly. Other things equal, one may expect private, solitary behaviors like many forms of exercise to be minimally influenced by social norms (although outcome goals may not). On the other hand, public behaviors often undertaken in and around others, such as smoking, are likely to be heavily influenced by group pressures. The response may also be related to other individual difference variables such as age and gender.

Finally, it is worth noting that group influences on individuals can operate both on the proposed behavior and on its competitors.

The latter is certainly the case for so-called problem behaviors such as drug use, smoking, and practicing unsafe sex. Here the pressure vectors are directed at the behaviors that others want stopped, not at their substitutes. That is, group pressures are on giving up a behavior. In some sense, the group does not care what the new behavior is (for example, whether the smoker takes up chewing gum or knitting), only whether the old behavior is abandoned.

On the other hand, social norms may have impacts on the new behavior. Thus, community pressures to get mothers to use ORS during episodes of diarrhea, or to feed their children Vitamin A, are directed at a new behavior. In each of these cases, there is really no important competitive behavior that the community would want to suppress (except perhaps in the case of ORS, where they may wish to discourage certain unhelpful traditional methods of treating diarrhea). And of course, there are behaviors where social pressures may be directed at both the old and new behaviors. This would be the case, for example, with changes in diet, where family members might bring pressures to bear on an overweight father to cut down on old high-cholesterol food items and also to substitute more fruits, grains, and vegetables in his diet.

Implications

The preceding discussion has several implications for social marketers. First of all, it is clear that for many individuals and for many behaviors, strategies that are solely aimed at changing cognitions about possible consequences (that is, influencing the individual's own attitude toward the act) will not be effective. Second, it obviously follows that an extremely important task during the formative stage of the strategic planning process is to gain an understanding of the extent to which interpersonal influences are likely to be important for one or more target groups.

If it is learned that group pressures are going to be important, then the next task for the social marketer is to learn the following:

- Which segments of the target population are likely to be most susceptible to this pressure?
- What are the most frequently mentioned groups that are likely to bring these kinds of pressures?

- What does the target market think that the groups of significant others want of them? That is, are others perceived as favoring or not favoring the behavior?
- What is the strength of the influence these significant others bring to bear?
- What is the relative likelihood that each group will have an influence on the target audience in the future?
- Just what do these target groups really think about the target behavior?

Once the fabric of the social influence structure is revealed to the social marketer, the next step is to put this component to use. Let us return to the example of the use of condoms by the partners of college women. Assume that research has revealed that the hypothetical Whitman College women pay attention to four groups in various areas of their lives: their parents, their close friends, other college women they perceive as resembling themselves, and their teachers. At many colleges and for many students, religious counselors would also be important, but I will simplify the discussion for the purposes of this example by considering only secular influences. Further, let us assume that the influence factors for this target market are those represented in Table 8.1.

With this information in hand, the social marketer can now consider a number of options in order to increase the likelihood that the target audience would undertake the desired behavior:

Table 8.1. Condom Use Influence Factors.

Group	Perceived Position	Actual Position	Degree of Pressure	Motivation to Comply
Parents	Against	For	Moderate	Low
Close friends	For	For	Moderate	High
Other women	For	For	Low	Moderate
Teachers	For	For	Very low	Low

- Change the perception of the parents' position from against to for (and then increase the students' motivation to comply).
- Change the perceived degree of pressure from other college women.
- Increase the motivation to comply with the wishes of teachers or other college women.

Assuming the social marketer chooses the second option, increasing the pressure from other college women, then a choice must be made as to whether to do so directly or indirectly. Direct pressure could be exerted though what is often called a *mobilization* campaign, where members of the target population are organized to achieve some important social goal.

Indirect pressure is often used in social marketing through effective media campaigns or through public relations. There are a number of possibilities:

- Identify one or more opinion leaders in the target populations and use them as spokespeople in advertisements, posters, brochures and the like.
- Use models in ads, posters, and the like who seem to be part of the influence group and have them offer opinions and advice that imply that this group strongly supports the use of condoms in sexual relations.
- Report statistics that indicate the extent to which other college women are engaging in the desired behavior and use this as a platform for urging the desired behavior.
- Create stories, films, soap operas, and the like showing members of the influence group actively supporting the desired behavior.

Increasing Perceived Behavioral Control

In order to induce individuals to move on to the Action Stage of the behavior-change process, marketers need to help them develop a sense that they can actually carry off the behavior. This is especially important during the Late Contemplation Stage, where individuals are getting closer and closer to taking action, or when they are in what Prochaska and DiClemente (1983) would call the

Preparation Stage. Many authors, beginning with Bandura (1977a), have called the sense that one can complete an action *perceived self-efficacy.* Others, such as Ajzen (1991), refer to it as *perceived behavioral control.*

Bandura (1986) defines perceived self-efficacy as "people's judgments of their capabilities to organize and execute courses of action required to attain designated types of performances" (p. 391). Bandura and his colleagues (Bandura, 1977a, 1977b, 1978, 1982, 1986; Bandura and Adams, 1982; Bandura, Adams, and Beyer, 1977) argue that self-efficacy is one of the most important prerequisites for behavior. Many other scholars recognize the importance of this factor (see Maddux and Rogers, 1983). For example, in 1988, Rosenstock, Strecher, and Becker decided to add the concept of self-efficacy to the well-known Health Belief Model (HBM) they had developed thirty years earlier. However, as Rosenstock notes (1990, p. 45), self-efficacy is not important for some behaviors of interest to social change specialists, particularly one-time behaviors that involve little more than being available to receive a service such as a vaccination against some important disease. The problem for marketers here is getting the person to show up for the vaccination. Marketers do not need to teach people skills about receiving injections!

On the other hand, the challenges are significantly greater for the consumer considering major lifestyle changes such as family planning or safe sex or considering giving up problem behaviors such as smoking, overeating, or alcohol abuse. In these cases, informal field research techniques such as focus groups or depth interviews can be used to induce consumers to reveal inadequacies that they may have difficulty either recognizing or articulating in more formal settings.

Field research will typically reveal that perceived behavioral control has two components. Balch (1974) labels these as *internal efficacy,* the person's sense of possessing the skills and knowledge to take the proposed action, and *external efficacy,* the person's perception that the action can actually take place, that is, that circumstances, the behavior of others, and so on will allow it to happen.

An absence of internal efficacy typically results from one or both of two deficiencies: lack of information or lack of skills. Action may not be undertaken because a consumer may not know where to obtain contraceptive products or how often and when to take birth control pills. A mother may not know the proper age for a child to be immunized. An overweight person may not know what foods are the most problematic. Even when consumers have this kind of information, they may lack the skill to use it. Action may not be taken because a man or woman may not know how to put on a condom (and take it off after sex). A mother may not know how to mix an oral rehydration solution and induce her child to drink the entire batch. A prostitute may not know how to negotiate with a client to get him to use condoms. A smoker may not have techniques to deal with the inevitable urge to resume smoking. In all cases, the problem is one of learning.

In the case of external efficacy—the consumer's sense that the environment will permit the behavior to happen—the barriers to action are relatively easier to deal with because they are often under the marketer's direct control. Condoms can be made available when college women need them. ORT solutions can be widely distributed in developing countries for mothers to get when their children have diarrhea. Health clinics can stay open during convenient hours and can have transportation available so mothers and patients can reach them easily. Formalities that stand in the way of immunizations and enrollments in drug counseling programs can be reduced. In each case, consumers must come to feel that none of these things will stand in the way of achieving mastery over the behavior.

However, there are many situations in which environmental conditions will prove effective barriers to action. When white U.S. southerners refused to provide vaccinations to blacks fifty years ago, there was little a social marketer—let alone the blacks themselves—could do to make the option possible. If curbside pickup of recyclables is not available in a community, efforts to encourage householders to recycle may not succeed because they will perceive that given their time constraints they will not be able to do it. In such cases, social marketers might do well to shift their definition of the target market from the individuals to the community.

A number of studies by Rotter (1966, 1982) and Kelley (1973) have shown that individuals who perceive that the locus of control for any proposed behavior is largely internal will more likely undertake it. And indeed, why should they try to undertake something if they really have no control over whether action will be successful and lead to desired outcomes? In such circumstances, it becomes the marketer's responsibility to make sure that the consumer has no excuse for concluding that he or she is not actually the one in charge.

Impersonal approaches can be used to provide crucial information and skills to increase consumers' sense of personal mastery. These approaches involve the use of the media both for advertisements and for public information campaigns. Print and radio sources are particularly good at communicating information that specifically addresses knowledge deficiencies. A number of social marketing campaigns have made extensive use of soap operas on radio and television as means of communicating important information to increase audience self-efficacy. Soap operas are extremely popular all over the world and carefully attended. Social marketers can use them not only to communicate information but also to change values and beliefs about outcomes (the focus of the previous chapter).

Social Learning Theory

Self-efficacy also comes about from learning specific skills. The media can also be used in skill development, although direct person-to-person training is usually best. The theory that underlies this approach is, again, associated with Albert Bandura, and is called *Social Learning Theory*. Up until the early 1960s, much of psychological learning theory rested upon the assumption that individuals had to practice behaviors personally and be rewarded for their efforts in order to become accomplished at some task. This approach was central to the work of B. F. Skinner and others. Bandura's contribution (Bandura and Walters, 1963) was to note that children seemed to learn new skills simply by watching other children. Children who observed others practicing the new skill and being rewarded for doing it often adopted the new skill themselves. Researchers were intrigued to discover that this sort of second-hand practice was sufficient to bring about behavior change all by itself!

Over the next twenty years, Bandura and others developed the Social Learning Theory (SLT) as an approach to bringing about desirable behavior changes. The theory has particular value in helping create increased self-efficacy, both personally and impersonally. SLT has been a major underlying framework for a number of well-known social marketing interventions, including the Stanford programs in California and the Pawtucket Heart Health Program in Rhode Island, which were described in detail in the Introduction.

In the preceding chapter, I discussed the role of individual expectations about outcomes and how these can determine behavior. SLT emphasizes the fact that the environment can also influence behavior both by communicating norms and by making it possible and easy to act.

SLT emphasizes the role that situational factors in the environment can play in influencing behavior. In the marketing literature, Kotler has emphasized the role of atmospherics on consumer behavior. He notes that consumers are likely to shop longer in pleasant environments painted in soothing colors. In the present context, it is clear that a cheery, brightly lit room with upbeat music is more likely to lead someone to exercise enthusiastically than is a dull, silent, cluttered room. Situational factors can also provide cues to—and opportunities for—behavior. On the negative side, the availability of drugs and easy money will increase the likelihood that a teenager will become a user or dealer. On the positive side, the availability of healthy snacks—fruits, vegetables, and the like—around a home or classroom will make it more likely that a child will learn healthy eating habits.

SLT proposes that learning of specific new behaviors takes place both directly and indirectly. For major changes in behavior or lifestyle, direct learning involves three major components: sequential approximation, repetition, and reinforcement. Sequential approximation refers to a point that I have been making throughout this book, namely that individuals do not instantly leap from not doing a behavior to doing it. They work their way up to it. Bandura and his colleagues emphasize the fact that this is also true of skill learning. One way of teaching smokers how to adopt a nonsmoking lifestyle is to reduce their consumption step by step, perhaps one cigarette at a time, starting with the easiest one to give up and working up to the most difficult. This process is called *shaping*. It works, in part, because it allows the target audience to adjust to the new behavior slowly. It lets them work out strategies for dealing with unexpected side effects. It lets them, if necessary, adjust their self-concept to the new lifestyle ("I'm an exerciser not a couch potato"). Among other effects, this slow adaptation allows individuals to manage their anxiety in dealing with the newness of the new behavior.

Of course, repetition is important. Traditional learning theory has demonstrated very clearly that the more times one practices a behavior, the more likely it will be done well and will become part of a permanent behavioral repertoire. And finally, reinforcement is essential if new behavior patterns are to be acquired and maintained. Research by Skinner and others on what has since come to be called *operant conditioning* has shown that people tend to repeat behaviors for which they are rewarded. The careful application of rewards, therefore, can significantly shape behavior. This topic will be discussed further in the next chapter.

Perry, Baranowski, and Parcel (1990) present another useful example of how the concepts of shaping and repetition can be used, in this case to teach diabetics how to learn self-injection. They propose that the self-injection process be broken down into a number of small steps that the target audience learns one at a time with many repetitions. Thus, diabetics can first learn how to fill the syringe with the proper amount of insulin while ensuring that the process is sterile and the liquid has no bubbles. Once they learn this, they can then move on to learn how to choose a bodily site for the injection, how to insert the needle and inject the fluid, and so on. As people become confident of their ability to handle one step, they move on to the next.

Heightened levels of self-control are synonymous with enhanced self-efficacy, which, I have argued, is essential for the new behavior to be taken on with the intention that it be permanent. Research (Kanfer and Goldstein, 1975; Locke, Bryan, and Kendall, 1968) suggests that self-control is most likely to be achieved if the individual (a) focuses on a very specific behavioral goal or series of goals (subsequent approximations), and (b) sets reachable goals. As a number of studies have shown (Stuart, 1977; Kanfer and Goldstein, 1975; Bandura, 1986), increased perceived self-control significantly improves behavioral learning and maintenance of learned behaviors.

Vicarious Learning

Individuals, as noted earlier, can learn new behaviors both directly and through vicarious or observational learning. *Observational learning* involves the use of role models who act out the desired behavior for the target audience. This audience not only learns the behaviors but can also observe the rewards that the role model achieves and thereby be vicariously reinforced to undertake the behavior on their own. Observational learning can be much more efficient than direct learning. By observing others either in person or through a movie or video, a target individual can experience a wide range of behavioral alternatives at one time and see a number of successful and unsuccessful change attempts, all without having to go through the trial-and-error process directly.

This process is often referred to as *modeling* the desired behavior. Modeling is used in many private sector marketing situations—a moment's reflection will recall ads showing customers how to take the car to Mr. Goodwrench, add Clorox to the wash water, speed through the airport to pick up a Hertz Rent-a-Car, start Jazzercizing, serve instant coffee to discerning guests, or a hundred other behaviors allegedly beneficial to the consumer and certainly beneficial to the sponsoring marketer.

Modeling can be very helpful in social marketing settings as well. It develops consumers' sense of self-efficacy, making it likelier that they will carry out desired behaviors. Social marketing television commercials have modeled many key behaviors. For example, an effective series of commercials prepared for the Partnership for a Drug-Free America shows (a) parents how to discuss drug use with their children and (b) children how to refuse an offer of drugs from one of their peers or classmates. Other commercials, produced by the beer industry, show young people taking away the car keys of inebriated friends under a slogan that "Friends Don't Let Friends Drive Drunk!"

Learning is often stimulated through the use of other media. For example, the AIDSCOM project in Mexico developed a series of comic books for sex workers featuring a character called Maritza showing them how to negotiate condom use with different types of men, including:

Julio, "El Ejecutivo" (The Business Man)

José, "El L'Avioso" (The Fast Talker)

Willie, "El Machista" (The Macho Man)

Nelson, "El Terco" (The Stubborn One)

Jaime, "El Indomable" (The Wild One)

In each case, Maritza was shown negotiating the use of a condom and achieving her dual goals of economic income and protection from AIDS and other STDs.

Regular movies and television programs also present opportunities to model important behaviors. In the 1970s, it was relatively common to see characters in television shows—including police—get into their automobiles without putting on their seat belts. After meetings with Hollywood and network producers and directors, this behavior was changed to model one that social marketers promoting seat belt use hoped everyone would come to see as normal. Similar efforts have been made to reduce or eliminate the amount of smoking (except by villains) and excessive drinking on television.

The performing arts community in the 1990s is particularly concerned about the AIDS epidemic, in part because it has claimed so many victims in their world. As a consequence, plays on Broadway and movies such as *Longtime Companion* and *Philadelphia* teach their audiences how to treat people with AIDS. The use of condoms as a normal part of lovemaking is now finding its way into more and more scripts. Jokes are made about who is responsible for providing the condoms, and not about whether condoms should be used at all. In a recent movie, an older actor (Lloyd Bridges) is about to reenter the dating game and, in a humorous aside, asks his ten- or twelve-year-old grandson for any last-minute advice. The grandson asks him if he has "protection." The grandfather then pulls a handful of condoms from his pocket. The implicit message here is intended to be: "Of course, every right-thinking person involved in the dating scene uses condoms these days."

Other Examples of Social Learning Theory

Two studies that have made extensive use of SLT are the Texas *A Su Salud* Project and the Minnesota Home Team Study (Perry,

Baranowski, and Parcel, 1990). The former was directed at the smoking behavior of lower-income Mexican-Americans. The study recognized that two barriers kept this target population from quitting smoking. First, there was the problem that individuals did not have the skills to quit. Second, they did not have the skills to cope with the stresses that are endemic to low-income lives that were, on the one hand, encouraging smoking behavior, and on the other, interrupting attempts to quit.

The program recruited people from the target community who could demonstrate skills and would report rewards of quitting, and put these people on television and radio. Next, they recruited networks of community members who would personally bring these modeling examples to the attention of smokers in the community. This network not only increased awareness of, and attention to, the role models but they also provided needed reinforcement for target smokers once they had engaged in the desired behavior. Research into the program indicated that both components were more effective in increasing the number of people who tried and maintained nonsmoking behavior than was the modeling activity by itself (McAllister and others, in press).

The Minnesota Home Team Approach applied SLT to the eating patterns of third-graders in thirty-one schools. The project was based on five weeks of direct mail activities carried out in the third-graders' homes with the parents' involvement. Each mailing contained an adventure book starring four characters, Hearty Heart, Dynamite Diet, Salt Sleuth, and Flash Fitness—all from Planet Strongheart—who modeled healthy lifestyles for the target audience. Each mailing contained games and challenges that induced students to read the books and to learn important information and healthy-diet skills. Children were required to label foods as healthy or not and to prepare a simple healthy snack recipe. Self-rewards were available through scorecards that the children kept at home and direct rewards were available through a contest that offered a winning team a trip to Disneyland. All of these activities were conducted with the involvement of the parents, who were, undoubtedly, providing additional rewards. At the end of the study, it was found that the Healthy Home project had a significant impact on the children's fat and complex carbohydrate consumption (Perry and others, 1988).

Coordinating Tactics

I have now put in place the key elements of a strategy designed to move a target consumer through the Contemplation Stage to Action. I have indicated that social marketers must develop a four-pronged approach. They must:

- Increase the perceived positive outcomes (benefits) from the proposed behavior.
- Decrease the perceived negative outcomes (costs) from the proposed behavior.
- Increase the pressure from influential groups or individuals in the target customers's social environment to carry out the desired behavior.
- Increase the target customers' sense of self-efficacy with respect to the behavior.

I have also suggested that benefit-based strategies should be emphasized for target audiences early in the Contemplation Stage while cost- and efficacy-based strategies should come increasingly to the fore as the audiences get closer to action. Interpersonal influence strategies can be employed throughout the campaign.

Finally, it is important to emphasize a characteristic that applies to the very best private sector strategies, namely *coordination*. Social marketing strategies inevitably will have many things going on at once. Soap operas may be created; posters may be printed and distributed. Articles may appear in the general press and in specialized magazines. Peers in the target audience's community may be recruited to bring information and pressure directly to bear on individual target consumers. All these spokespeople and vehicles will be carrying messages to the target audience. There exist, therefore, plenty of chances for different messages (coming at the target audience at the same time) to cancel each other out—or at least lose the synergy that can happen when all of the elements are well synchronized. Thus, if it is assumed that the target audience is early in the Contemplation Stage, it is important that everything that goes out from the campaign emphasize the benefits of the proposed behavior. As research has shown, individuals at this early stage are less likely to be interested in cost information. Indeed, if a campaign decides to try to minimize perceived costs too early, it is entirely possible that this will only heighten the importance of cost considerations and interfere with the target audience's perception of the benefits. In a worst-case scenario, premature discussion of costs may boomerang and throw the target audience member back into the Precontemplation Stage.

The same is true of premature discussion of skill issues. If a target consumer who has not yet absorbed the benefits of the new behavior is confronted with a discussion of what may be seen as difficult skills, this may have the effect of turning the customer away from the desired outcome.

On the other hand, as the campaign progresses and target customers are moving closer to the desired behavior, it becomes important that everyone switch gears and begin working on diminishing costs and increasing self-efficacy. At this stage, it will be wasteful to talk about benefits. Consumers will already know these and will want to get on to other issues. Irrelevant messages that emphasize benefits may cause the consumer to lose interest in the behavior because the proper momentum is not kept up. Marketers must focus on giving consumers the information and skills that they need to carry out the behavior. The marketers must also make sure that their lack of attention to matters of distribution and the training of key intermediary personnel is not reducing perceived self-efficacy.

The trickiest element here is the use of direct group pressure. Group pressure that is brought to bear indirectly through advertisements and public relations tactics can be controlled by the marketer and, if there is close attention to timing and coordination, be precisely coordinated with the overall message strategy. However, people not directly under the marketer's control, for example health workers, social service agencies, counselors, volunteers trying to reach difficult cases in ghettos or remote villages in developing countries, and so on, may present serious coordination problems. The only solutions here are careful training and monitoring, issues that we shall return to later.

Summary

The second set of challenges facing a social marketer at the Contemplation Stage involves bringing social pressure to bear and ensuring that the target audience sees that it has the behavioral control to make the behavior happen. Social pressure can take many forms. Other individuals can serve as information sources. It has been well documented that people often learn about new ideas or learn new facts about old ideas not directly from the source of the ideas but from others in their social network as part of a "two-step flow of communications." The intermediaries in this process are called opinion leaders, and they not only provide facts but also serve as role models for innovative behaviors. It is important for social marketers to identify such opinion leaders, who are significant forces for (and sometimes against) change, because working through them can be much more cost-effective than attempting mass marketing or communications campaigns.

Spokespeople can often be recruited by social marketers to serve as opinion leaders in specific media campaigns. While it is helpful to have a spokesperson who is well known and instantly recognizable, it is also critical that he or she have at least the qualifications of expertise, trustworthiness, or empathy.

Groups can have very important roles to play in pressuring consumer decisions. In some cases, groups are part of the decision process itself and some sort of group consensus must be reached for action to take place. In other cases, where the individual is eager to act (especially in some socially aberrant way), group permission may be required for the new behaviors to take place. In some instances, not just permission but approval may be required. Finally, there are situations in which the individual does not want to act but the group does. In such a case, direct social pressure will be brought to bear. Such pressure may have little effect on those consumers who are Inner-Directed and relatively impervious to social influence. However, consumers who are Other-Directed and very much sensitive to what they read others as preferring will react strongly to social pressure.

Social marketers cannot ignore group influence. For each target audience, they must understand which groups are important, what the target audience thinks the groups want, what the groups really want, and how motivated the target audience is to comply with each group's wishes. This can form the basis for a communication campaign changing perceptions of what others want or changing what others actually want. In many cases, mobilization campaigns can prove particularly effective in bringing community social influence directly to bear.

People will also not undertake new behaviors if they think they cannot succeed. Lack of a sense of behavioral control can be very inhibiting, especially in the Late Contemplation Stage. Behavioral control is a function of two factors: *internal efficacy,* the person's sense of possessing the skills and knowledge to take the proposed action, and *external efficacy,* the person's perception that the action can take place, that is, that environmental circumstances will permit it to happen. Internal efficacy can be increased by providing the consumer with information about the action (how, when, where, and so forth) and skills to carry it out. External efficacy can be improved somewhat more easily by improving the ease with which the behavior can take place. This is often a function of improved distribution, hours of operation, and so on.

Social learning theory can prove very helpful in increasing individuals' sense of internal efficacy. Individuals can be helped to learn specific information and skills through sequential approximation, repetition, and reinforcement. Particularly useful is the technique of shaping, whereby the individual is moved step by step toward a desired outcome. Where consumers cannot be reached one-on-one, the process of vicarious learning can be effective. Here, the target individual sees others performing the behavior and, through these observations, learns to do it. Others are in effect modeling the desired behavior. Television, including regular entertainment fare, can provide very effective vehicles for modeling desired behaviors.

Efforts to bring social influence to bear and increase the consumer's sense of behavioral control must be coordinated carefully with other tactics designed to improve the benefit-cost trade-off. While all four elements may be present at any time, it is clear that benefits should be emphasized to those in the Early Contemplation Stage, whereas costs and social pressure should be introduced as the audience moves into the Late Contemplation Stage. In many cases, behavioral control may prove to be the final barrier to preparation and action.

Chapter Nine

Inducing Action and Ensuring Maintenance

Once a consumer has completed the Contemplation Stage and has come to the conclusion that he or she should undertake the recommended action and, in fact, intends to do so, the social marketer's task is not complete. First, the consumer's intention must be translated into action. Then, where appropriate, actions must be repeated, improved, and, in many cases, made a permanent part of a new lifestyle. Actions promoted by social marketing can be thought of as four types:

- *One-time actions,* such as having a vasectomy or donating a human organ for transplant
- *Repeated but finite actions,* which require repeated behaviors but have a definite end point, such as getting a child immunized or participating in a drug withdrawal program
- *Permanent lifestyle changes,* such as recycling, getting regular exercise, or stopping smoking
- *Situational actions* where a socially desired behavior is to be undertaken in certain situations, such as designating a driver when drinking alcohol or using ORT when a child has diarrhea

The principal challenge in the first two cases can be seen as primarily to develop action strategies. In the latter two, the challenge is both action and maintenance. In some cases, maintenance can involve not only repeating the behavior, but also improving it, for example, as when mothers get better at administering ORT.

Inducing Action

The problem of how to get someone to initiate action has received limited attention in the behavior-change literature (Kuhl and Beckmann, 1985). What is it that makes people who intend to act, actually act? And on the other hand, what keeps individuals who intend to act from doing so? Somewhat more is known about *barriers* to action than about *triggers* to action. The barriers to action cited by researchers like Weinstein (1988) and others fall into five broad categories:

1. *Impossible.* Some behaviors cannot be carried out because circumstances in the target audience's life or in the broader marketplace do not permit it.
2. *Too Complex.* The customer may be overwhelmed by the apparent difficulty of the activities involved in carrying out the recommended behavior.
3. *Require too much time.* Customers often feel they do not have time to carry out the recommended behavior.
4. *Lack priority.* In many cases, target audiences have many other commitments and choose not to bother with the recommended behavior.
5. *Forgotten.* Many people do not act simply because they forget the new behavior or no one suggests it.

Each of these barriers to action has a relatively straightforward solution.

1. *Make the impossible possible.* A behavior must be feasible to be adopted. Any impediments that the social marketer can control must be attacked directly. For example, *availability* is an essential ingredient of virtually every social marketing program, but it is often neglected by marketers who are too fixated on the communications aspect of the strategy. Good social marketers realize that one must make opportunities for behavior as convenient and painless as possible. This means making social marketing products such as ORS packets, oral contraceptives, and condoms available in every locality and at every outlet feasible, making them as accessible and convenient as chewing gum and cigarettes. Indeed, experts at SOMARC, one of the pioneers in contraceptive social market-

ing, believe that distribution is one of the most important parts of their programs and one of the single most difficult parts to achieve. They and others like them recognize that all the advertising and promotion in the world can only get customers interested and excited. If people cannot get the advertised product or service, all of that effort will be wasted!

Availability is important not only for products but also for services. Social marketers must attempt, as much as possible, to bring services to the people rather than vice versa. Health clinics should be available locally or health workers should travel to the community on a regular basis. Making mothers travel to distant locations for services with intangible future benefits (like vaccination or growth monitoring) will be a very hard sell.

Economic cost is a second important barrier where products or services must be purchased. In such cases, sliding scale fees or prices should be considered as a central tactical element.

2.   *Make the complex simple.* Many behaviors that social marketers recommend are too complicated and have too many steps for the target audience to carry out. Graeff, Elder, and Booth (1993) cite a hand-washing program in Guatemala, where the planning team proposed that mothers wash their hands twenty-six times a day using up to two minutes and over half a liter of water every time—a major burden to women who often must pump and carry water by hand. In cases like this, the prudent social marketer will sit down and reanalyze the required behavior to see what can be eliminated or cut back. In Guatemala, the researchers discovered after talking with the local epidemiologist that focusing on only two hand-washing occasions would have a significant impact on diarrhea morbidity: hand-washing before preparing meals and hand-washing before administering food to children under three years old.

If the task cannot be made simple, then social marketers should attempt to develop a gradual approach by which the behavior could be adopted in steps. Where the marketer helps guide this step-by-step behavior, the technique is called *shaping*. Shaping was described in the previous chapter as a means of increasing consumers' sense of behavioral control. It can be very helpful when old, hard-to-break patterns of behavior must be extinguished and new patterns adopted. Smoking is a good example. Rather than have someone quit "cold turkey," the marketer can help the smoker cut down in stages. One approach is to have the target smoker inventory the current cigarette occasions and rate each in terms of importance. The smoker would then gradually give up smoking on the easiest occasions step by step, perhaps with the encouragement of a group leader, until even the last and toughest occasion is smoke free. Extensive external or internal reward systems are essential for this shaping to occur.

A variation on shaping is called the *foot-in-the-door* technique. Here, researchers have found that someone who has agreed to make a small commitment first will be much more likely to make a larger commitment later on. For example, Scott (1977) found that people were more likely to make a larger volunteer commitment for a recycling program if they had earlier agreed to a simpler task. This foot-in-the-door approach, according to Scott, can be effective when the behavior is not too large and when requests are made in person.

3.   *Minimize the time inconvenience.* Simplifying the target behaviors will inevitably cut down the time commitment, as will making products and services available close at hand. In addition, for services where the audience must go somewhere to be served, social marketers should ensure that operating hours are as long as possible—or at least that they are designed to fit the audience's schedule and not that of the marketing staff. (I can recall a blood donation drive that expected late-shift plant workers to come in before their shift to give blood rather than inconvenience the volunteers who would have to stay late to collect the blood during the shift.) Also, it is critical that the service hours be adhered to faithfully. There is nothing more frustrating to a well-meaning client than to find that the clinic is not open when its sponsor said it would be or that the recycled materials are not collected as scheduled.

4.   *Increase the urgency.* Private sector salespeople know how important it is to close a sale. Once a customer is committed to an act—that is, has moved into the Action Stage—the salesperson should get the contract signed and product or service bought. Similarly, in many social marketing settings, once the target customer has reached the Action Stage it is also important to get a commitment to the desired action on the spot while urgency can be made

clear. If customers fail to act at the moment, they may well forget to act later. Of course, increasing urgency is a complex problem. If an audience member is still in the Contemplation Stage, say because the necessary sense of behavioral control is missing (for example, a woman who thinks she cannot get her partner to use a condom) stressing urgency will simply not work.

Repeated exhortations to act—through the media, by public figures and celebrities, and, best of all, by friends, family, and co-workers—have proven most effective in heightening a sense of urgency during the Action Stage.

5.   *Abolish forgetting.* An extremely important technique for social marketing programs to overcome forgetting is the provision of cues and reminders for action—preferably at a point where the customer might be able to undertake the necessary behavior. This is what Wells refers to as an *aperture*—a window of opportunity where the target audience member is receptive to the social marketer's influence. Of course, reminder ads ("Don't forget to take your blood pressure pills!") are an excellent tool—if the budget can afford it. Point-of-sale material in retail outlets or service centers can also be very effective. The bright orange banners that Woodward's puts up in Pakistani pharmacies are very dramatic reminders that "Condoms are available here." A similar function is served by posters in clinics that remind mothers to get their child immunized or to pick up a growth monitoring chart. Brochures or stick-up wall posters given to school children to take home can remind parents to stock up on Vitamin A or serve more leafy green vegetables.

In the "Five-a-Day for Better Health" campaign of the National Cancer Institute, two simple techniques were found useful in inducing people who wanted to eat five fruits and vegetables a day to do so more often. One was to put a magnet on the refrigerator reminding people to eat more fruits and vegetables. The other was simply to have cut-up fruits and vegetables at the front of the refrigerator (or on the counter) where the hungry consumer would be sure to see them.

Maintaining Action

As I noted in Chapter Four, during the Contemplation Stage, consumers think about positive and negative consequences, social influences, and perceived behavioral control. As a result of that thinking process, they form intentions to act and then act for the first time. Now they have experience. In the Maintenance Stage, they undertake what marketers call *postpurchase evaluation* (Andreasen, 1982). This evaluation consists of a comparison between the expectations they formed during the Contemplation Stage and the reality (as they perceive it) during the Action and early Maintenance Stage (Oliver, 1980). The outcome of this evaluation will play a very strong role in influencing whether they are likely to repeat the behavior.

This is one of the very important reasons why monitoring of customer satisfaction is so critical in social marketing programs, especially in their early months, as described in Chapter Three. Private sector marketers have long ago learned that waiting for customers to stop buying or patronizing a service before taking action on a problem is extremely poor management. A flawed product or service not corrected quickly enough can lead not only to lost customers—who are hard to get back—but also to unflattering word-of-mouth that can have a highly damaging ripple effect. The marketing literature makes it very clear that, while consumers may tell two or three others about a pleasant consumption experience, they may tell from ten to fifteen people about an unpleasant one! Constant customer satisfaction measurement should thus be a central component of any marketing strategy where maintenance of behavior is especially crucial.

Sources of Disappointment

What could go wrong? There are possibilities within each of the four topic areas consumers think about in the Contemplation Stage (see Slovic, Fischhoff, and Lichtenstein, 1979; Graeff, Elder, and Booth, 1993, p. 76).

1. *Unsatisfactory positive consequences.* The outcome could turn out to be less wonderful than the target consumer thought for one of the following reasons:

- Expectations were raised too high. The consumer thought that ORS would stop the diarrhea but it did not.
- The positive outcomes were hard to detect. The consumer expected the new exercise and eating regime to reduce

cholesterol levels but now sees no change and feels no different.

- The positive outcomes are deferred. Stopping smoking will eventually clear up the lungs but, in the short run, nothing will be observed. Recycling or driving fifty-five miles per hour will eventually lead to less pollution but the effects are invisible today.
- The positive outcomes are only the absence of something. Vaccinations keep polio from happening—but unvaccinated children often stay healthy. How is a person to know if the vaccination did anything?

2. *Excessive negative consequences.* The outcome could turn out worse than expected for one of the following reasons:

- The negative consequences were underestimated. Waiting times were much longer than anticipated. Condoms were too expensive. Recycling took many more hours each week.
- Unexpected negative consequences appeared. The woman suggested to her male friend that he use a condom and he became very angry and accusatory. The mother went to the clinic to get a first vaccination and was treated like a dumb peasant by the snobbish nurse and then she met a doctor who criticized her for waiting so long to bring the child in for a first shot.

3. *Important people provided negative feedback.* The target audience member thought that husband, in-laws, and traditional healers would support the new behavior, but they do not. The mother-in-law criticizes the new weaning foods. The traditional healer disparages the value of Vitamin A capsules. The husband complains when the mother gets the child vaccinated but neglects his meal.

4. *Behavioral control was less than expected.* The behavior did not turn out to be as easy to do as the consumer expected due to either of the following factors:

- *The System.* The clinic did not stay open at convenient hours. Condoms were not available. No one could be found to babysit other children.

- *The Consumer.* The consumer might have believed that putting on a condom in the middle of love-making would be relatively easy and nondisruptive, but without the proper skills, it turned out to be awkward and very disruptive.

Marketing Support

Given all these ways in which the experience could turn out to be unsatisfactory, what is a social marketer to do? There are five broad classes of actions to take to increase the prospects that new behaviors will be maintained:

1. *Control expectations.* If consumers are not to be discouraged by their experience, they need to have reasonable expectations of both positive and negative consequences. Thus, mass communications messages should not imply that ORT cures diarrhea—which it doesn't. Mothers should not be told that waiting times at clinics are short if they are not. Women should be told of the likely side-effects of certain medicines they take (such as Depo-Provera) so they are not shocked by them when they occur.

2. *Make hidden benefits visible.* The availability of blood pressure kits in the home and in the shopping mall can do a lot to provide feedback to patients who have undertaken cholesterol-reducing behaviors. Mothers can be given a calendar on which to write how much a sick child is eating each day as a way of making visible the results of improved feeding practices (Graeff, Elder, and Booth, 1993, p. 77).

3. *Improve the system.* Clearly, if there is something wrong with the product or service that the marketer can control, then it should be instantly fixed. Thus, nurses and doctors can be alerted to the effect of their behavior on patients and trained in more customer-friendly techniques. Condom prices can be dropped or subsidized for some groups. Recycling systems can be streamlined. Availabilities of products and services can be increased.

4. *Enlist the support of significant others.* Social marketing campaigns should not be directed solely at target consumers, but should also encourage others in the target's social environment to be supportive. Thus, as Graeff, Elder, and Booth (1993) point out, husbands can be encouraged to praise their wives' extraordinary child care efforts. Mothers-in-law can be taught the values of the

new practices being urged on their sons' wives and told to congratulate them on their performance. Traditional healers could be recruited and paid to help promote the new behavior.

5.   *Redouble skills training.* Where consumers must take action but are frustrated when they cannot do it well, marketers must develop new and more imaginative training components for their behavior-change program. Parents should be shown new ways to make fruits and vegetables "fun foods." Householders should be shown simple recycling techniques. Dieters should be shown how to choose low calorie options in fast food outlets or on airplanes.

Using Extrinsic Rewards

Social marketers can play important roles in creating rewards for consumers as they undertake new behaviors. If the target audience's evaluation of the proposed behavior has at least some chance of being unfavorable, social marketers are wise to consider adding extrinsic rewards to the intrinsic rewards of the behavioral outcome. *Intrinsic rewards* are those that are inherent in the behavior—the sense of safety one gets from wearing seat belts, the pleasing mirror image from weight loss. *Extrinsic rewards* are rewards that are unrelated (or marginally related) to the behavior in question. Extrinsic rewards have been used in many social marketing projects. They can be tangible things like diplomas or awards or they can be intangibles such as praise from a health worker or from an authority figure on the radio or television. Robert Gillespie of Population Communications once arranged for a number of pharmacies in an Asian country to give discounts to families pledging to keep their families to one or two children (1985). Delauriers and Everett (1977) found that ten-cent tokens given to bus riders increased public bus usage in the United States. The Academy for Educational Development found that vaccination certificates in the PREMI program mentioned in the Introduction encouraged repeat behavior by Ecuadoran mothers. They also found that a lottery in The Gambia helped improve mothers' skills at mixing oral rehydration solutions.

Gillespie cites a number of other rewards that have been used by family planning programs in developing countries. For example, provincial governors in Indonesia gave awards of acclamation to villages that were successful in achieving a two-child-per-family goal. Mothers clubs in Korea provided social support to couples committed to having one or two children, and also offered health, education, and financial assistance. Green cards in India and Bangladesh afforded couples with one or two children priority health and educational opportunities. In Kerala state, India, non-pregnant women received money deposits every six months, with withdrawal privileges after three years. And in Gujarat, India, a bag of cement was given to the village council for every vasectomy performed in the village. Note how some of these rewards went to communities rather than to individuals, providing an incentive to increase social pressure for the recommended behavior.

Social marketers must be very cautious in using positive extrinsic rewards. A practical reason is that such rewards can wear out quickly. A prize offered every week soon loses its salience and effectiveness. A variety of rewards usually has more impact. Further, it may turn out that consumers come to carry out the behavior just to achieve the reward and not because the behavior is internally satisfying. This is especially the case if the reward is perceived by the consumer to be excessive for the behavior being rewarded. Overjustification of behavior can lead consumers to believe that a behavior is less intrinsically rewarding in the future (Lepper and Green, 1978).

But a more serious problem with positive extrinsic rewards is the potential ethical dilemma they raise. Their purpose is to help induce socially-desirable behaviors—but for the wrong reasons. That is, they seek behavior not so much for the inherent or intrinsic value to the consumer but for some secondary reward. If the extrinsic reward is the main reason for action, we clearly have a case of manipulation. This is not what the best social marketing is all about. Social marketing is a win-win technology because it meets people's basic needs while meeting program goals. But if an extrinsic reward induces people to do something that they would not otherwise do—and will regret doing once they have done it—then this is not good social marketing. It is unethical, because it meets the program's needs while subverting the consumer's needs. Positive extrinsic rewards pose less of an ethical problem in the following circumstances:

- When they are used to overcome inertia to start someone trying a new behavior that is likely to be satisfying in itself once begun.

- When they are just one of many positive consequences the consumer sees for trying a behavior.
- When they induce behaviors that are reversible. If a free radio induces someone to use condoms to prevent unwanted pregnancies, this behavior can be reversed if the target audience member finds the outcome unsatisfactory. However, if the radio is given for a vasectomy, this is unethical manipulation because the behavior is not normally reversible.

Negative extrinsic rewards (that is, punishments for continuing the old behavior) are also sometimes effective, especially for governments. For example, Singapore places a lot of stress on punishment as a means of controlling social behavior, dealing out fines and other penalties for infractions of its social norms. In the area of family planning, couples in Singapore with three or more children pay higher taxes and are excluded from government housing, and the third child cannot go to the same school as the first two (Gillespie, 1985).

Consumers can be also be taught to reward themselves. McGuire (1989) has long been an advocate of teaching self-persuasion to consumers. He argues that consumers can be trained to counterargue against others who might dissuade them from a course of action, and should be taught how to handle others who disparage their actions. This is particularly valuable to teenagers, who are often subject to intense peer pressure should they decide to go against group norms, for example, by not doing drugs, by remaining a virgin, or by quitting smoking.

Consumers can be taught to praise themselves when they do something right. This can be an internal monologue that says "I am doing the right thing." It can also involve the provision of concrete rewards and punishments. One approach suggested for smoking cessation is to have the consumer put a significant sum of money in an envelope and take out twenty-five cents every time they do not smoke on prespecified occasions. After a fixed time period, the remaining funds are donated to a detested group (such as the Ku Klux Klan). Smokers are torn between two decidedly mixed outcomes—pleasurable smoking plus supporting the KKK versus cutting out smoking and not helping the KKK. Very often the latter combination wins out!

A Caution

One implication of the preceding discussion is that a clear understanding of what will go on during the Action and Maintenance Stages of the behavior-change process must be achieved early in the planning process. Potential problems that could crop up at either level should be dealt with in advance, not treated after the fact. Program managers must anticipate what might go wrong with postpurchase evaluations and seek to preempt the occurrence or impact of the problem. Very often this will mean great emphasis on availability and better training of critical intermediaries. Marketers must also ensure that the target audience members face constant reminders to repeat their good behavior. And finally, the social marketer must seriously consider the use of a wide range of reward systems that will add positive value to behaviors that may have very many natural disincentives.

Summary

An intention to act is not an action. Marketers must ensure that first and subsequent steps transpire. Typical barriers to action are that the consumer finds the behavior too difficult, too complex, too time-consuming, too low in priority, and/or too easy to forget. The solutions are relatively straightforward.

The social marketer needs to make the behavior possible by increasing availability of opportunities to act and by making them convenient. Where economic costs are a factor, ways must be found to reduce monetary outlays—in total or each time period.

Too many recommended behaviors are too complicated. They need to be simplified and consumers need to be helped to learn to perform them through such techniques as shaping. Opportunities to take the action need to be made convenient for the customer, not for the marketer. A sense of urgency should be introduced to motivate first steps. Cues for action and reminders must be put in place to overcome forgetting and to trigger initial and repeat actions.

Maintaining action is crucial in many social marketing campaigns. Marketers must closely monitor the postbehavior evaluation process. This evaluation process involves a comparison between prior expectations and how the behavior actually turned out. Several things can go wrong. The positive consequences can turn out to be unsatisfactory, perhaps because expectations were too high or because positive outcomes were hard to detect. Or there can be excessive negative consequences, including some not anticipated. Important people may provide negative feedback. Finally, behavioral control may be less than expected because the system broke down or because the consumer lacked the necessary knowledge or skills.

Solutions for the social marketer include controlling expectations so that they are realistic, enhancing benefit visibility, improving delivery systems, enlisting the support of significant others, and redoubling skills training.

Selective use of rewards can help ensure that consumers repeat desirable behaviors. These rewards can be intrinsic or extrinsic. They can be provided by the social marketer or by the consumer in the form of self-rewards. In using marketer-provided extrinsic rewards, social marketers must take special care that they are acting ethically. In particular, they must be especially cautious about the use of extrinsic rewards to induce consumers to undertake irrevocable actions that society deems to be desirable but that the consumer might personally wish to avoid.

Chapter Ten

Creating Strategic Partnerships: Marketing to Other Publics

In the preceding chapters, I have described the critical role that other individuals in the target consumer's social network can play in inducing initial action and then making sure it is reinforced and maintained. This points to the fact that, to achieve success, social marketing programs must obtain the help and assistance of a wide range of individuals and groups, those that Kotler and Andreasen, in their text on marketing for nonprofit organizations (1991), refer to as *other publics*. Here is a partial list of other publics that can influence social marketing success:

- Commercial sector distributors
- Commercial sector research agencies
- Commercial sector advertising agencies
- Public agencies (for example, Ministries of Health)
- The media
- Retailers
- Funding organizations (for example, the U.S. Agency for International Development)
- Volunteers
- Paid staff
- Other nonprofit organizations
- Corporations
- Other intermediaries (for example, health clinics and their staffs)

In each of these cases, the social marketer needs the public to perform certain behaviors that will help make the program successful. For example, for vaccination programs to be fully effective, health clinic workers must treat mothers well, must take advantage of all vaccination opportunities when young children come to the clinic for other reasons, and must reward the mother with praise so that she will return for other vaccinations and will spread positive word-of-mouth to other mothers.

For an AIDS program to be successful, pharmacies must be influenced to carry condoms and display them prominently along with banners and point-of-sale display cards. Bar owners must be encouraged to stock bowls of condoms for easy access. Brothel managers must make condoms available to sex workers and insist that they be used. The social marketer's own staff and volunteers must be convinced to go out into seedy neighborhoods and very remote villages to talk to local leaders, distribute information, and put up posters. Newspapers have to write articles on the dangers of AIDS and how to protect oneself against it. Ministries of Health need to stock condoms in their clinics, urge their use and permit politically risky advertising of condoms in the media. Radio and television stations must agree to carry public service announcements and advertisements on AIDS, weave AIDS themes into their soap operas, and have discussion shows on safe sex. Doctors and traditional healers need to tell their clients about the AIDS problem. Corporations, government organizations, and nonprofits need to put up AIDS posters at their workplaces, carry AIDS articles in their newsletters, and possibly hold AIDS information meetings for their workers.

Social marketing does not consist of the social marketer just talking directly to the target customer. Many more people must be involved to make it work (Smith and Schechter, 1992)!

But how is a social marketer to induce the enthusiastic cooperation of these other groups and individuals in carrying out actions that are in the program's interests? The reader will not be surprised to learn that the answer is simply to apply the very same concepts and techniques I have been discussing throughout this volume to these challenges. This is because, in each case, the problem is plainly to get someone to take a voluntary action or actions that will serve the program's interests. This is just another marketing task—no different from getting ultimate consumers to lose weight, stop smoking, or get their children vaccinated.

When dealing with any public, the marketer must carry out formative research, even if it is very informal (say, holding conversations with key members of the target public). Then the marketer needs to plan a behavior-change strategy that depends on whether the target audience (say, the physicians or the brothel managers or the volunteers) is in the Precontemplation, Contemplation, Action, or Maintenance Stage. And if the target is found to be in the Contemplation Stage, the social marketer should think of ways to:

- Increase the positive consequences of cooperating
- Decrease the perceived costs and barriers
- Bring social pressure to bear
- Make sure that the target public feels confident that the actual behavior or behaviors can be accomplished

For targets at the Action or Maintenance Stages, the social marketer should be concerned with how they have evaluated their experience, what rewards they are receiving, and whether other (extrinsic) rewards should be brought into play to maintain their behavior or whether reminder communications are needed for continuing participation. In all cases, the social marketer must put the target audience's needs, wants, and perceptions first and not those of its own organization. That is, the social marketer must urge cooperation because it is in the other public's interest, not because it is in the marketer's interest. Never say, "Do it for the good of the program—your help will make us even more effective!"

To understand how the social marketing paradigm can be stretched to these other situations, I will consider a selected few of these key publics. As the reader will see, in each case, I am simply using many of the principles outlined in Chapters One through Nine.

Attracting Commercial Sector Support

A great many of the most successful social marketing programs around the world make extensive use of commercial sector help in carrying out their missions. These organizations supply products (such as condoms, pills, or ORS packets), conduct marketing research, create advertising, distribute and promote merchandise, run clinics, and so on. They have helped reduce family sizes in developing countries, reduce drug use in the United States, and improve maternal and child health in the Middle East. Commercial participants have ranged from pioneering organizations such as Porter/Novelli in Washington, D.C., which has been a central player in social marketing for more than twenty years, to local distributors and advertising and research agencies in Egypt, the Philippines, and the Dominican Republic. These collaborations have proved difficult at times but they can be rewarding for all sides (Saunders and others, 1993).

Over the years, the one area in which there has been consistent commercial sector involvement in social marketing programs is advertising. Probably the best known example is the participation of advertising agencies working through the Ad Council in the United States in a wide range of social marketing projects. For example, in one year (1987–1988), they developed very effective social marketing campaigns with the following themes:

- "Help stop AIDS. Use a condom." (Scali, McCabe, Sloves, Inc.)
- "You can learn a lot from a dummy—buckle your safety belt." (Leo Burnett U.S.A.)
- "Take time out. Don't take it out on your kid." (Lintas: Campbell-Ewald)
- "Take a bite out of crime." (Saatchi & Saatchi)
- "Just Say No [to drugs]" (DDB Needham Worldwide, Inc.)
- "Smokey says: Only you can prevent forest fires." (Foote, Cone & Belding Communications)
- "The toughest job you'll ever love [the Peace Corps]." (Baker Spielvogel Bates Worldwide, Inc.)
- "Bad guys abuse public lands. Good guys save them." (W.B. Doner and Company Advertising)

Increased participation by commercial sector organizations like these advertising agencies at the international and local level is essential for two reasons. First, social marketing organizations need the talent. Today, we simply do not have enough people trained in the mindset and techniques of social marketing to go around. Importing commercial sector skills is a way of getting instant sophistication. (However, it is important to note that just because a commercial sector organization claims to do marketing, it does not mean that they follow the principles outlined in this book—that is, that they do it well!) Second, if social marketing programs are to be sustainable for the long run beyond the initial infusion of outside funding and support, more commercial sector organizations must be induced to take them over or to collaborate in major ways with public or nonprofit agencies that do social marketing.

How then does one go about inducing a commercial sector organization to become involved in social marketing? What inspires a profit-oriented business to create ads for an AIDS campaign, for example, or to distribute ORS packets, conduct focus groups for a recycling program, or take over the management of a health clinic?

As was made clear earlier, the first step is to find out whether the commercial sector organization is aware of the opportunity to become involved. Assuming that the target organization is aware and is in the Contemplation Stage, how might they be induced to cooperate? Taking the hypothetical case of a potential commercial sector condom distributor, the challenges are to heighten the positive consequences the distributor might see flowing from cooperation, minimize any perceived costs, point out how others important to the distributor would support their participation, and show how easy it is to move forward.

Increasing Positive Consequences

There are likely to be three broad sets of positive consequences that a commercial sector organization might see in participating in a social marketing program. These include increased revenue and profits directly arising from sale of the social marketing products and services, other profit-related benefits to the organization outside the social marketing program (such as increased contact with potential customers, public goodwill, and so on), and personal satisfaction from helping with a major social problem in the country.

With respect to profitability, there do indeed appear to be real profit possibilities for commercial sector organizations participating in marketing programs. In many parts of the world, there has been a good deal of successful privatization of public services such as sanitation, prison management, and the like, where commercial sector organizations have found that they could make a reasonable return on investment while providing public services. This line of thinking can equally apply to social marketing in such areas as ORT or contraceptive marketing, where commercial sector marketers may be able to do a job that a public enterprise finds not cost-effective and make it profitable.

How does the commercial sector make social marketing programs profitable? Take production and distribution. Woodward's, a major distributor of over-the-counter drug products (including "Gripe Water," a general purpose tonic taken for a variety of real or imagined ailments), carries the major responsibility for distribution and promotion of condoms in Pakistan for both family planning and AIDS programs. Woodward's brings considerable marketing savvy that has a major impact on program costs and effectiveness. Because Woodward's already deals with the kinds of outlets in which the social marketing project wants distribution, they can reduce the costs of establishing initial distribution—they know where the outlets are and are already serving them. They can also increase the percent coverage of available outlets (market penetration)—many social marketing organizations have difficulty cracking distribution outlets such as the major pharmacy chains where Woodward's has considerable clout—and they can reduce the per-unit carrying and delivery costs, because they are already going to outlets with their regular line and the cost of adding the social marketing product line is relatively tiny!

However, it is often difficult to get the commercial sector to take on this kind of responsibility. The major reason is that social sector products are typically very low priced. Even where the basic product to be sold is provided free, as in condom distribution programs sponsored by the U.S. Agency for International Development, the margins have historically seemed too small to justify commercial sector involvement from a purely economic standpoint. However, recent evidence suggests the exciting possibility that it is possible to make contraceptive social marketing (CSM) self-sufficient. In an extensive 1992 study of projects in seven countries, The Futures Group's SOMARC program found that projects in four countries were producing total cost recovery (Stover and Wagman, 1992). As the authors conclude:

> In four of the longest running projects—Mexico (condom), the Dominican Republic (orals), Indonesia (condom), and Barbados (condom)—long term sustainability is already assured. In Mexico, the Protector condom project became operationally self-sufficient in 1990 and purchased its first commercial supply of condoms in 1991. In the Dominican Republic, sales and associated marketing activities of the oral contraceptive are totally self-sufficient. Marketing of the original DuaLima Red condom in Indonesia is also being completely supported by the commercial sector. In Barbados, the Panther Condom project has achieved complete self-sufficiency, and the distributor purchased the first commercial supply of commodities in late 1991 using project-generated funds [Stover and Wagman, 1992, p. 5].

In March 1994, SOMARC further announced that condom projects in Morocco and Turkey had also achieved complete self-sufficiency "with all marketing activities, including product procurement, packaging, advertising, promotions, public relations, and market research, now solely funded from revenue from condom sales." SOMARC further notes that it "has drastically shortened the timeframe in which it graduates social marketing products to self-sufficiency; whereas it previously has taken five to six years to graduate a product to self-sufficiency, SOMARC can now conduct the process far more quickly, graduating products in as little as two-and-a-half years. This is due in large part to SOMARC's having required its commercial partners to make substantial initial investments of resources in the project. Developing this kind of commitment in the partner often allows a project to shift very rapidly to self-sufficiency" (SOMARC III, 1994, p. 1).

Even where involvement does not provide direct profit, there are other positive consequences for businesses that can be used to encourage hesitant commercial sector managers to become involved. These arguments speak to their specific needs and wants—not those of the public sector or nonprofit organizations that would like them to become involved:

- *Participation can sometimes open up new opportunities.* Social marketing programs often have an aura about them that opens doors. A condom distribution program sponsored (even indirectly) by a government agency like a Ministry of Health may be very welcome in outlets where the distributor has not been able to establish sales. Introducing the social marketing product in the field can be a way to make initial inroads.

- *Participation can often build up significant goodwill,* especially if there is government involvement in the program. As noted earlier, one of the reasons that major multinational marketers such as Unilever and Brooke Bond Tea Company became distributors of the Nirodh condom throughout India in the 1970s was that they hoped it would cause the government to look favorably upon them in the future, reducing the difficulties often encountered by foreign companies operating in the country.

- *Participation can sometimes lead to the learning of new skills* that will benefit the commercial sector organization elsewhere in its business. One of the benefits that Woodward's saw from its involvement with the USAID-sponsored condom distribution program in Pakistan was that it exposed local Woodward's management to advanced marketing techniques. For example, it was in the social marketing project that they first learned about focus groups—a technique they now use to great advantage to learn more about their traditional commercial sector markets.

In the case of advertising agencies that volunteer their services to create ads for social marketing programs, there are other potential positive consequences (Kotler and Andreasen, 1991, p. 319):

- Potential business contacts with important community leaders who are also volunteering to help the program
- Public goodwill that may help recruit top-flight staff in future
- Psychic benefits for agency executives and staff, derived from working on important social issues rather than just "selling soap"
- Opportunities for individual and agency creativity that may be considerably greater than when a paying client is calling the tune (and the agency may see a chance to make a major public impression with a highly innovative campaign)

- Opportunities to give experience to junior staff people where a major client is not at risk

While this assistance can be very valuable for social marketing programs, social marketers may find advertising agency help a mixed blessing. For example, the agency may cut costs if the campaign is too expensive. Junior people may not do particularly good work. And the agency may focus most of its energies on being creative—hoping to win a major award for its work—and, in the process, lose sight of the program's basic strategy. Many agencies seem to take on the campaigns in order to win creativity awards. This is not necessarily good for the program. The solution is to treat the volunteering agency as one would treat any volunteer group, that is as professionals, and require that they perform as professionals.

Decreasing Negative Consequences

The negative consequences that commercial sector marketers are likely to consider are not unlike those in any other business investment. Thus, social marketers need to make efforts to minimize the investment that the commercial sector organization would have to make in the joint venture. They would also need to provide realistic estimates of sufficient volume and reasonable costs that would indicate that profits will be forthcoming or that downside losses will be acceptable.

There are also a number of potential costs unique to the social marketing setting that may inhibit commercial sector marketers. Potential commercial sector marketers may be concerned that they will be put under the glare of public scrutiny of their actions (though this may be a plus for some organizations) and any seeming wastes of public or donated funds may be held up to criticism that would be unreasonable in the commercial sector. They may worry that budgets will not be adequate for carrying out their activities. And—given the unfortunate image of their craft in some circles—they may also worry about working with people who do not understand marketing and, indeed, may be hostile to it. In each of these cases, social marketers must seek to minimize costs as much as possible.

Increasing Social Pressure

Social pressure can be a very important factor in securing commercial sector involvement in social marketing ventures. In some cases, as in India, government pressure may make participation close to mandatory. Thus, in the early days of contraceptive social marketing in India, participation by major international convenience goods marketers in distributing condoms to remote reaches of the country was suggested by the government as something these marketers ought to do in the public interest. The fact that import licenses for many of the bread-and-butter products of these firms were under government control undoubtedly influenced the firms' willingness to assist. Similarly, the participation of major polluters in recycling programs in the United States is also close to mandatory if they do not wish to risk further sanctions.

However, it is also often possible to bring into play competitive pressures. Commercial sector firms are always on the lookout for ways to differentiate themselves from competitors. This may be a good argument for involvement in social marketing. For example, recent research on homebuilders (Andreasen and Tyson, 1993) showed that those who intended to plant or save more trees on their prospective homesites to help the environment did so because they liked to think of themselves as being ahead of their competition in their approach to building and development. Clearly, one of the reasons Porter/Novelli and The Futures Group continue to be so active in the area of social marketing is that it makes them quite distinctive in the highly competitive worlds in which they operate.

Increasing Behavioral Control

As indicated in Chapter One, one of the major differences between the commercial sector and social marketing is that there are often serious restrictions on what a marketer is allowed to do in social marketing. Thus, a commercial sector marketer may feel that there is a potential for helping out and feel social pressure to do so. However, they may also be unwilling to become involved because they fear that they will not have full freedom to do whatever it takes to achieve success. They may feel that they will not be allowed to ask certain research questions or use certain advertising themes, or that they will face other restrictions because of political and social concerns. These limitations on their behavioral control must be reduced as much as possible.

Involving the Media

The public media are an extremely important component of any social marketing campaign, but especially during the Precontemplation Stage. There is much that the media can do to communicate program messages—and there is also much they can do that can be counterproductive. The media can tell the public much about AIDS and what to do to prevent it. They can point out the dangers of pollution and the benefits of recycling. They can alert mothers to the need for vaccinations and report the hours at which vaccination centers are open. They can publicize rallies that social marketers organize to inform communities about needed behavior changes.

Over several years of working with social marketing organizations, I have found that a great many of them do not know how to deal effectively with the media. They often do not get the coverage they want—and they often get coverage they do not want. The major problem is that they have not learned to apply the marketing mindset discussed in Chapter One to this problem (Andreasen, 1989). That is, most public relations specialists in nonprofit organizations are selling-oriented; they are not customer-driven.

In trying to get a story covered, the selling-oriented PR specialist begins by assuming that he or she has a great story, and that the general public would be really interested if only the media would cover it. If the media are reluctant to run the story, then it is likely to be either because they do not fully appreciate how truly interesting it is and how much their audience would like to be exposed to it or because they have some sort of bias against the topic or the organization. The PR specialist thinks he or she knows how journalists think. Getting coverage is just a matter of convincing them what a wonderful story the PR person has. Thus, getting the story out is just a matter of writing a press release, sending it to the appropriate people, and following up with a hard sell to get the story in print or on the air. And the PR person uses basically the same approach for everyone.

How then would the approach advocated in this book be different?

First, one can assume that any journalist asked to help out with a social marketing project will at least consider it—but there will be a great deal of competition for the journalist's attention and for the media space or time. Second, because the journalists will be in Contemplation mode, the social marketer would need to:

1. *Emphasize the positive consequences of covering the topic for the journalist and the medium.* Most social marketers emphasize the benefits to the social marketer or to the society at large if only the problem is solved. But as we have seen, what drives journalists is what's in it for them. Thus, the social marketer needs to find out what their needs and wants are. Investigation is likely to discover that the journalists and media want to cover stories that:

Fit their own mission

Sell papers or attract audiences (for example, to newscasts)—that is, that appeal to their own customers

Are easy to translate into colorful stories—preferably with dramatic pictures

Meet deadlines

It will also be clear that each journalist and each medium will have their own particular needs and wants, and thus a single approach will not meet everyone's needs—an effective PR strategy will have to be segmented. Some journalists and media will only want stories with a human interest angle. Some reporters will only be interested if they themselves can get involved in the story and become its star (getting a lot of television "face time"). Some will want prepackaged stories or videos that they can run as is; others will want to do their own digging and put their own spin on it.

2. *Minimize the costs of coverage* by assuring the media that there are no downsides to coverage—especially where the issue involved is controversial.

3. *Bring social pressure to bear.* Showing that other media are going to cover the issue can be a compelling motivation—although it is sometimes helpful to offer key media some sort of exclusive angle on some stories. Stories that contain comments from public

figures showing their support for the issue can also be effective as a source of pressure-to-publish for the media.

4. *Make coverage easy* by having all the necessary facts, phone numbers, and key names available. Set up photo or video shoots in advance. Prepackage materials in the style the journalist or medium uses wherever possible.

Involving Other Publics

As indicated in the preceding two extended examples, the key to securing cooperation is to treat it as another challenge for marketing. And in each case, one needs to show the target audience that doing what the social marketer wants will meet the target audience's needs and wants. Let us see how this might apply to critical challenges involving some of the other important publics whose help is needed to make social marketing programs effective.

Staff and Volunteers

There are two key problems in attracting and keeping staff and volunteers for social marketing programs. They might be labeled quantity and quality problems. The *quantity* problem is one of getting enough people to carry out the complex and socially important tasks of a social marketing program. The *quality* problem is one of getting personnel with the right kinds of skills, in our case, marketing skills. A major source of both problems is the low level of funding of most social marketing programs, particularly during the start-up phase, making it hard to provide the needed outreach and the level of support necessary to keep personnel happy.

Recruiting

In attracting volunteers or staff, the secret is to find ways to make the job seem to be meeting the target audience's needs and wants. One must not talk about why the organization needs the volunteer or staff member and how much better off the organization would be if the person joined up. Instead, one must talk about the target individual's needs and wants and how joining the organization will meet them.

Once volunteers are on board, experience has shown that they are more likely to maintain their new behavior if they are treated like other staff members. This means training them carefully, setting specific standards for their performance, and holding them accountable for achieving specific goals. This will ensure that they will carry out program guidelines carefully. The latter is particularly important when the program manager wants the volunteers to follow the same kinds of customer-centered guidelines that would be given to staff.

Training

There are many elements of social marketing programs that involve contact between representatives of the social marketing program and target customers. These representatives could be the organization's own staff and volunteers. Or they could be health workers at a clinic who process mothers having their children vaccinated, or community outreach workers who go from house to house to inform families about nutrition, AIDS, the need for immunizations, and so on. Each instance where these representatives come in contact with a target customer is what Jan Carlzon of Scandinavian Airlines called a "moment of truth" (Carlzon, 1987). Each of these encounters is an occasion on which a representative can have an important positive effect on the target audience—or can effectively sabotage the program. The easiest way for the latter to happen is if it becomes clear to the target audience that the representative does not have the consumer's needs and wants at heart.

Unfortunately, too many social marketing moments of truth are between customers and representatives who are recruited from social classes above the clientele to whom they are supposed to provide services. In such encounters, the natural inclinations of the nurses, doctors, or volunteers may well make them quite patronizing and even disdainful of the attitudes and behaviors of the people they are supposed to help and influence.

It is essential, therefore, that these representatives learn the rudiments of the basic approach developed in this book. They must be trained to quickly assess what stage the target audience is in with respect to the proposed behavior. They need to get a quick fix on the target's principal needs and wants, and understand how to use the information as the basis of a persuasive strategy to move the target to the next stage (Action or Maintenance). All the while, the most important challenge is to have the target customer understand as clearly and as deeply as possible that the representative has the customer's interests first in mind—not organizational or personal interests! This applies not only to behavior-change encounters but also to encounters where the contacts are more perfunctory, such as vaccination administration or condom sales. In both kinds of situations, workers would have much to learn from companies like Nordstrom's and Ritz Carlton in the United States.

How does one get these representatives to adopt the appropriate mindset and orientation? There are basically three approaches:

- *Use power:* Set rules, enforce them, punish those who do not follow guidelines.
- *Use rewards:* Develop a measuring system, say, postencounter interviews, and reward workers on how well they are rated. Many retailers throughout the world do this with their sales staffs.
- *Use self-interest:* Show them how it serves their own needs and desires.

Obviously the last approach is the one that a marketer would recommend. It involves finding out what motivates each of these workers and establishing that a customer orientation is the best way to achieve these ends. This will be most effective when the worker's goals are reasonably well aligned with those of the social marketer. That is, people who want to be really good at community outreach will be happy to learn that the greatest number of village mothers will change their behavior if the worker develops a customer-driven persuasion approach. Similarly, people who want to be really good nurses can be shown that they will be more effective in, say, getting mothers to return for all their children's vaccinations if the mothers perceive that the nurses really have the mothers' interests at heart.

And of course, one must pay attention to perceived costs, social influence, and behavioral control. One concern that community outreach workers or nurses will have is that this customer-friendly stuff will just take up too much time—and they are very busy! It is important to point out to them that, at minimum, all you are asking for is an attitude, a way of talking to target audiences, that tells them you care. At maximum, it requires only a little more time to determine customers' readiness to change and their principal needs and wants. But again, one should emphasize that the time is more than justified by the greater payoffs it achieves.

It is, of course, also important to bring social pressure to bear by showing that others—particularly respected others—have adopted the new approach. And careful training in the techniques of customer assessment and customer-friendly response styles will give the workers the sense of self-efficacy so that they will believe that they can make the new approach a reality.

Workplace Owners and Managers

Workplace settings are often very effective for carrying out social marketing programs (Kaur, 1988; Rinehart, Blackburn, and Moore, 1987). In the factory or the office, one can lecture, show videos, pass out materials, and schedule follow-up contacts during or after working hours and reach large numbers of people all at one time. Workplaces have been the sites of efforts to increase ride-sharing, decrease smoking and drug use, increase tolerance of minorities, and so on. Workers in job sites tend to be excellent behavior-change targets for several reasons:

- They often are of above-average education and literacy.
- They are often upwardly mobile and interested in ways in which they can make their lives better.
- They often have migrated to larger cities to seek better lives and so are temporarily freed from inhibiting village norms.
- They see factory supervisors and bosses as role models and so the latter can have important effects through modeling and social influence.
- They find it harder to avoid social marketing messages in the workplace than it would be at home or in the village.
- They are more likely to attend a lecture and be at least attentive if they are given time off from work to come.

Managers and owners are likely to participate in such programs if they see it as in their interests, if they perceive social pressure to do so, and if the social marketer minimizes efficacy concerns by helping out with (or taking over) the work. A recent study summarized some of the benefits employers could receive if they participated in workplace-based family planning programs (Rinehart, Blackburn, and Moore, 1987):

- Healthier workers stay on the job longer, take less sick leave, and perform better.
- Fewer pregnancies mean less need for maternity benefits.
- Employment-based family planning programs may improve labor-management relations.
- Additional health benefits can encourage workers to stay with one employer rather than shift to another, a major factor where labor is in short supply.

It is a listing of these positive consequences for employers that will most likely carry the day—not platitudes from the social marketer about the way participation in the program will help the country.

Communities and Families

Much of the approach taken in this book has focused on individuals as the ultimate target market for a social marketing program. Hornik and others have argued that we may want to think about the larger community as the focus of attention, especially after the social marketing program is well along in its life cycle. Both the Stanford and Pawtucket interventions described in the Introduction took a community orientation. It can be argued that, if one makes behavior change a community objective, the program can have more impact—and more efficiency—than if it tries to bring about change one person at a time. This is the rationale behind efforts to turn whole cities like Los Angeles into smoke-free zones (at least in public spaces) or efforts to beautify small towns. The effort to get the United States to cut gasoline consumption after the oil crisis of the 1970s was a community-based approach, as was the effort in Palo Alto in the 1960s to get the entire community to conserve water.

The customer-driven approach advocated here can also work

in these larger groups, although it is more awkward. It is harder to define a community or family as being at a given stage of the behavior-change process, since members will differ. However, the average (modal) stage of the parties is a useful way to begin. If the group is mostly at the Contemplation Stage, then the effort must turn to promoting benefits, decreasing costs, bringing social pressure to bear, and increasing the group's sense of behavioral control. In community settings, social pressure may well be the most effective of the four components. A bandwagon effect can prove to be particularly powerful in convincing late majority and laggards to adopt a new practice lest they get left behind (E. M. Rogers, 1983).

Summary

Target audiences are not the only groups—or publics—toward which social marketers must direct their efforts. Help is typically needed from staff, volunteers, donors, intermediaries, researchers, and advertising professionals. In each case, the marketer's challenge is to induce cooperative behavior. And since behavior is the bottom line again here, this is just another opportunity to apply social marketing principles. Marketers need to increase the positive benefits of cooperation and decrease the costs. They must bring social pressure to bear and make cooperation easy, just as with their main message.

Many of the most effective social marketing campaigns have been successful at least in part because of the contributions of the commercial sector. These include the many efforts of the U.S. Advertising Council, family planning programs in developing countries, and the Partnership for a Drug Free America. The positive benefits that the commercial sector typically seeks include increased direct revenue and profits, other profit-related benefits such as increased contact with potential customers and public goodwill, and personal satisfaction from helping with a major social problem. Privatization of some aspects of social marketing campaigns is often a way of increasing commercial profits and helping the program achieve long-run sustainability. Social marketers, however, must be cautious—if the positive benefits turn out to be below expectations, the cooperating commercial sector advertising agency, distributor, or researcher may lose interest, substitute inexperienced staffers, and otherwise not stay on top of the campaign. There is also always the danger that the commercial organization will divert campaign objectives to meet their own needs.

Costs that may inhibit commercial partners include potential negative publicity (for example, from appearing to waste donated money), inadequate budgets, and working with people who do not understand marketing. Social pressure, however, can be important in overcoming worries about costs. The government and the media can often be effective in bringing needed pressure to bear, as can the commercial organization's peers. A final concern will be perceived behavioral control. Commercial marketers may have a hard time adapting to many of the restrictions on their actions outlined in Chapter One. Social marketers must do their best to minimize these constraints as much as possible.

Another form of cooperation that is essential to any effective social marketing program—especially at the Precontemplation Stage—is with the media. In dealing with the media, social marketing organizations too often revert to the undesirable selling mindset described in Chapter One. They try to persuade the media to tell the social marketer's story, rather than seeing that their task is to meet the needs and wants of the media first so that they will want to tell the story. Like any social marketing task, marketers need to show media gatekeepers that doing what the social marketer wants will meet the media person's own goals. They need to reduce potential costs to the media, such as adverse public reaction. They need to learn how to bring social pressure to bear, possibly by pointing out that competitors in the media will be cooperating even if the gatekeeper being addressed does not. Finally, they must maximize the media's sense of behavioral control by making it easy to cooperate.

Volunteers are essential to most social marketing programs. Attracting and keeping them is a matter of making sure the volunteer experience produces positive benefits that are important to the volunteer—not just to the organization. Volunteers must see few personal costs, some amount of social pressure, and an experience that they can easily handle. Teaching customer satisfaction skills is an extremely important part of the training of volunteers and staff. These individuals are often the ones who are closest to customers and whose interpersonal skills can make or break a social marketing campaign. While training can use power or rewards to achieve the desired behavior, it is better to simply show the trainee that the desired action will serve the trainee's own interests.

Workplaces are often very important sites for social marketing programs because the target audiences there are usually more literate, upscale, and open to change than the general population. Lectures can be held, supervisors can be used as role models, and various places and media can be used for effective program messages. Again, managers and owners of these sites need to see that cooperation in the social marketing program is in their own interest.

Finally, communities and families can be the focus of some social marketing efforts. Many behaviors of interest require couples (as with AIDS) or whole cities (as with recycling) to take the final action. Using the community as the target of the campaign may yield significant efficiencies as compared to working one person at a time. However, using a customer-driven approach is more difficult when one is dealing with groups. Still, focus on the four major behavioral determinants emphasized throughout this book can prove very powerful—like individuals, groups see benefits and costs, respond to social pressure, and need to perceive themselves as able to act.

Central Principles of the New Social Marketing Paradigm

This has been a book about a new approach to bringing about voluntary changes in individual behavior that can have dramatic benefits for both individuals and society. It uses marketing approaches perfected in the commercial sector to address difficult problems affecting health, safety, education, employment, and the environment. It is different from other approaches to these problems such as social advertising and health education. But it has much in common with them.

The book has not been intended as a comprehensive text on every aspect of social marketing. I have given only limited treatment to such topics as how to organize a social marketing program or an entire organization or how to carry out many tactical elements of social marketing campaigns. There is little on creating specific advertisements, brochures, packages, and products, or on determining prices, choosing distributors, and so on.

Rather, I have attempted to present a serviceable broad strategic approach to the behavior-change challenges facing social marketing managers. By *serviceable,* I mean that the approach is simple and portable, that is, easy to carry around mentally. By *broad,* I mean that the approach is sufficiently flexible to be used in a wide range of behavior-change settings. Finally, by *strategic,* I mean that it is intended for use in guiding general courses of action—and not, as I have said, narrow tactical choices. Tactical help is already available in basic marketing texts (such as Kotler and Armstrong,

1994) and in a wide range of equally serviceable social marketing sources. (See Recommended Reading at the end of this book.)

A New Paradigm

It is, perhaps, not immodest to refer to this approach as a new paradigm for social marketing. As I argued at the outset, although social marketing has been around for some time, it has not had a conceptual underpinning of its own. It lacked a paradigm (Kuhn, 1970). The new paradigm outlined in this book has twelve central principles:

1. Social marketing has as its bottom line the influence of behavior, not providing information or changing attitudes.
2. To be effective, social marketing programs must be guided by an underlying mindset that puts the target customer at the center of every strategic decision. That is, social marketing programs must be customer driven.
3. Strategic planning for a customer-driven social marketing program must constantly listen to customers; thus, strategic planning involves a cycle of six steps:
   Formative listening to target customers (and other environmental sources)
   Planning a specific strategy and set of tactics
   Developing an organizational structure and a set of control systems to carry out the plan
   Pretesting the strategy and tactics
   Implementation
   Monitoring and adjusting
4. To carry out formative listening during the first step of the strategic planning process—and to plan subsequent strategies—one must have a model or framework for understanding how consumers make decisions and take action.
5. The framework of understanding proposed here makes clear that consumers come to take and maintain action through a series of four stages. These are labeled:
   Precontemplation
   Contemplation (divided into Early and Late Contemplation)
   Action
   Maintenance

6. Social marketing strategies must be adapted for the stage at which each target audience is found.

7. At the Precontemplation Stage, the major social marketing challenge is to overcome consumer's tendencies to selectively ignore or screen out social marketing messages. The techniques of education, propaganda, and media advocacy may be particularly helpful here.

8. After the Precontemplation Stage, behavior is driven and maintained by many factors, the most important four of which are:
Perceived benefits
Perceived costs
Perceived social influences
Perceived behavioral control

9. To get consumers to move from the Contemplation Stage to Action and Maintenance, marketers must:
Increase perceived benefits
Decrease perceived costs
Increase perceived social pressure
Increase perceived behavioral control

10. To maintain new behavioral patterns, consumers must feel rewarded. They must also be subject to regular reminders until the new behaviors become an ingrained way of life.

11. Target consumers are not all the same and so segmenting markets will improve program effectiveness and efficiency.

12. The social marketing paradigm can be applied not only to target consumers, but also to the behaviors of a wide range of other publics whose assistance and cooperation are essential for the success of the social marketing program.

These twelve principles can serve as a checklist for practitioners. They can also serve as a starting point for those academic thinkers who may wish to extend the conceptual underpinnings of this important discipline—or to challenge some of the principles themselves.

Social Marketing Successes

Although social marketing as a discipline is not very old, it can already claim a number of successes. In the last ten years, it has been introduced into an increasingly wide range of policy domains from health to education to the environment. It has proven itself to be cost-effective in at least one area, contraceptive social marketing. And along with a number of other intervention strategies, social marketing has had a major positive effect on specific social problems, many of which were described in the Introduction.

One need only look at the problem of child survival to see significant progress. As indicated in the Preface, children around the world today are faced with very great risks of illness and death from afflictions and problems we know how to deal with—measles, malaria, malnutrition, overpopulation, and the like. But it is also true that, using social marketing and many other intervention strategies, we have made significant strides in ameliorating these problems in the last ten years. Some statistics tell the story:

- The World Health Organization announced that, by 1990, 80 percent of the world's infants had complete vaccination coverage against the six vaccine-preventable childhood diseases—measles, diphtheria, whooping cough, tetanus, polio, and tuberculosis. By contrast, in 1984, only 10 percent were covered for measles and 25 percent for the other five diseases.
- Between 1984 and 1991, use of oral rehydration therapy worldwide tripled from 12 percent of cases to 36 percent. Access to ORS packets more than doubled from 35 percent to 79 percent.
- Overall, infant mortality fell from 106 per thousand in 1980 to 83 per thousand in 1991; deaths among children under five fell from 167 to 130 per thousand (U.S. Agency for International Development, 1992).

On the domestic front, we can take a sense of pride in the fact that, over the last decade, cigarette consumption is down significantly in almost all age and gender groups. More party-goers are opting to have a designated driver when planning to drink excessively. Teenagers are increasing their use of contraceptives (Vobejda, 1994). We have made important reductions in use of illicit drugs on the part of secondary and college students and young adults, and in alcohol use among high school seniors (Johnston, O'Malley, and Bachman, 1992). The high blood pressure program has been a major success and more people are recycling.

The intellectual underpinnings of social marketing have also grown enormously. We have developed a significant and still growing body of research and other scholarly literature—cited throughout this volume—and substantial field experience in the form of case studies. We have trained a small but growing cadre of top-flight social marketing professionals. And there is now a small group of educational institutions providing courses and workshops where one can learn more about this promising new approach.

Some Remaining Practical Challenges

There is, of course, a great deal that still remains to be done on both the practical and intellectual sides if social marketing is to attain its full potential. A recent review of child survival projects offers an indication of the practical and intellectual challenges (U.S. Agency for International Development, 1992). Among the issues that USAID believes we need to address are the following:

- *Sustainability.* Most social marketing programs have limited lifetimes and limited funding—although there are exceptions like the twenty-two-year-old National High Blood Pressure Education Program described in the Introduction. Yet, if social marketing is to have lasting effects, someone must carry on the work. Programs must be made sustainable. We have made a start on solving this problem. Some family planning programs have already proven cost-effective (Stover and Wagman, 1992). But more must be done. In a recent review of health communication programs in developing countries, Bossert (1990) identified five factors that increase the chances of long-term sustainability:

Develop programs from the start with the participation of host governments, institutions, or agencies.

Make successes visible.

Integrate programs with existing delivery structures such as Ministry of Health departments or programs.

Secure alternative funding before the end of the program.

Give careful and extensive training to people who will be working in the program area after the formal end of the program.

To the extent that sustainability requires specific actions on the part of commercial sector collaborators, other nonprofit organizations, and government agencies, the social marketing approach itself can be brought directly to bear. Chapter Ten offers a number of specific recommendations.

For many programs, there is a tendency to think that, if they are to be sustainable, some sort of government agency should take principal responsibility. However, not all social marketers agree that government institutions ought to be the ones to sustain social marketing programs. Government bureaucrats often have agendas that either oppose the social marketing effort or support it only in the current political climate. Bureaucrats' commitment is typically more closely tied to their own personal goals.

Sustainability may be more likely where programs are shifted to the commercial sector, as in the case of the Partnership for a Drug Free America program, and there is ownership by an institution that sees direct benefits for itself from continuation of the program. It also enhances sustainability when programs involve alliances or coalitions with local groups who can eventually take over, as in the CDC Planned Approach to Community Health (PATCH) program (Hanson, 1988–89). And the most hope of sustainability may lie with programs that are community-based and are begun only after community ownership of the program already exists, an approach that is hard to achieve but very valuable (Green and Kreuter, 1991). It is an approach being adopted by the Centers for Disease Control and Prevention in its Prevention Marketing Initiative focusing on HIV/AIDS among youth in five cities.

•   *Documenting results.* There are many more social marketing successes than have appeared in the public literature. And among those evaluations that have appeared, researchers have had limited success in separating out the specific effects of what social marketers have done from what other players have done. We need more future projects with careful published evaluations—and more of these evaluations should involve quasi-experimental designs where the effects of social marketing interventions can be isolated.

•   *Service and supply.* Social marketers need to increase their emphasis on access to services and service quality as components of their programs. It remains the case today that too many observers—and too many practitioners—still think of social marketing as advertising. But as I have noted throughout this book, the real success of a great many interventions can be attributed to the access of target consumers to services and to the quality of those services—rather than to mere communications. For example, in the area of child health:

> One of the most significant accomplishment of the 1980s is the simple fact that more than 80 percent of the world's children now have access to at least some health services. . . . Having access to services, however, does not mean that people fully utilize the services or that service providers offer the best and most effective care possible. Studies by USAID and the World Health Organization show that health care workers can improve the effectiveness of the basic child survival interventions by, for example, screening children more consistently who may be at risk for more serious diarrhea than the watery diarrhea that ORT can address, advising mothers to continue feeding children during diarrheal episodes, ensuring that mothers understand how to administer ORT, advising about follow-up treatments or return visits, and take advantage of all opportunities to complete the immunization series of children brought to the clinic for other reasons [U.S. Agency for International Development, 1992, p. 20].

Much more attention in future programs must be paid to non-communications elements of social marketing. The emphasis in this book on consumer efficacy and on the potential negative impacts of postpurchase evaluations make the need for this emphasis very clear.

• *Program monitoring*. It is still the case in many social marketing programs that managers and researchers tend to emphasize end-of-program evaluations over monitoring. However, as noted in Chapter Three, commercial sector marketers place heavy emphasis on regular tracking of program progress as a means of correcting ineffective program elements and of adjusting to changes in the marketing environment. Social marketers must become equally zealous in their insistence on such feedback systems.

Intellectual Research and Development

Social marketing needs better implementation and better documentation of that implementation. But implementation can only be as good as the present state of the art in social marketing. If the discipline is to grow, then academics, researchers, and farsighted practitioners must make research-and-development investments in the basic paradigm on which social marketing is grounded. There are a number of challenges that are immediately apparent:

• *We need to learn more about how consumers turn intentions into actions.* We know a reasonable amount about how intentions are formed at the end of the Contemplation Stage. Yet too often intentions remain unfilled even though barriers to action have been effectively removed. We need to learn what triggers action—and how social marketers can pull those triggers more often.

• *We need to understand the nature of the emotional investments consumers make in their existing behaviors.* The paradigm proposed here is highly cognitive. It presupposes that the relevant decisions to act are highly involving. We assume that consumers in the Contemplation Stage engage in a good deal of thinking before taking action. Yet, we know that many of the behavioral categories that social marketing addresses have a large emotional component, for example drug use, child care, and weight reduction. Future revisions of the basic paradigm should develop a role for the concept of emotions. We also need to know how social marketers can use emotional messages to move consumers through the four stages, particularly in triggering action.

We also need to know how to contend with the negative effects that emotions can have on programs. Consumers have expressive needs that can interfere with "rational" actions. Many cases of STD or HIV infection can be traced to momentary rushes of emotion that got in the way of risk-reducing behavior. We know little about how to allow for or minimize these factors.

• *We need to explore more complex bases for segmenting markets for social marketing programs.* Lifestyle or psychographic research (Riche, 1989) is commonly used in commercial sector marketing to segment households and individuals in terms of their activities, interests, and opinions. It permits the social marketer to separate consumers who are, say, active party-goers and socialites from those who bowl and tinker with their cars. The American Cancer Society has been exploring the use of a geographically-based lifestyle segmentation system (PRIZM) as a way of developing more customer-sensitive cancer-prevention strategies. These segmentation bases allow one to couch consumer messages about benefits and costs in terms of a target audience's general behavior patterns and interests. It is an approach that should be explored further—including in urban areas of developing countries.

•   *We need more research designed to discover clues to individual readiness-to-change* to the next stage of the behavior-change process. It would be ideal if, in specific social marketing contexts, we could identify a half dozen measures of (say) demographics, past behavior, and present behavior that would mark those in a given stage who are more likely to change than others. By allowing social marketers to carefully target such individuals, considerable increases in impact and efficiency could be obtained.

•   *We need to develop standardized measures of the major components of the consumer framework developed in this book.* These could be used routinely in future KAPB studies around the world, as well as in more informal studies and focus groups in specific programs. To the extent that this research measures such critical factors as perceived consequences, social influence, and perceived behavioral control in the same way in many, many different contexts, we could begin to develop research benchmarks or norms. Such norms would allow program managers to categorize consumers instantly into the four behavioral stages (Prochaska and DiClemente, 1983) and to point to influence factors (such as improved self-efficacy) that would have the maximum impact in changing their behavior. (For other suggestions for future research and modeling, see Andreasen, 1992.)

A Reminder About Ethics

As I said at the beginning of this book, marketing is a very powerful technology for change. In the private sector, it has had many profound effects on our lives through the products and services it has brought us, the advertisements it has created to tell us about ourselves (see Pollay, 1986), and the values it has promoted that tell us what is important. Social marketing is also potentially very powerful. And those who plan to use it have a special obligation to use the technology responsibly. Their obligation to behave ethically is well beyond that of their commercial sector counterparts (Smith, 1993).

As I said in the Introduction, the most fundamental ethical

problem in social marketing follows from the fact that social marketing is designed to further social ends. But who is to decide what is a proper social end? Should the majority define what is a proper application of social marketing? But what if the majority is wrong or evil—as in the case of Nazi Germany? Is the social marketing practitioner or scholar to abet this activity? Or stand up and declare that it is not right?

And what of tactics and strategies? Suppose the objective of a campaign seems right and responsible. Are all means justified? Can one use free radios as a premium for vasectomies because the goal of population control is a noble one? Is it permissible to withhold information about the side effects of birth control pills or injectable contraceptives from mothers in developing countries because it would only confuse them? If those side effects are known to be very rare, is it all right not to mention them given that most members of the target audience are poorly educated and do not have the ability to appreciate the true risks? (Certainly, they would still have the free choice not to act!)

In private sector marketing, unethical behavior has a good chance of being found out and eliminated by external forces. Citizens—even very young children—are suspicious of business people. They don't trust ads. And if citizens don't complain, competitors will. Finally, there are often government and private sector watchdog agencies around to make sure that there is "truth in advertising" and "truth in labeling."

But there are no such automatic checks and balances in social marketing. There are no competitors who will complain if a clinic is misinforming patients or marketers are seducing people into actions that they might not otherwise want to take by offering trinkets as rewards. There are no government watchdogs that say that ads from the Partnership for a Drug Free America or the American Cancer Society distort the truth. Except where there is a counter-lobby (like the tobacco industry for antismoking programs), those who are purportedly acting in the public interest are rarely challenged.

But why not just let marketers' consciences be their guide? Unfortunately, there is a very real personal danger that an individual's sense of right and wrong will be clouded by the overwhelming urge to "do good." In the private sector, employees who offer bribes to foreign governments know this is wrong but they go ahead because they think it is necessary in competition or to get ahead in their careers. In social marketing, it is tempting to move ahead with whatever it takes and not question the action because one's heart is in the right place. This is indeed a slippery slope, down which we must not let practitioners slide. A little deception to achieve a small change can very soon become a big deception that achieves a big change. Again, the Nazi experience is very instructive.

Ethics are especially important for social marketers to consider when deciding on courses of action. Theirs is a public trust. By definition, they are trying to do things that society wants them to do. But unlike commercial managers and private sector employees, they are not called to account by a specific group like the stockholders or the management committee. They work for the *society*. But the society is a vague and amorphous thing. Society is not down the hall. It doesn't meet in Orlando every February to vote on organization practices.

So, *social marketers must internalize society's conscience.* Not only must they do social marketing right—they must also do the right thing! They must ask again and again: Am I doing what is ultimately best for my stakeholders—the society? Am I respecting the rights and integrity of my target audiences? Am I resisting the temptation to cut corners even though it means I will bring about a better world a little later?

There is no universal set of rules spelling out ethical social marketing behavior. Ethical behavior can only come from individual social marketers developing an internal compass that forces them to ask again and again: Are my goals right? And are the paths to achieve them moral ones?

Conclusion

The prospects for social marketing in the next decade are impressive. It is my hope that this book has provided those who are wondering what social marketing is all about a better sense of its core concepts and its potential power. Further, I hope that the integrated paradigm set out here provides those practicing in the field a simpler and clearer framework by which they can achieve their bottom-line behavior-change goals.

Many people look upon commercial sector marketing, with its "ring around the collar" advertising and its obnoxious salespeople, as one of the more undesirable characteristics of economically developed cultures. Yet, as I have tried to show in this volume, the very best marketing concepts and techniques can have a profound effect on the world's major social problems. Marketing provides a true win-win scenario: social marketers get what they want (major social impacts) and consumers get what they want (because marketers start by trying to meet consumer needs and wants). I only hope that more social innovators discover this lesson and learn how to apply it.

Perhaps this volume will help.

References

Achenbaum, A. R. "Market Testing: Using the Marketplace as a Laboratory." In R. Ferber (ed.), *Handbook of Marketing Research.* New York: McGraw-Hill, 1975.

Ajzen, I. "From Intentions to Actions: A Theory of Planned Behavior." In J. Kuhl and J. Beckmann (eds.), *Action Control: From Cognition to Behavior.* Berlin: Springer-Verlag, 1985.

Ajzen, I. "The Theory of Planned Behavior: Some Unresolved Issues." *Organizational Behavior and Human Decision Processes,* 1991, *50,* 179–211.

Ajzen, I., and Fishbein, M. *Understanding Attitudes and Predicting Social Behavior.* Englewood Cliffs, N.J.: Prentice Hall, 1980.

Albrecht, K. *The Only Thing that Matters: Bringing the Customer to the Center of Your Business.* New York: Harper Business, 1992.

Albrecht, K., and Zemke, R. *Service America: Doing Business in the New Economy.* Homewood, IL: Dow Jones-Irwin, 1985.

Andreasen, A. R. "Non-Profits: Check Your Attention to Customers." *Harvard Business Review,* 1982, *60*(3), 105–110.

Andreasen, A. R. "Life Status Changes and Changes in Consumer Preferences and Satisfaction." *Journal of Consumer Research,* 1984, *11,* 784–794.

Andreasen, A. R. "'Backward' Marketing Research." *Harvard Business Review,* 1985, *63*(3), 176–182.

Andreasen, A. R. *Conducting an Effective Retail Audit.* Washington, D.C.: SOMARC/The Futures Group, 1988a.

Andreasen, A. R. "Alternative Growth Strategies for Contraceptive Social Marketing Programs." *Journal of Health Care Marketing,* 1988b, *8*(2), 38–46.

Andreasen, A. R. *Cheap but Good Marketing Research.* Homewood, Ill.: Business One-Irwin, 1988c.

Andreasen, A. R. "Communicating by Listening." *NonProfit Issues and Opportunities,* 1989, *1*(5), 1–4.

Andreasen, A. R. *Strategic Marketing Planning Workbook.* Alexandria, Va: United Way of America, 1990.

Andreasen, A. R. *The Strategic Marketing Planning Guidebook*. Atlanta: American Cancer Society, 1992.

Andreasen, A. R. "Presidential Address: A Social Marketing Research Agenda for Consumer Behavior Researchers." In M. Rothschild and L. McAlister (eds.), *Advances in Consumer Research*, Vol. 20, conference proceedings, Association for Consumer Research, 1993, pp. 1–6.

Andreasen, A. R. "Social Marketing: Definition and Domain," *Journal of Marketing and Public Policy*, Spring 1994, pp. 108–114.

Andreasen, A. R., and Manning, J. "Culture Conflict in Health Care Marketing." *Journal of Health Care Marketing*, 1987, 7(1), 2–8.

Andreasen, A. R., and Tyson, C. B. *Improving Tree Management Practices of Homebuilders: A Social Marketing Approach*. Washington, D.C.: American Forests, 1993.

Asch, S. E. "Effects of Group Pressure upon the Modification and Distortion of Judgments." In G. E. Swanson, T. M. Newcomb, and E. L. Hartley (eds.), *Readings in Social Psychology* (rev. ed.). New York: Holt, 1952, 2–11.

Assael, H. "Perceptual Mapping to Reposition Brands." *Journal of Advertising Research*, 1971, *2*, 39–42.

Atkin, C. K., and Freimuth, V. "Formative Evaluation Research in Campaign Design." In R. E. Rice and C. K. Atkin (eds.), *Public Communications Campaigns*. Newbury Park, Calif.: Sage, 1989.

Atkin, C. K., and Wallack, L. *Mass Communication and Public Health: Complexities and Conflicts*. Newbury Park, Calif.: Sage, 1990.

Averill, J. R. "The Role of Emotional and Psychological Defense in Self-Protective Behavior." In N. D. Weinstein (ed.), *Taking Care: Understanding and Encouraging Self-Protective Behavior*. New York: Cambridge University Press, 1987.

Backer, T. E., Rogers, E. M., and Sopory, P. *Designing Health Communications Campaigns: What Works?* Newbury Park, Calif.: Sage, 1992.

Bagozzi, R. P. "Marketing as Exchange: A Theory of Transactions in the Marketplace." *American Behavioral Science*, March-April 1978, pp. 535–556.

Bagozzi, R. P., and Warshaw, P. "Trying to Consume," *Journal of Consumer Research*, 1990, *17*, 127–140.

Baker, S. A. "An Application of the Fishbein Model for Predicting Behavioral Intentions to Use Condoms in a Sexually Transmitted Disease Clinic Population." Unpublished doctoral dissertation, University of Washington, 1988. Quoted in Carter, W. B. "Health Behavior as a Rational Process: Theory of Reasoned Action and Multiattribute

Utility Theory." In K. Glanz, F. M. Lewis, and B. K. Rimer (eds.), *Health Behavior and Health Education*. San Francisco, Calif.: Jossey-Bass, 1990, pp. 63–91.

Balch, G. I. "Multiple Indicators in Survey Research: The Concept of 'Sense of Political Efficacy.'" *Political Methodology*, 1974, *1*(2), 1–44.

Bandura, A. "Self-Efficacy: Toward a Unifying Theory of Behavior Change," *Psychological Review*, 1977a, *84*, 191–215.

Bandura, A. *Social Learning Theory*. Englewood Cliffs, N.J.: Prentice Hall, 1977b.

Bandura, A. "The Self System in Reciprocal Determinism." *American Psychologist*, 1978, *33*, 344–358.

Bandura, A. "Self-Efficacy Mechanism in Human Agency." *American Psychologist*, 1982, *37*, 121–147.

Bandura, A. *Social Foundation of Thought and Action*. Englewood Cliffs, N.J.: Prentice Hall, 1986.

Bandura, A., and Adams, N. E. "Analysis of Self-Efficacy Theory of Behavioral Change." *Cognitive Therapy and Research*, 1982, *1*, 287–310.

Bandura, A., and Walters, R. H. *Social Learning and Personality Development*. New York: Holt, Rinehart & Winston, 1963.

Bandura, A., Adams, N. E., and Beyer, J. "Cognitive Processes Mediating Behavioral Change." *Journal of Personality and Social Psychology*, 1977, *35*, 125–139.

Baranowski, T. "Beliefs as Motivational Influences at Stages in Behavior Change." *International Quarterly of Health Education*, 1992–93, *13*(1), 3–29.

Baranowski, T., and Jenkins, C. D. "Reciprocal Determinism at the Stages of Behavior Change: An Integration of Community, Personal, and Behavioral Perspectives." *International Quarterly of Health Education*, 1989–90, *10*(4), 297–327.

Baume, C. "Developing a Questionnaire for an Acute Respiratory Infection Pilot Study." In R. E. Seidel (ed.), *Notes from the Field in Communication for Child Survival*. Washington, D.C.: Academy for Educational Development, 1993.

Bearden, W. O., and Etzel, M. J. "Reference Group Influences on Product and Brand Purchase Decisions." *Journal of Consumer Research*, 1982, *9*, 181–186.

Becker, M. H. (ed.). "The Health Belief Model and Personal Health Behavior," *Health Education Monographs*, 1974, *2*(4), 324–473.

Bennett, C. A., and Lumsdaine, A. A. (eds.). *Evaluation and Experimentation: Some Critical Issues in Assessing Social Programs*. New York: Academic Press, 1975.

Bloom, P., and Novelli, W. D. "Problems and Challenges in Social Marketing," *Journal of Marketing*, 1981, *45*(2), 79–88.

Bossert, T. J. "Can They Get Along Without Us? Sustainability of Donor-Supported Health Projects in Central America and Africa." *Social Science and Medicine*, 1990, *30*(9), 1015–1023.

Brehm, J. W., and Cohen, A. R. *Explorations of Cognitive Dissonance.* New York: Wiley, 1962.

Brokenshaw, D., MacQueen, K., and Stess, L. *Anthropological Perspectives on AIDS in Africa.* Research Triangle Park, N.C.: AIDSTECH Project, 1988.

Bush, R. P., Ortinau, D. J., and Bush, A. P. "Personal Value Structures and AIDS Prevention." *Journal of Health Care Marketing*, 1994, *14*(1), 12–20.

Campbell, D. T., and Stanley, J. C. *Experimental and Quasiexperimental Designs for Research.* Chicago: Rand-McNally, 1966.

Carlaw, R. W., Mittlemark, M., Bracht, N., and Luepker, R. "Organization for a Community Cardiovascular Health Program: Experiences from the Minnesota Heart Health Program." *Health Education Quarterly*, 1984, *11*, 243–252.

Carlzon, J. *Moments of Truth.* Boston: Ballinger Books, 1987.

Celsi, R. L., and Olson, J. C. "The Role of Involvement in Attention and Comprehension Processes," *Journal of Consumer Research*, 1988, *15*, 210–224.

Cisneros, H. *MacNeil-Lehrer Newshour,* comments broadcast May 17, 1995.

Coreil, J., and Mull, D. "Introduction: Anthropological Studies of Diarrheal Illness." *Social Science and Medicine*, 1988, *27*(1), 1–3.

Davidson, A. R., and Jaccard, J. J. "Population Psychology: A New Look at an Old Problem." *Journal of Personality and Social Psychology*, 1975, *37*, 1073–1082.

DDB Needham Worldwide. *Directory of Advertising Testing Services*, 1989.

Debus, M. *Methodological Review: A Handbook for Excellence in Focus Group Research.* Washington, D.C.: HealthCom, Academy for Educational Development, n.d.

Debus, M. *Lessons Learned from the Dualima Condom Test Market.* Washington, D.C.: SOMARC/The Futures Group, 1987.

de Fossard, E. "Radio Broadcasts on Immunization to Schools in Swaziland." In R. Seidel (ed.), *Notes from the Field in Commmunication for Child Survival.* Washington, D.C.: Academy for Educational Development, 1993, 129–136.

Delauriers, B. C., and Everett, P. B. "Effects of Intermittent and Continuing Token Reinforcement on Bus Ridership." *Journal of Applied Psychology*, 1977, *62*(4), 369–375.

Deutsch, J., and Liebermann, Y. "Effects of Public Advertising Campaign on Consumer Behavior in a Demarketing Situation." *International Journal of Research in Marketing,* 1985, *2,* 287–290.

Dickson, P. R. "Person-Situation: Segmentation's Missing Link." *Journal of Marketing,* 1982, *46,* 56–64.

Eisenberg, L. "Disease and Illness." *Culture, Medicine, and Psychiatry,* 1977, *1,* 9–23.

Elliott, B. J. *A Re-Examination of the Social Marketing Concept.* Sydney: Elliott & Shanahan Research, 1991.

Engel, J. F. "The Psychological Consequences of a Major Purchase Decision." In W. S. Decker (ed.), *Marketing in Transition.* Chicago: American Marketing Association, 1963.

Farquar, J. W., and others. "The Stanford Five-City Project: Design and Methods," *American Journal of Epidemiology,* 1985, *122,* 323–334.

Fine, S. "Toward a Theory of Segmentation by Objectives in Social Marketing." *Journal of Consumer Research,* 1980, *7,* 1–13.

Fine, S. *The Marketing of Ideas and Social Issues.* New York: Praeger, 1981.

Fine, S. (ed.). *Social Marketing: Promoting the Causes of Public and Nonprofit Agencies.* Needham Heights, Mass.: Allyn & Bacon, 1990.

Fishbein, M., and Ajzen, I. *Belief, Attitude, Intention, and Behavior: An Introduction to Theory and Research.* Reading, Mass.: Addison-Wesley, 1975.

Fisher, J. D., and Fisher, W. A. "Changing AIDS-Risk Behavior." *Psychological Bulletin,* 1992, *111*(3), 455–474.

Fox, K.F.A., and Kotler, P. "The Marketing of Social Causes: The First Ten Years." *Journal of Marketing,* 1980, *44,* 24–33.

Frank, R. F., Massy, W. F., and Wind, Y. *Market Segmentation.* Englewood Cliffs, N.J.: Prentice-Hall, 1972.

Gengler, C., Oglethorpe, J., and Mulvey, M. "A Qualitative Analysis of Infant Feeding Decisions." Paper presented to the Marketing and Public Policy Conference, Atlanta, Georgia, 1995.

Gillespie, R. W. *A Review of Incentives and Disincentives in Developing Countries.* Unpublished working paper. Pasadena, Calif: Population Communications, 1985.

Glanz, K. "Perspectives on Group, Organization, and Community Interventions." In K. Glanz, F. M. Lewis, and B. K. Rimer (eds.), *Health Behavior and Health Education: Theory, Research, and Practice.* San Francisco: Jossey-Bass, 1990.

Glanz, K., Lewis, F. M., and Rimer, B. K. (eds.). *Health Behavior and Health Education: Theory, Research, and Practice.* San Francisco: Jossey-Bass, 1990.

Good, C. *Ethnomedical Systems in Africa.* New York: Guilford Press, 1987.

Gortmaker, S. L., and Izazola, J. A. "The Role of Quantitative Behavioral

Research in AIDS Prevention." In J. Sepulveda, H. Fineberg, and J. Mann (eds.), *AIDS Prevention Through Education: A World View.* New York: Oxford University Press, 1992.

Graeff, J. A., Elder, J. P., and Booth, E. M. *Communication for Health and Behavior Change: A Developing Country Perspective.* San Francisco: Jossey-Bass, 1993.

Green, L. W., and Kreuter, M. W. *Health Promotion Planning: An Educational and Environmental Approach.* (2nd ed.) Mountain View, Calif.: Mayfield, 1991.

Green, L. W., and Lewis, F. M. *Measurement and Evaluation in Health Education and Health Promotion.* Mountain View, Calif.: Mayfield, 1986.

Green, P., and Krieger, A. M. "Segmenting Markets with Conjoint Analysis." *Journal of Marketing,* 1991, *55*(4), 20–31.

Green, P. E., and Srinivasan, V. "Conjoint Analysis in Consumer Research: Issues and Outlook." *Journal of Consumer Research,* 1978, *5,* 103–123.

Green, P. E., and Wind, J. "New Ways to Measure Consumer Judgments." *Harvard Business Review,* 1975, *53,* 107–117.

Hale, J. L., and Dillard, J. P. "Fear Appeals in Health Promotion Campaigns: Too Much, Too Little, or Just Right?." In E. W. Maibach and R. L. Parrott (eds.), *Designing Health Messages.* Newbury Park, Calif.: Sage, 1995.

Hanson, P. "Citizen Involvement in Community Health Promotion: A Rural Application of CDC's PATCH Model." *International Quarterly of Health Education,* 1988–89, *9,* 177–186.

Helquist, M. J., and Rosenbaum, J. "Hotlines: Providing Anonymous Help and Support." In W. A. Smith and others, (eds.), *A World Against AIDS: Communication for Behavior Change.* Washington, D.C.: Academy for Educational Development, 1993.

Hernandez, J.F.S., de Guzman, E. M., Cabañero-Verzosa, C., and Seidel, R. "From Idea to Mass Media: Teaching Mothers the Concept of Dehydration." In Seidel, R. (ed.), *Notes from the Field in Commmunication for Child Survival.* Washington, D.C.: Academy for Educational Development, 1993, 69–78.

Hochbaum, G. M. *Public Participation in Medical Screening Programs: A Sociopsychological Study.* (*Public Health Service Publication no. 572.*) Washington, D.C.: U.S. Government Printing Office, 1958.

Holland, J., and Skinner, B. *The Analysis of Behavior.* New York: McGraw-Hill, 1961.

Holtgrave, D. R., Tinsley, B. J., and Kay, L. S. "Encouraging Risk Reduction: A Decision-Making Approach to Message Design." In E. W. Maibach and R. L. Parrott (eds.), *Designing Health Messages.* Newbury Park, Calif.: Sage, 1995.

Homer, P. M., and Kahle, L. R. "A Structural Equation Analysis of the Value-Attitude-Behavior Hierarchy." *Journal of Personality and Social Psychology*, 1988, *54*, 638–646.

Hornik, R. "Alternative Models of Behavior Change." In J. Wasserheit, K. Holmes, and S. Aral (eds.), *Research Issues in Human Behavior and Sexually Transmitted Disease in the AIDS Era*. Washington, D.C.: American Society for Microbiology, 1992.

Hornik, R., Zimicki, S., and Less, M. B. *The HealthCom Project in the Philippines: The National Urban Immunization Program 1989–1990*. Washington, D.C.: Academy for Educational Development, 1991.

Hornik, R., and others. *Results for the Evaluation of the PREMI/HealthCom Project in Ecuador 1985–1988*. Washington, D.C.: Academy for Educational Development, 1991.

Jaccard, J. J., and Davidson, A. R. "Toward an Understanding of Family Planning Behavior: An Initial Investigation." *Journal of Applied Social Psychology*, 1972, *2*, 228–235.

Janis, I. L. "Effects of Fear Arousal on Attitude Change: Recent Developments in Theory and Experimental Research." In L. Berkowitz (ed.), *Advances in Experimental Social Psychology*, Vol. 4. New York: Academic, 1967.

Janis, I. L., and Mann, L. *Decision Making*. New York: Free Press, 1977.

Janz, N. K., and Becker, M. H. "The Health Belief Model: A Decade Later." *Health Education Quarterly*, 1984, *11*(1), 1–47.

Johnston, L. D., O'Malley, P. M., and Bachman, J. G. *Smoking, Drinking, and Illicit Drug Use Among American Secondary School Students, College Students, and Young Adults, 1975–1991*. Washington, D.C.: National Institute on Drug Abuse, 1992.

Judd, C. M., and Kenny, D. A. *Estimating the Effects of Social Interventions*. Cambridge, England: Cambridge University Press, 1980.

Kahle, L. "The Values of Americans: Implications for Consumer Adaptation." In R. E. Pitts, Jr., and A. G. Woodside (eds.), *Personal Values and Consumer Psychology*. Lexington, Mass.: Lexington Books, 1984.

Kanfer, F. H., and Goldstein, A. P. (eds.) *Helping People Change*. Elmsford, N.Y.: Pergamon Press, 1975.

Kaur, S. "Employment-Based Family Planning Programs in Mexico." *Employee Benefits Journal*, 1988, *13*(4), 24–29.

Kelley, H. H. "The Processes of Causal Attribution." *American Psychologist*, 1973, *28*, 107–128.

Kincaid, D. L., Jara, J. R., Coleman, P., and Segura, F. *Getting the Message: The Communications for Young People Project*. Evaluation Study 56. Washington, D.C.: U.S. Agency for International Development, 1988.

King, A. C., Flora, J. A., Portman, P., and Taylor, C. B. "Smokers' Challenge: Immediate and Long-Term Findings of a Community Smoking Cessation Contest." *American Journal of Public Health*, 1987, *77*, 1341–1342.

Kinnear, T. C., and Taylor, J. R. *Marketing Research: An Applied Approach*. New York: McGraw-Hill, 1991.

Kotler, P. "Strategies for Introducing Marketing into Nonprofit Organizations." *Journal of Marketing*, 1979, *43*, 37–44.

Kotler, P., and Andreasen, A. R. *Strategic Marketing for Nonprofit Organizations*. (4th ed.) Englewood Cliffs, N.J.: Prentice Hall, 1991.

Kotler, P., and Armstrong, G. *Principles of Marketing*. (6th ed.) Englewood Cliffs, N.J.: Prentice Hall, 1994.

Kotler, P., and Levy, S. "Broadening the Concept of Marketing." *Journal of Marketing*, 1969, *33*, 10–15.

Kotler, P., and Levy, S. "Demarketing, Yes, Demarketing." *Harvard Business Review*, 1971, 49(6), 74–80.

Kotler, P., and Roberto, E. *Social Marketing: Strategies for Changing Public Behavior*. New York: Free Press, 1989.

Kotler, P., and Zaltman, G. "Social Marketing: An Approach to Planned Social Change." *Journal of Marketing*, 1971, *35*, 3–12.

Kuhl, J. "Volitional Mediators of Cognitive-Behavior Consistency: Self-Regulatory Processes and Action Versus State Orientation." In J. Kuhl and J. Beckmann (eds.), *Action Control: From Cognition to Behavior*. Berlin: Springer-Verlag, 1985.

Kuhl, J., and Beckmann, J. (eds.). *Action Control: From Cognition to Behavior*. Berlin: Springer-Verlag, 1985.

Kuhn, T. *The Structure of Scientific Revolutions*. Chicago: University of Chicago Press, 1970.

Kunreuther, H., Sanderson, W., and Vetschera, R. "A Behavioral Model of the Adoption of Protective Activities." *Journal of Economic Behavior and Organization*, 1985, *6*, 1–15.

Laurent, G., and Kapferer, J. N. "Measuring Consumer Involvement Profiles." *Journal of Marketing Research*, 1985, *22*, 41–53.

Lavidge, R. J., and Steiner, G. A. "A Model for Predictive Measurements of Advertising Effectiveness." *Journal of Marketing*, 1961, *25*, 59–62.

Lazarsfeld, P. F., Berelson, B., and Gaudet, H. *The People's Choice*. New York: Duell, Sloan, and Pierce, 1944.

Lefebvre, R. C., and Flora, J. A. "Social Marketing and Public Health Intervention." *Health Education Quarterly*, 1988, *15*(3), 299–315.

Lefebvre, R. C., Lasater, T. M., Carleton, R. A., and Peterson, G. "Theory and Delivery of Health Programming in the Community: The Pawtucket Heart Health Program." *Preventive Medicine*, 1987, *16*, 80–95.

Lefebvre, R. C., and others. "Characteristics of Participants in Community Health Programs: Four Year Results." *American Journal of Public Health*, 1987, 77, 1342–1344.

Lefebvre, R. C., and others. "Use of Database Marketing and Consumer-Based Health Communications in Message Design: An Example from the Office of Cancer Communications' 'Five a Day for Better Health' Program." In E. W. Maibach and R. L. Parrott (eds.), *Designing Health Messages*. Newbury Park, Calif.: Sage, 1995.

Lepper, M. R., and Green, D. (eds.). *The Hidden Costs of Reward: New Perspectives on the Psychology of Human Motivation*. Hillsdale, N.J.: Erlbaum, 1978.

Lewin, K. *A Dynamic Theory of Personality*. New York: McGraw-Hill, 1935.

Locke, E. A., Bryan, J. F., and Kendall, L. M. "Goals and Intentions as Mediators of the Effects of Monetary Incentives on Behavior." *Journal of Applied Psychology*, 1968, 542, 104–126.

Lovelock, C. H. "A Market Segmentation Approach to Transit Planning, Modeling and Management." *Proceedings of the Sixteenth Annual Meeting, Transportation Research Forum*, 1975.

Luck, D. J. "Social Marketing: Confusion Compounded." *Journal of Marketing*, 1974, 38, 70–72.

McAlister, A., and others. "Three-Year Panel Study of Health Promotion and Smoking Cessation in Three Southwest Texas Border Communities." In K. Glanz, F. M. Lewis, and B. K. Rimer, (eds.), *Health Behavior and Health Education*. San Francisco: Jossey-Bass, 1990.

McCarthy, E. J., and Perrault, W. D. *Basic Marketing*. (11th ed.) Homewood, Ill.: Irwin, 1993.

Maccoby, N., and Farquar, J. W. "Communicating for Health: Unselling Heart Disease." *Journal of Communications*, Summer 1975, 114–126.

McDivitt, J. A., and McDowell, J. *Results from the Evaluation of the Health-Com Project in Central Java 1988–1989*. Washington, D.C.: Academy for Educational Development, 1991.

McDivitt, J. A., McDowell, J., and Zhou, F. *Evaluation of the HealthCom Project in West Java: Results from Surveys of Mothers and Volunteer Health Workers*. Washington, D.C.: Academy for Educational Development, 1991.

McElroy, K. R., Gottlieb, N. H., and Burdine, J. N. "The Business of Health Promotion: Ethical Issues and Professional Responsibilities." *Health Education Quarterly*, 1987, 14, 91–109.

McGuire, W. J. "Some Internal Psychological Factors Influencing Consumer Choice." *Journal of Consumer Research*, 1976, 2, 302–319.

McGuire, W. J. "Public Communication as a Strategy for Inducing Health-Promoting Behavior Change." *Preventive Medicine*, 1984, 13, 299–319.

McGuire, W. J. "Theoretical Foundations of Campaigns." In R. E. Rice and C. K. Atkin (eds.), *Public Communications Campaigns.* Newbury Park, Calif.: Sage, 1989, pp. 43–66.

MacStravic, R. E. *Marketing Health Care.* Germantown, Md.: Aspen Systems, 1977.

Maddux, J. E., and Rogers, R. W. "Protection Motivation, and Self-Efficacy: A Revised Theory of Fear Appeals and Attitude Change." *Journal of Experimental Social Psychology,* 1983, *19,* 469–479.

Maibach, E. W., and Cotton, D. "Moving People to Behavior Change: A Staged Social Cognitive Approach to Message Design." In E. W. Maibach, and R. L. Parrott (eds.), *Designing Health Messages.* Newbury Park, Calif.: Sage, 1995.

Malafarina, K., and Loken, B. "Progress and Limitations of Social Marketing: A Review of Empirical Literature on the Consumption of Social Ideas." In M. Rothschild and L. McAlister (eds.), *Advances in Consumer Research,* Vol. 20. Conference proceedings, Association for Consumer Research, 1993.

Manoff, R. K. *Social Marketing.* New York: Praeger, 1985.

Mecklenburg, R. E., and others. *How to Help Your Patients Stop Using Tobacco: A National Cancer Institute Manual for the Oral Health Team.* (NIH Publication No. 91–3191.) Bethesda, Md.: National Cancer Institute, National Institutes of Health, 1990.

Miller, D., and Friesen, P. H. "Longitudinal Study of the Corporate Life Cycle." *Management Science,* 1984, *30*(10), 1161–1183.

Minkler, M. "Improving Health Through Community Organization." In K. Glanz, F. M. Lewis, and B. K. Rimer (eds.), *Health Behavior and Health Education: Theory, Research, and Practice.* San Francisco: Jossey-Bass, 1990.

Mizerski, R. W., Golden, L. L., and Kernan, J. B. "The Attribution Process in Consumer Decision Making." *Journal of Consumer Research,* Sept. 1979, pp. 123–140.

Monahan, J. L. "Thinking Positively: Using Positive Affect When Designing Health Messages." In E. Maibach and R. L. Parrott (eds.), *Designing Health Messages.* Thousand Oaks, Calif.: Sage, 1995, 81–113.

Montgomery, K. *Target Prime-Time.* New York: Oxford University Press, 1988.

Murphy, P., and Bloom, P. "Ethical issues in Social Marketing." In S. Fine (ed.), *Social Marketing: Promoting the Causes of Public and Nonprofit Agencies.* Needham Heights, Mass.: Allyn & Bacon, 1990.

National Cancer Institute. *Pretesting in Health Communications.* Bethesda, Md.: National Cancer Institute, 1981.

National Heart, Lung, and Blood Institute. *The Public and High Blood Pres-*

sure: A Survey. DHEW Publication No. 73–356. Bethesda, Md.: National Heart, Lung, and Blood Institute, 1973.

National Heart, Lung, and Blood Institute. *Public Perceptions of High Blood Pressure and Sodium.* NIH Publication No. 86–2730. Bethesda, Md.: National Heart, Lung, and Blood Institute, 1986.

National Heart, Lung, and Blood Institute. *The Fifth Report of the Joint National Committee on Detection, Evaluation, and Treatment of High Blood Pressure.* Bethesda, Md.: National Heart, Lung, and Blood Institute, 1992.

Netemeyer, R. G., Burton, S., and Johnston, M. "A Comparison of Two Models for the Prediction of Volitional and Goal-Directed Behavior: A Confirmatory Analysis Approach." *Social Psychology Quarterly,* 1991, *54*(2), 87–100.

Novelli, W. D. "Applying Social Marketing to Health Promotion and Disease Prevention." In K. Glanz, F. M. Lewis, and B. K. Rimer (eds.), *Health Behavior and Health Education: Theory, Research, and Practice.* San Francisco: Jossey-Bass, 1990.

Nyswander, D. "The Open Society: Its Implications for Health Educators." *Health Education Monographs,* 1966, *1,* 3–13.

Oliver, R. L. "A Cognitive Model of the Antecedents and Consequences of Satisfaction Decisions." *Journal of Marketing Research,* November 1980, pp. 460–69.

O'Rand, A. M., and Krecker, M. L. "Concepts of the Life Cycle: Their History, Meanings, and Uses in the Social Sciences, *Annual Review of Sociology,* 1990, *16,* 241–262.

Pareja, R., and Salazar, E. "Production of a Child Flipchart, by and for the Community." In R. Seidel (ed.), *Notes from the Field in Commmunication for Child Survival.* Washington, D.C.: Academy for Educational Development, 1993, 119–128.

Perloff, L. S., and Fetzer, B. K. "Self-Other Judgments and Perceived Vulnerability to Victimization." *Journal of Personality and Social Psychology,* 1986, *50,* 502–511.

Perry, C. L., Baranowski, T., and Parcel, G. S. "How Individuals, Environments, and Health Behavior Interact: Social Learning Theory." In K. Glanz, F. M. Lewis, and B. K. Rimer (eds.), *Health Behavior and Health Education.* San Francisco: Jossey-Bass, 1990, 161–186.

Perry, C. L., and others. "Parent Involvement with Children's Health Promotion: The Minnesota Home Team." *American Journal of Public Health,* 1988, *78,* 1156–1160.

Peter, J. P., and Olson, J. *Consumer Behavior.* Homewood, Ill.: Irwin, 1993.

Peters, T. J., and Waterman, R. H. *In Search of Excellence: Lessons from America's Best Run Companies.* New York: HarperCollins, 1982.

Petty, R. E., Cacioppo, J. T., and Schumann, D. W. "Central and Peripheral Routes to Advertising Effectiveness: The Moderating Role of Involvement." *Journal of Consumer Research,* 1983, 10, 134–148.

Plummer, J. T. "The Concept and Application of Life Style Segmentation," *Journal of Marketing,* 1974, *38*(1), 33–37.

Pollay, R. W. "The Distorted Mirror: Reflections on the Unintended Consequences of Advertising." *Journal of Marketing,* Spring 1986, *50,* 18–36.

Prochaska, J. O., and DiClemente, C. C. "Stages and Processes of Self-Change of Smoking: Toward an Integrative Model of Change." *Journal of Consulting and Clinical Psychology,* 1983, *51,* 390–395.

Prochaska, J. O., and DiClemente, C. C. "Self-Change Processes, Self-Efficacy and Decisional Balance Across Five Stages of Smoking Cessation." In P. F. Anderson, L. E. Mortenson, and L. E. Epstein (eds.), *Advance in Cancer Control.* New York: Liss, 1984a.

Prochaska, J. O., and DiClemente, C. C. *The Transtheoretical Approach: Crossing the Traditional Boundaries of Therapy.* Homewood, Ill.: Dow Jones-Irwin, 1984b.

Prochaska, J. O., and DiClemente, C. C. "Common Processes of Change in Smoking, Weight Control, and Psychological Distress." In S. Shiffman and T. A. Wills (eds.), *Coping and Substance Abuse.* New York: Plenum, 1985.

Prochaska, J. O., and DiClemente, C. C. "Toward a Comprehensive Model of Change." In W. R. Miller and N. Heather (eds.), *Treating Addictive Behaviors: Processes of Change.* New York: Plenum, 1986.

A Program Manager's Guide to Media Planning. Washington, D.C.: SOMARC/The Futures Group, n.d.

Ramah, M., and Cassidy, C. M. *Social Marketing and the Prevention of AIDS.* Washington, D.C.: AIDSCOM, Academy for Educational Development, 1992.

Rangun, V. K., and Karim, S. *Teaching Note: Focusing the Concept of Social Marketing.* Cambridge: Harvard Business School, 1991.

Rasmuson, M., Seidel, R. E., Smith, W. A., and Booth, E. M. *Communication for Child Survival.* Washington, D.C.: U.S. Agency for International Development, Bureau of Science and Technology, Office of Health and Office of Education, 1988.

Reynolds, T. J., and Gutman, J. "Laddering Theory: Method, Analysis, and Interpretation." *Journal of Advertising Research,* Feb./March) 1988, *28,* 11–31.

Rice, R. E., and Atkin, C. K. (eds.). *Public Communications Campaigns.* Newbury Park, Calif.: Sage, 1989.

Riche, M. F. "Psychographics for the 1990s." *American Demographics,* 1989, *11*(7), 24–31.

Rinehart, W., Blackburn, R., and Moore, S. H. "Employment-Based Family Planning Programs." *Population Reports,* Family Planning Programs. Population Information Program, Series J, Number 34. Baltimore: Johns Hopkins University, Sept.-Oct. 1987.

Roberts, A. H., and Seidel, R. "Breastfeeding Practices in Jordan: Designing Effective Messages." In R. Seidel (ed.), *Notes from the Field in Commmunication for Child Survival.* Washington, D.C.: Academy for Educational Development, 1993, 51–68.

Robertson, T. S. "The Process of Innovation and the Diffusion of Innovations." *Journal of Marketing,* 1967, *31*(1), 14–19.

Robinson, J. *The Economics of Imperfect Competition.* London: Macmillan, 1954.

Roccella, E. J., Bowler, A. E., Ames, M. V., and Horan, M. J. "Hypertension Knowledge, Attitudes, and Behavior: 1985 NHIS Findings." *Public Health Reports,* 1986, *101,* 599–606.

Rogers, E. M. *Diffusion of Innovations.* New York: Free Press, 1962.

Rogers, E. M. *Diffusion of Innovations.* (3rd ed.) New York: Free Press, 1983.

Rogers, E. M., and Singhal, A. "The Academic Perspective." In C. Atkin and L. Wallack (eds.), *Mass Communication and Public Health.* Newbury Park, Calif.: Sage, 1990.

Rogers, E. M., and Storey, J. D. "Communications Campaigns." In C. R. Berger and S. H. Chaffee (eds.), *Handbook of Communication Science.* Newbury Park, Calif.: Sage, 1988.

Rogers, E. M., and others. *Proceedings from the Conference on Entertainment-Education for Social Change.* Los Angeles: Annenberg School of Communications, 1989.

Rogers, R. W. "A Protective Motivation Theory of Fear Appeals and Altitude Change." *Journal of Psychology,* 1975, *91,* 93–114.

Rogers, R. W. "Cognitive and Psychological Processes in Fear Appeals and Attitude Change: A Revised Theory of Protection Motivation." In J. T. Cacioppo and R. E. Petty (eds.), *Social Psychophysiology.* New York: Guilford, 1983.

Rokeach, M. *The Nature of Human Values.* New York: Free Press, 1973.

Rosenstock, I. M. "What Research in Motivation Suggests for Public Health." *American Journal of Public Health,* 1960, *50,* 295–302.

Rosenstock, I. M. "Why People Use Health Services." *Milbank Memorial Fund Quarterly,* 1966, *44,* 94–127.

Rosenstock, I. M. "Historical Origins of the Health Belief Model." *Health Education Monographs,* 1974, *2,* 328–335.

Rosenstock, I. M. "The Health Belief Model: Explaining Health Behavior Through Expectancies." In K. Glanz, F. M. Lewis, and B. K. Rimer (eds.), *Health Behavior and Health Education: Theory, Research, and Practice.* San Francisco: Jossey-Bass, 1990.

Rosenstock, I. M., and Kirscht, J. P. "The Health Belief Model and Personal Health Behavior." *Health Education Monographs*, 1974, *2*, 470–473.

Rosenstock, I. M., Strecher, V. J., and Becker, M. H. "Social Learning Theory and the Health Belief Model." *Health Education Quarterly*, 1988, *15*, 175–183.

Rothschild, M. D. "Marketing Communications in Nonbusiness Situations or Why It's So Hard to Sell Brotherhood Like Soap." *Journal of Marketing*, Spring 1979, pp. 11–20.

Rotter, J. B. "Generalized Expectancies of Internal vs. External Control of Reinforcement." *Psychological Monographs*, 1966, *80*, 1–28.

Rotter, J. B. *Social Learning and Clinical Psychology.* New York: Praeger, 1982.

Salmon, C. (ed.). *Public Information Campaigns.* Newbury Park, Calif.: Sage, 1990.

Saunders, S. G., and others. "Public and Private Sector Collaboration for the Commercial Marketing of ORS in Honduras." In R. E. Seidel (ed.), *Notes from the Field in Communication for Child Survival.* Washington, D.C.: Academy for Educational Development, 1993.

Scott, C. A. "Modifying Socially Conscious Behavior: The Foot-in-the-Door Technique," *Journal of Consumer Research*, 1977, *4*, 156–164.

Seidel, R. (ed.). *Notes from the Field in Communication for Child Survival.* Washington, D.C.: Academy for Educational Development, 1993.

Sheth, J. N. "Segmenting the Health Care Market." In S. Fine (ed.), *Social Marketing: Promoting the Causes of Public and Nonprofit Agencies.* Needham Heights, Mass.: Allyn & Bacon, 1990.

Shimp, T. A., and Bearden, W. O. "Warranty and Other Extrinsic Cue Effects on Consumer Risk Perceptions." *Journal of Consumer Research*, 1982, *9*, 38–46.

Simon, J. "Some 'Marketing Correct' Recommendations for Family Planning Campaigns." *Demography*, 1968, *5*, 504–507.

Slater, M. D. "Choosing Audience Segmentation Strategies and Methods for Health Communications." In E. W. Maibach and R. L. Parrott (eds.), *Designing Health Messages.* Newbury Park, Calif.: Sage, 1995.

Slovic, P., Fischhoff, B., and Lichtenstein, S. "Accident Probabilities and Seat Belt Usage: A Psychological Perspective." *Accident Analysis and Prevention*, 1979, *10*, 281–285.

Smith, N. C. "Ethics and the Marketing Manager." In N. C. Smith and J. A. Quelch, *Ethics in Marketing.* Homewood, Ill.: Irwin, 1993.

Smith, W. A. *Consumer Demand and Satisfaction: The Hidden Key to Successful Privatization.* Washington, D.C.: Academy for Educational Development, HealthCom Project, n.d.

Smith, W. A. *Lifestyles for Survival: The Role of Social Marketing in Mass Education.* Washington, D.C.: Academy for Educational Development, 1989.

Smith, W. A. *Environmental Education and Communications.* Washington, D.C.: Academy for Educational Development, 1993.

Smith, W. A., and Schechter, C. *Organizing the Health Communication Function: A Program Manager's Perspective.* Washington, D.C.: Academy for Educational Development, 1992.

Smith, W. A., and others. *A World Against AIDS: Communication for Behavior Change.* Washington, D.C.: Academy for Educational Development, 1993.

Snyder, L. B. "The Impact of the Surgeon General's 'Understanding AIDS' Pamphlet in Connecticut." *Health Communication,* 1991, *31*(1), 37–57.

SOMARC III. "SOMARC's Condom Projects in Morocco and Turkey Achieve Complete Self-Sufficiency." *SOMARC III Highlights,* 10, March 1994.

Stover, J., and Wagman, A. *The Cost of Contraceptive Social Marketing Programs Implemented Through the SOMARC Project,* Special Study #1. Washington, D.C.: SOMARC/The Futures Group, June 1992.

Stuart, R. B. (ed.). *Behavioral Self-Management: Strategies, Techniques, and Outcomes.* New York: Brunner/Mazel, 1977.

Substance Abuse and Mental Health Services Administration. *National Household Survey on Drug Abuse: Highlights 1991.* Washington, D.C.: U.S. Department of Health and Human Services, February 1993.

Sudman, S. *Applied Sampling.* New York: Academic Press, 1976.

Sudman, S., and Bradburn, N. *Asking Questions: A Practical Guide to Questionnaire Design.* San Francisco: Jossey-Bass, 1972.

Sudman, S., and Ferber, R. *Consumer Panels.* Chicago: American Marketing Association, 1979.

Summary Report Technical Advisory Group Meeting. Washington, D.C.: Academy for Educational Development, HealthCom, April 2, 1992.

Sutton, S. M., Balch, G. I., and Lefebvre, R. C. "Strategic Questions for Consumer-Based Health Communications." *Public Health Reports,* in press.

Svenson, O., Fischhoff, B., and MacGregor, D. "Perceived Driving Safety and Seatbelt Usage." *Accident Analysis and Prevention,* 1985, *17,* 119–133.

U.S. Agency for International Development. *Child Survival: A Seventh Report to the Congress on the USAID Program.* Washington, D.C.: U.S. Agency for International Development, April 1992.

Vobedja, B. "Teens Improve on Prevention of Pregnancy." *The Washington Post,* June 7, 1994, p. A-1.

Wallack, L. "Media Advocacy: Promoting Health Through Mass Communication." K. Glanz, F. M. Lewis, and B. K. Rimer (eds.), *Health Behavior and Health Education: Theory, Research, and Practice.* San Francisco: Jossey-Bass, 1990.

Wallack, L., Dorfman, L., Jernigan, D., and Themba, M. *Media Advocacy and Public Health.* Newbury Park, Calif.: Sage, 1993.

Weibe, G. D. "Merchandising Commodities and Citizenship on Television." *Public Opinion Quarterly,* 1951–52, *15,* 679–691.

Weinstein, N. D. "Unrealistic Optimism About Future Life Events." *Journal of Personality and Social Psychology,* 1980, *39,* 806–820.

Weinstein, N. D. "Reducing Unrealistic Optimism About Illness Susceptibility." *Health Psychology,* 1983, *2,* 11–20.

Weinstein, N. D. "Why It Won't Happen to Me: Perceptions of Risk Factors and Illness Susceptibility." *Health Psychology,* 1984, *3,* 431–457.

Weinstein, N. D. "Unrealistic Optimism About Illness Susceptibility: Conclusions from a Community-Wide Sample." *Journal of Behavioral Medicine,* 1987, *10,* 481–500.

Weinstein, N. D. "The Precaution Adoption Process," *Health Psychology,* 1988, *7,* 355–386.

Wells, W. D. *Planning for R.O.I.: Effective Advertising Strategy.* Englewood Cliffs, N.J.: Prentice Hall, 1989.

Whitely, R. C. *The Customer Driven Company.* Reading, Mass.: Addison-Wesley, 1991.

Wilkie, W. D., and Pessemeir, E. A. "Issues in Marketing's Use of Multi-Attribute Attitude Models," *Journal of Marketing Research,* 1973, *10,* 428–441.

Wilkie, W. L. *Consumer Behavior* (2nd ed.) New York: Wiley, 1990.

Williams, G., Grant, B., Harford, T., and Noble, J. "Population Projections Using DSM-III Criteria: Alcohol Abuse and Dependence, 1990–2000," *Alcohol Health and Research World,* 1989, *13,* 366–370.

Wind, J., Rao, V. R., and Green, P. E. "Behavioral Methods." In T. S. Robertson and H. H. Kassarjian, *Handbook of Consumer Behavior.* Englewood Cliffs, N.J.: Prentice Hall, 1991, pp. 507–532.

Wind, Y., Douglas, S. P., and Perlmutter, H. "Guidelines for Developing International Marketing Strategy," *Journal of Marketing,* April 1973, *37,* 14–23.

Windsor, R., Baranowski, T., Clark, N., and Cutter, G. *Evaluation of Health Promotion and Education Programs.* Mountain View, Calif.: Mayfield, 1984.

Winnard, K., Rimon, J., and Convisser, J. "The Impact of Television on the Family Planning Attitudes of an Urban Nigerian Audience." Paper presented to the American Health Association, 1987 (referenced in Atkin and Wallack, 1990, p. 178).

Winston, J. A. *The Designated Driver Campaign Developed Nationally by the Harvard Alcohol Project.* Cambridge, Mass.: Harvard University School of Public Health, 1990.

Witt, R. E., and Bruce, G. D. "Group Influence and Brand Choice," *Journal of Marketing Research,* Nov. 1972, *9,* 440–443.

World Bank. *World Development Report 1993: Investing in Health.* New York: Oxford University Press, 1993.

Wright, P., and Weitz, B. "Time Horizon Effects on Product Evaluation Strategies." *Journal of Marketing Research,* 1977, *14,* 429–443.

Yoder, P. S., and Oke, E. A. *Ethnomedical Research For Formative Purposes: An Example From Nigeria.* Working paper, Center for International Health and Development Communication, Annenberg School of Communications, University of Pennsylvania, May 1989.

Yoder, P. S., Oke, E. A., and Yanka, B. "Ethnomedical Research for Developmental Purposes: Examples from Nigeria and Zaire." In R. Seidel (ed.), *Notes from the Field in Commmunication for Child Survival.* Washington, D.C.: Academy for Educational Development, 1993, 17–26.

Yoder, P. S., and Zheng, Z. *HealthCom in Lesotho: Final Evaluation Report.* Center for International Health and Development Communication, Annenberg School for Communication, University of Pennsylvania, Working Paper #1005, 1991.

Yoder, P. S., Zheng, Z., and Zhou, F. *Results of the HealthCom Evaluation in Lubumbashi, Zaire, 1988–1990.* Washington, D.C.: Academy for Educational Development, 1991.

Zaichkowsky, J. L. "Students' Attitudes Towards Use of Condoms." *Public and Nonprofit Marketing: Cases and Readings.* Palo Alto: Scientific Press, 1990, 125–132.

Name Index

Subject Index

A

Academy for Educational Development, 220, 284

Accessibility and availability issues, 15–16, 277–278, 283, 315

Advertising. *See* Communications program

Advertising agencies, social marketing involvement, 292

AIDS prevention project(s), 45–46, 82, 91–92, 109, 127, 247, 248, 269–270, 290; hypothetical, segmentation strategy in, 184–188, 189, 192–193, 194–196

American Cancer Society, 72, 316

American Forests, 102–104

Apple Computer, 54–55, 69, 258

B

Behavior change: as bottom line in social marketing, 8, 13–14; and education and propaganda, 9–11, 149–150; and extrinsic rewards, 247–249, 284–286; and forgetfulness, 280; and individual's status change, 187; long-term, 61–62; persuasion approach to, 11; versus "raised awareness," 78; reinforcement of desired behavior in, 165–166; role of significant others in, 157–160; shaping in, 267–268, 278–279; social influence approach to, 12–13; and social pressure, 10, 159–160, 257–263, 273; sources of disappointment in, 281–283; and target's stage, 182–183; traditional approach to, 2–3;

and vicarious learning, 269–270. *See also* Consumer behavior model

Behavior modeling, 162, 269–270

Behavior modification theory, 12, 165–166

Behavioral control: and action efficacy, 161; and constructive blame, 162–163; and self-efficacy, 161, 264–266, 268; perceived, 263–271

Benchmarking, 87–88

Benefit-based strategy(ies), 226–238; added inducements as, 246–249; attributes data in, 227–228; benefit segmentation as, 232–236; as combination of costs and benefits, 242–246; in Contemplation Stage, 272–273; laddering research as, 230; values research in, 229–230

Benefits: invisible nature of, 60, 283; third party, 61

C

Campaigns, defined, 70

Centers for Disease Control and Prevention (CDC): HIV/AIDS prevention, 44, 45–46, 82, 314; Planned Approach to Community Health (PATCH) program, 314

Child survival programs. *See* Health-Com projects

Cognitive theories of behavior, 259–260

Commercial sector, 3–5, 38; communications programs, 200; Communications Test, 122; negative image, 28–29, 40–41; targeted marketing in, 174, 175

348